Bottoms Up!

Bottoms Up!

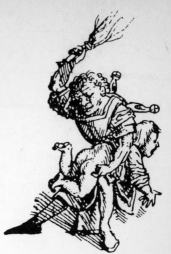

A Pathologist's Essays on
Medicine and the Humanities

William B. Ober, M.D.

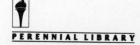

PERENNIAL LIBRARY

Harper & Row, Publishers, New York
Cambridge, Philadelphia, San Francisco
London, Mexico City, São Paulo, Singapore, Sydney

First PERENNIAL LIBRARY edition published 1988.

LIBRARY OF CONGRESS CATALOG CARD NUMBER: 88-45120

ISBN: 0-06-097188-6 (pbk.)

88 89 90 91 92 FG 10 9 8 7 6 5 4 3 2 1

Contents

Figures

Preface

The kind reception given to *Boswell's Clap and Other Essays* has encouraged me to assemble another collection of essays. All but one have appeared in medical journals that do not reach a general readership, but their substance as well as the approach should be of wider interest. The former collection was limited to the medical afflictions of literary men. In the present collection I have broadened the scope to what may loosely be called "Medicine and the Humanities," including not only literary subjects but those taken from music, the fine arts, history, and anthropology, all seen through a medical eye.

The past decade has witnessed increasing awareness by educators that it is not enough to teach doctors the theory and practice of medicine. Medical education involves two major processes, first the transmission of information and skills, second the development of an attitude. The technological explosion after World War II created a large body of new information and new techniques. Such technological progress is not to be dismissed lightly; it is the lifeblood of advances in medical science and their application to patients' needs. Nor would anyone gainsay the importance of acquiring a fund of medical knowledge. But it has become apparent that medical schools and graduate training programs are turning out physicians who are test oriented and procedure oriented rather than patient oriented; the public perceives these physicians as being less responsive to their patients as human beings. Announcing proposals to reform the medical school curriculum, President Derek Bok of Harvard pointed out that what seems to be essential information that must be transmitted to students today will be outmoded tomorrow, and he quotes Dean Burwell's semifacetious remark to Harvard medical students: "Half of what we have taught you is wrong. Unfortunately, we do not know which half." With respect to inculcating an attitude, both to patients and to the profession, one recalls President James B. Conant's formula in awarding the M.D. degree at Commencement: "I confer upon you the degree of Doctor of Medicine and welcome you to the merciful calling of medicine." If medicine is not a merciful calling, we cannot justify its existence.

Writing on the relationship between medicine and literature, Dr. Edmund Pellegrino of Catholic University notes that medicine and literature are united in an unremitting paradox: the need simultaneously to stand back from, yet share in, the struggle for human life. In recent years many medical schools have begun to offer courses in literature, and they serve several goals: "teaching empathy with the ill person, giving insight into the peculiarities of the medical life and the doctor's place in society and culture, underscoring the dilemmas of medical morals, and improving the narrative form of history taking." These are no small matters. Can anyone believe that a physician who has read Tolstoy's *The Death of Ivan Ilyich* is not better equipped to understand the sufferings of a patient with incurable cancer than one who has not?

Dr. Lewis Thomas has written that the impact of medical schools on the undergraduate curriculum is "baleful and malign." Too many premedical students choose to study the sciences at the expense of the humanities. Norman Cousins, the distinguished editor and engaging writer, tells us: "The result is that many graduates are deprived of their rightful cultural heritage. . . . It affects the total ability of the physician to deal with the complex equation that is represented by an individual patient's illness. . . . [T]he wise physician understands the ease with which modern society transfers its malaises to the individual. He comprehends the variations of stress in modern family life and in relationships in general. He understands disappointments, rejection, blocked exits. He has an appreciation of what is required to make an individual whole again." To paraphrase Matthew Arnold, the good doctor must see his patient clearly and see him whole.

It is comforting to know that these prominent intellectual figures agree that a well-rounded education is valuable for physicians and are preaching that doctrine to the unenlightened members of medical faculties. More and more medical schools are adding courses in the humanities to their curricula. Indeed, one of Norman Cousins' many hats is the title Adjuvant Professor in the UCLA School of Medicine program in Medical Law and Human Values, and many other qualified scholars are actively teaching literature, philosophy, ethics, medical history, and socioeconomics as recognized and useful courses in medical schools. One does not like to throw cold water on a cause in which one strongly believes and has espoused for more than three decades, but I must point out that we do not have an objective test to prove that a doctor whose education in the humanities has been well rounded is any better a doctor—that is, more proficient, more caring, more compassionate—than one who is not. My acquaintanceship includes any number of competent, caring, compassionate doctors whose chief recreation is golf and whose reading does not rise above the level of the daily newspaper or *Time* magazine. But when one looks at members of medical school faculties, supposedly the elite of the profession, one does find that the majority are cultivated, well read, familiar with literature, the fine arts, music, philosophy. The breadth of their intellectual background does enable them to reason and argue cogently, to debate questions of medical ethics and responsibility, and to relate what they have read or seen in humane disciplines to the clinical problems of their patients—and perhaps that is for the better. Even in the empirical world of medical science some matters must be taken as articles of faith. Emily Dickinson's comment on the paradox is worth remembering:

> "Faith" is a fine invention
> When Gentlemen can *see*—
> But *Microscopes* are prudent
> In an Emergency.

The judgment remains subjective. The essays collected here can be taken as case histories from the notebooks of a practicing medical humanist who uses the microscope when it is prudent to do so.

Georges Simenon, certainly a successful writer, has said, "Writing is not a profession, but a vocation of unhappiness." I cannot accept his point of view. Perhaps it is a craft rather than a profession, but there is no unhappiness. It may be a self-indulgence, but few of my activities have given me greater pleasure than writing sentences and constructing paragraphs. When I was a schoolboy, my teachers placed great importance on learning how to write expository prose, and it occurs to me that I may not have learned much since then. I cannot deny the impeachment that I have used every opportunity to transform a scientific discipline into a literary one.

Choosing a title for this collection has been difficult. Initially, I wanted to call it *Laertes' Shroud.* The allusion is to Penelope's ruse to put off her suitors; she would weave her father's shroud by day and unravel it at night. That is a fair metaphor for my *métier;* I practice pathology by day and try to unravel questions in the humanities at night. But most casual readers coming upon such a title would think of the wrong Laertes, the one familiar to them from *Hamlet,* not Penelope's father. I also entertained the idea of calling the collection *Weighing the Heart,* part of the title of one of the essays and descriptive of what every pathologist does in the course of an autopsy. It also connotes the affection with which the essays were written, the pleasure I take in the methods of my specialty, and the warm feelings I have for my subjects. But we finally settled on *Bottoms Up!* It may seem a bit ambiguous, perhaps even frivolous; someone might mistake it for a book of after-dinner toasts or even an account of shipwrecks. But it has the virtue of being eye-catching and it echoes the crisp snap of the opening *B* and closing *p* of *Boswell's Clap.*

Many audiences have asked me how or why I select my subjects for investigation, and the *incipits* are variable. Clearly, the essays on František Koczwara's death and the trial of Spencer Cowper derive from my regular work in forensic pathology. Among the many causes of death that a medical examiner views are autoerotic asphyxia and drowning. Likewise, the essays on placentophagy and on infertility in the Bible relate to my subspecialty in obstetrical and gynecological pathology. The study of Johnson and Boswell as melancholics stems in part from my previous essay on Boswell but more immediately from a lengthy essay on melancholia in eighteenth-century literature, "Eighteenth-Century Spleen." I wanted to use Johnson and Boswell as contrasting case histories of the malady, but the section became too long and out of proportion to the rest. Therefore, I wrenched it out and wrote it as a separate piece, leaving the body to be published elsewhere.

The study of Carlo Gesualdo and the survey of the iconography of flagellation are by-products of a long essay on Swinburne's masochism, published in *Boswell's Clap.* As I waded through the muddy literature of sadomasochism, I became aware of Gesualdo's violent life, and a recording of his madrigals demonstrated how he translated his feelings into music. Also, as I read this literature, I came across many representations of the flagellatory scene. I had my hospital photographer make copies and tossed them into a manila folder. When the essay on Swinburne was published, the folder went into a filing cabinet, and I forgot about it. Cleaning out the cabinet some seven years later, I came across the manila folder, riffled through it, and could see the title essay taking shape.

The study of Rimbaud and his many problems took root in my undergraduate days, when I was first exposed to the poems of Baudelaire, Verlaine, Mallarmé, and Rimbaud. Their imagery and use of language were intoxicating to an adolescent whose previous acquaintance with

French poetry was limited to the measured alexandrines of Racine and selections from Victor Hugo and his contemporaries. The intoxication has diminished over the years, but my interest in the poets has not. How was I at seventeen to know that three of the four poets were psychopaths? The reader will note that psychopathology occupies a prominent place in these essays—melancholia, masochism, hysteria, autoerotic asphyxia, and other dinner-table topics. I have spent much of my life as a witness to *peccata mundi* and their consequences. It took me many years to recognize that in this world there is more psychopathology than anatomic pathology. The essay on Margery Kempe also takes its origin from my undergraduate years. Her *Book* had only recently been published, and it created a modest stir of interest in her unusual personality and religious experiences. My friend Howard Nemerov wrote a poem about her, part of which I use as an epigraph, and Margery's problems lurked in the back of my mind for half a century. Whether I have reconciled mysticism with hysteria I cannot judge, but at least I have given her a thorough medical examination.

"Can the Leper Change His Spots?" is owed to my friend Dr. A. Bernard Ackerman, the distinguished dermatopathologist, who invited me to write an article for the journal he was then editing. I protested my lack of expertise in dermatopathology, but he made it clear he wanted an article on an historical subject. At the time I had on my desk some slides from a case of leprosy, a skin biopsy taken at my own hospital. Leprosy is very rare in Bergen County, and the case served as the point of departure for a "grand rounds" devoted to the disease. Wishing to present something more than photomicrographs of the biopsy, I had my hospital photographer prepare projection slides from illustrations in books from my own library to show how the disease was represented in medieval and Renaissance art. I suggested the iconography of leprosy as a suitable topic, and Dr. Ackerman approved. Little did I know that this kind invitation would lead to three years of visiting libraries and museums, enjoyable excursions that took my wife and me from Istanbul to Honolulu and from Bergen, Norway, to Palermo and to our own national leprosarium at Carville, Louisiana. I trust the reader will notice that the essay does not tell him anything about leprosy as a disease; a large corpus of medical literature exists that serves that purpose far better than I could attempt. What I have tried to accomplish is to show how leprosy was depicted in art and how many nonmedical considerations shaped the way it was represented.

The idea for the essay "Weighing the Heart against the Feather of

Truth" came during a visit to the National Museum at Cairo. In the museum's bookshop I found a postcard captioned "Horus Weighing the Heart" from a wall painting in an Eighteenth Dynasty tomb at Thebes. Why Horus was performing an act that every pathologist does at the autopsy table intrigued me, and I resolved to investigate. The incident led me to explore aspects of ancient Egyptian religion and burial practices, and the result was the essay.

I have been lucky with libraries. No one searches the literature unaided, and I owe much to the many libraries I have used. The Library of the New York Academy of Medicine, now under the expert direction of Brett Kirkpatrick and his associate Anne Pascarelli, has been most accommodating in retrieving materials. The Reading Room of the British Library (formerly the British Museum) has sheltered me on many occasions and provided excellent service. On one occasion the Bayerische Staatsbibliothek at Munich retrieved an 1863 volume of *Sitzungsberichte* in a mere twenty minutes, and I was able to locate a transcription of Ibn al-Khatib's mid-fourteenth-century manuscript on bubonic plague. The organization of interlibrary loan services is so efficient that I have never had to do without the specific book or manuscript I required. But my chief debt is to the dozens of unnamed reference librarians, overworked and underpaid, who are the scholar's lifeline to the past. They have put their special knowledge at my disposal with efficiency and goodwill. All I had to do was ask, and it was given unto me. In like fashion staff members of any number of museums have been helpful, and their institutions have been acknowledged under the illustrations.

The assistance and advice of most of the individuals who have come to my rescue have been acknowledged at the time of primary publication of these essays. But a few debts require more than that. I must thank my former resident Dr. Nabil Alloush, who came to me from Aleppo, for providing a literal translation of the Arabic text of Ibn al-Khatib's essay on bubonic plague. I have nothing but praise for the skills of Mr. Walter Goddard, my hospital photographer. The essay on the iconography of *Fanny Hill* has not been published elsewhere, and I must thank Janice Wrench of the North Library in the British Library for putting most of the materials I used at my disposal. In preparing the essay I received useful information and advice from Dr. James Basker and Dr. Hugh Amory of Harvard as well as from Dr. John Riely of Boston University.

Two of these essays were presented as formal lectures. "Can the Leper Change His Spots?" was the fifteenth Ernest J. and Elena Bruno Memorial Lecture, given at Lenox Hill Hospital in November 1982. It gave me great pleasure to participate in this series, established by my close friend Dr. Michael S. Bruno to honor his father and mother. "Reuben's Mandrakes: Infertility in the Bible" was given as the Paul Klemperer Memorial Lecture at Mount Sinai Hospital in June 1983, and I was pleased to be invited to honor the memory of that distinguished pathologist and scholar, whose company was always illuminating. Those essays that have appeared in the *Bulletin of the New York Academy of Medicine* have profited from the editorial skills of my fellow pathologist Dr. William D. Sharpe.

For the continuing encouragement of my work from valued friends within my own specialty—Dr. Harold L. Stewart of Bethesda, Maryland, Dr. Hugh G. Grady of Norristown, Pennsylvania, Dr. Melvin B. Black of San Francisco, and Dr. John H. Edgcomb of New York—I am indeed grateful. Dr. Madeleine Pelner Cosman of Tenafly, New Jersey, has provided sound advice when my essays involved medieval and Renaissance matters. Dr. Robert C. Wallach of New York has been unfailingly supportive; Dr. Lawrence J. Denson of Hackensack, New Jersey, has provided words of wisdom when required; Dr. Howard M. Spiro of New Haven, Connecticut, has also helped give shape to my ideas. Friends who have made my frequent forays to England comfortable and hospitable include Professor and Mrs. Kenneth D. Bagshawe of London and Chilham, Kent; Dr. and Mrs. A. John Beale of Sissinghurst, Kent; Mr. and Mrs. Richard C. Wheeler-Bennett of London and Calne, Wiltshire; Dr. and Mrs. Henry Pleasants of London; and Dr. Hugh L'Etang of London.

But my greatest debt is to my wife, an incalculable obligation, not only for time stolen from her society, but for anticipating my needs, for sharing the rigors and companionship of travel, and for providing a well-ordered household in which I could pursue my avocation. It is to her that I dedicate this book.

Tenafly, N.J.   William B. Ober, M.D.
October 1986

Acknowledgments

I would like to express my gratitude to the following journals:

Bulletin of the New York Academy of Medicine for permission to reprint "Carlo Gesualdo, Prince of Venosa: Murder, Madrigals, and Masochism," 49 (1973): 634–45; "Notes on Placentophagy," 55 (1979): 591–99; "Weighing the Heart against the Feather of Truth," 55 (1979): 636–51; "The Plague at Granada: Ibn al-Khatib and Ideas of Contagion," 58 (1982): 418–24; "Johnson and Boswell: 'Vile Melancholy' and 'The Hypochondriack,'" 61 (1985): 657–78.

The American Journal of Dermatopathology for permission to reprint "Can the Leper Change his Spots?: The Iconography of Leprosy," 5 (1983): 43–55, 173–86; "Bottoms Up! The Fine Arts and Flagellation," 6 (1984): 451–60, 541–52.

The American Journal of Forensic Medicine and Pathology for permission to reprint "The Sticky End of František Koczwara, Composer of *The Battle of Prague*," 5 (1984): 145–49; "The Trial of Spencer Cowper: Expert Witnesses to the Rescue," 8 (1987): 172–78.

New York State Journal of Medicine for permission to reprint "Robert Musil: What Price Homosexual Sadism?" 72 (1972): 1071–76.

The International Journal of Gynecological Pathology for permission to reprint "Reuben's Mandrakes: Infertility in the Bible," 3 (1984): 299–317.

Literature and Medicine for permission to reprint "Margery Kempe: Hysteria and Mysticism Reconciled," 4 (1985): 24–40.

Medical Heritage for permission to reprint "All the Colours of the Rimbaud," 2 (1986): 187–207.

Credits to museums and libraries for permission to reproduce illustrations from their collections are acknowledged in the captions below the illustrations.

Part
One
Perversion

Anatomized

1
Bottoms Up! The Fine Arts and Flagellation

*T*he story of man's inhumanity to man is older than recorded history. Ancient Egyptian wall paintings illustrate the beating of slave laborers who worked on the pyramids and other public works. Boys were beaten in ancient Greece at Sparta in the festival of Artemis Orthia, and naked men ran through the streets of ancient Rome with straps to beat whatever women they encountered. At Pompeii, the murals in the House of Mysteries remind us that ritual flagellation was an essential element in the initiation ceremonies of a Dionysiac cult. In the medieval church, disobedient members of the clergy were punished by flagellation, and self-flagellation was practiced as an efficacious means of penance. Following the Black Death of the mid-fourteenth century, flagellant brotherhoods, first organized in Italy, led processions of laymen and laywomen for mutual flagellation. The movement spread through Europe, partly because the moral corruption of the church impelled people to use their own efforts to mitigate the divine judgment they felt was at hand. Flogging and whipping were readily added to the list of punishments meted out by the judiciary, an easy transfer from practices invoked in the name of religion for sins of commission. The end result of these flagellations was to produce a condition common in dermatopathology, the classical *rubor, tumor, calor, et dolor* of a transient, reversible vascular and inflammatory response.

Iconographic representation of the foregoing is abundant, and recapitulation unnecessary. The *locus classicus* for flagellation in Western Christian art is the flagellation of Christ. Paintings, engravings, and drawings of the scene usually show Christ bound to a pillar and being beaten by two men with whips. He is usually depicted looking heavenward with a look of pious resignation; the mild expression usually seen on the faces of the flagellators belies what must have happened in the actual event. Exceptions are found in the realism of Northern European painting after the fifteenth century, but they are not numerous. An outstanding exception is a flagellation of Christ by the fifteenth-century Catalan painter Luis Borrassá, now in the Musée Goya at Castres, France, which clearly displays the sexual sadism involved. The whip handles are penile, and the thongs can be taken as seminal emissions.[1] But the conventional image is usually bland; only in a few representations does Christ's body exhibit the marks of scourging.

This essay will not attempt to catalogue religious or judicial flagellatory icons, nor will it deal, except in passing, with depictions of flagellation for pornographic purposes. The exposition will be largely confined to secular flagellation or, in the euphemism now current, "domestic discipline." The raw material includes frescoes in churches, carved choir stalls, engravings in connoisseurs' cabinets, caricatures, and even the hebdomadal chastisement of the Katzenjammer Kids, bottoms up in the Sunday comic strip. There is no need to be encyclopedic about a subject whose thematic material is limited and unvarying. The nineteenth-century verses about Keate, the flogging headmaster of Eton, apply. An old Etonian encountered Keate at a social gathering and was dismayed that his former mentor did not recognize him:

> "You've flogged me oft I wot,
> And yet it seems that me you've quite forgot."
> "E'en now," said Keate, "I cannot guess your name
> —Boys' bottoms are so very much the same."

Incidents involving flagellation have found their way into literature, even in a "respectable" guise. Rousseau's erotic response to being spanked as a boy is well known, and Swinburne's obsessive verses are equally familiar.[2] That schoolboy flogging was a quotidian event at Rugby is clear from *Tom Brown's Schooldays* (1857), though no actual description is given. In Hugh Walpole's novel *Fortitude* (1913), Peter Wescott, the disobedient twelve-year-old boy hero, is whipped by his sadistic father in an early chapter to give substance to the novel's motto, "'Tisn't life that matters, 'tis the courage you bring to it." In a less idealistic vein, Christopher Isherwood's camera eye catches Mr. Norris taking his pleasure in being beaten by a Berlin madam who seems quite expe-

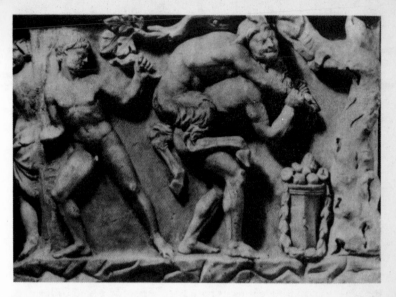

Figure 1.1. Two satyrs punishing Pan for inebriety. Detail from a second-century Roman sarcophagus. British Museum 2298C.

rienced at the job. In Aldous Huxley's *Time Must Have a Stop* (1944), we witness the English expatriate and voluptuary Eustace Barnack spanked by one of his *filles de joie,* and that reminds him of the two smacks given by his nursemaid Fräulein Anna when he failed to "do Töpfchen" before she went to fetch the *Spritze.*

Except for those associated with Dionysiac cults, icons of flagellation are rare in classical Greek, Roman, or Hellenistic art. The initiation scene in Pompeii's House of Mysteries is the most familiar example and has been frequently reproduced. Less well known is a detail from a second-century Roman sarcophagus at the British Museum (BM 2298) showing a triumphal procession of Bacchus and Ariadne decorated with many figures in relief.[3] One vignette displays two satyrs punishing Pan, presumably for inebriety; he is horsed on the back of one while the other holds up his tail and birches him (fig. 1.1). The scene found a responsive chord in several minor Italian Renaissance artists. Amico Aspertini's drawing (ca. 1500), executed while the sarcophagus was at S. Maria Maggiore, depicts it without much modification, as do similar works by Battista Naldi (ca. 1560), an anonymous North Italian artist (ca. 1460), an even earlier Central Italian artist (ca. 1420–30), and others.

A popular legend in the late medieval period was the story of Aristotle and Phyllis. The fable tells how Alexander the Great neglected affairs of state to devote himself to his pretty young wife (in some accounts, his mistress), Phyllis. The nobles of his council sent his former tutor Aristotle to remonstrate with the king. Aristotle's reasoning was so cogent that the young king turned his mind back to the business of government. Phyllis was displeased and resolved to revenge herself upon the aging philosopher. She vamped, made advances, and soon Aristotle was infatuated with her. When he pressed her to satisfy his love, she insisted he must prove it by letting her ride upon his back. He agreed, and she placed a saddle on his back, a bit in his mouth, and rode him around the palace garden with the reins in her hand, having previously told Alexander to watch the horseplay. When the game was over, Alexander summoned Aristotle and asked him to explain how his behavior was so different from his advice. Aristotle is said to have replied, "If a woman can make such a fool of so old and wise a man as I, how much more dangerous it is for a younger, less experienced man like yourself." The moral of the fable is the risk of submitting to the attractions of the female sex: consider Samson and Delilah, David and Bathsheba, even Falstaff and the merry wives of Windsor.

Georges Sarton has traced the theme of the legend to comparable stories in Indian, Arabic, and Oriental sources.[4] It appeared in European literature in the first half of the thirteenth century, more or less coevally, in a French *fabliau* by Henri d'Andeli and an anonymous German tale titled "Aristoteles und Fillis." Sarton lists some of the iconographic representations of the story, chiefly from the last quarter of the fifteenth through the first quarter of the sixteenth century, citing ivory carvings and sculptured reliefs as well as a number of drawings and engravings, four of which he reproduces, including one by Lucas van Leyden. In all but one of the cited examples and in all that Sarton chose to publish, both Artistotle and Phyllis are fully clothed, the latter somewhat sumptuously, as befits a king's wife (or mistress). Phyllis is shown astride Aristotle's back as he crouches on all fours, and in all of them she holds a whip. Sarton mentions but does not reproduce the woodcut by Hans Baldung Gruen (1484/5–1545) which shows them both nude (fig. 1.2). Perhaps that distinguished scholar was hesitant to

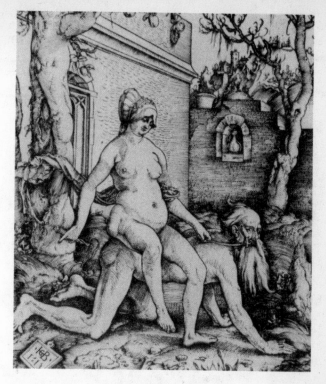

Figure 1.2. Aristotle and Phyllis. Hans Baldung Gruen, 1513. Woodcut.

reproduce, even in a learned journal, a picture in which nudity made the sexual element so explicit. The intellectual and moral climate was somewhat more prim fifty years ago.

Gruen supplies several extra dimensions to this cautionary tale about the dominating female. The jug in the niche of the garden wall suggests a jug of wine (are we to supply, *pace* Omar Khayyam, "And thou astride me in the wilderness?"), perhaps loss of reason following inebriety. One tree is fruitful and bears apples, the emblem of man's first disobedience; the other is barren, unproductive like the relationship between Aristotle and Phyllis. Alexander peeping over a parapet lends a suggestion of voyeurism. Perhaps he enjoyed the scene, for as Yeats reminds us in "Among Schoolchildren," "Soldier Aristotle played the tawse/Upon the bottom of a king of kings." But the focus is on the naked couple, Aristotle tense and apprehensive, Phyllis a bit overripe and wearing a

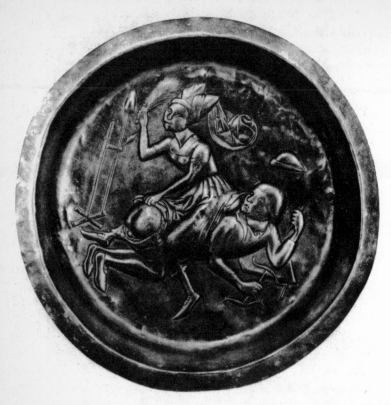

Figure 1.3. Aristotle and Phyllis. Dutch/Walloon copper plate, ca. 1480.

self-indulgent smile. She hardly presents as a young beauty who would distract the young Alexander; her breasts are about to decline, and her paunch gives promise that in a few years she may become the Venus de Kilo. Yet Gruen could draw lithe, supple women in sexually provocative postures; compare his drawing "Three Witches" in the Albertina at Vienna or his painting "Three Graces" in the Prado. The woodcut of Aristotle and Phyllis is dated 1513, but its moral message is one that has echoed through the centuries: Carnal lust degrades man's dignity.

The Aristotle-Phyllis legend found its way into lesser art forms, for example a bronze aquamanile (French, ca. 1400) with both figures fully clad and Phyllis sans whip, and a copper plate (fig. 1.3) of Dutch or Walloon workmanship dating from circa 1480. In the latter, Artistotle is interrupted by Phyllis while he is spinning thread, clearly a woman's task to which he has been subjugated. The ball of raw wool is on a stand at the left, and Aristotle on all fours holds a spindle in one hand while he and Phyllis are wearing peasant-style plebeian clothing. She is fully dressed, but his trousers are pulled down at the rear, exposing his buttocks, which Phyllis is beating with a stylized sheaf. A comical touch is provided by his hat flying off, and exposure of his scrotum supplies a note of domestic lubricity. What does one do with such a plate? Cover it with a doily and serve cookies? A somewhat more conventional treatment of the subject is seen in a carved thirteenth-century choir stall in the cathedral at Lausanne. Underneath a trefoil Gothic arch Phyllis, whip in hand, bestrides a bearded Aristotle, both fully clothed; the significance of a pair of wrestling men above the arch is elusive.

But scenes of flagellation were not always restricted to engravings for the cabinets of wealthy collectors or domestic utensils for the well-to-do. One finds them in places of public accommodation, even churches. One of the walls in the Collegiate Church at San Gimigniano is decorated by a fresco by Taddeo di Bartolo (ca. 1360–ca. 1420), one of the last great Sienese painters of the trecento. Executed in 1393, the full fresco displays the variety of punishments meted out in hell to sinners. A detail (fig. 1.4) shows a woman being birched for her adultery by demons, while below a homosexual is impaled on a pole from anus to mouth; the end of the pole is in the mouth of another homosexual seated on the left, his hands tied behind his back. The brutality speaks for itself, but the fresco was designed as a religious painting with a moral message: The punishment fits the crime. There is no evidence that such admonitory icons had any effect on sexual mores in San Gimigniano or that adultery or homosexuality were practiced any less there than in any other Italian city of the time. One recalls the maxim: Lust knows few checks, but some are better left uncashed.

Also at San Gimigniano and only a shade less savage is the first of seventeen panels illustrating the life of St. Augustine, painted in 1463–65 for the Church of S. Agostino by Benozzo Gozzoli (1420–97), the Florentine best known for his frescos in the chapel of the Medici palace. The panel (fig. 1.5) shows the future bishop of Hippo being taken to his first school at Tagaste. At the left foreground his well-dressed parents entrust their bright-eyed son, a lad of perhaps eight years, to the schoolmaster. The school, with many students busy at their lessons, is an open loggia occupying the right middle distance. At

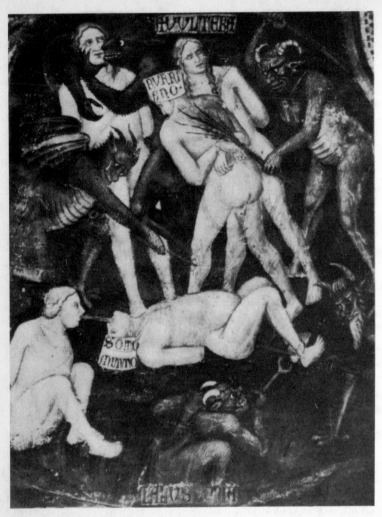

Figure 1.4. The Punishments of Hell. Taddeo di Bartolo, 1393. Fresco, Collegiate Church, San Gimigniano.

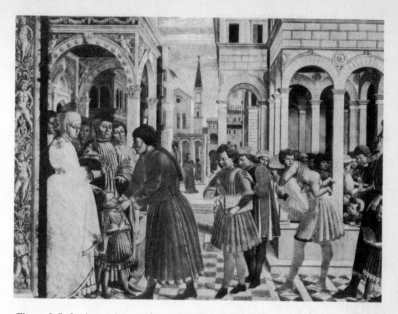

Figure 1.5. St. Augustine at school. Benozzo Gozzoli, 1463–65. Fresco, Chiesa S. Agostino, San Gimigniano.

the right foreground stand the schoolmaster and the young Augustine, whose eyes are on his hornbook. The schoolmaster's left hand points a warning signal to the studious lad while he holds a whip in his right hand and is flogging a young boy not more than four or five years old, naked from the waist down, horsed on the back of an older pupil. That Italian schoolmasters chastised their students is historically true, but it was never a major feature of the schoolroom as it was in English public schools, especially those of the eighteenth and nineteenth centuries. St. Augustine's *Confessions* do not record schoolboy floggings; he was an apt pupil, much liked by his masters. The placement of the scene is disturbing; a discreet reminder in the background would have sufficed as a comment on schoolboy discipline, but here the whipping is shown front and center, as the principal action in the fresco. Biographical information about Gozzoli's private life is meager, and one is first tempted to question how he treated his apprentices. But Michael Baxandall points out that patrons had a good deal to say about the content of such com-

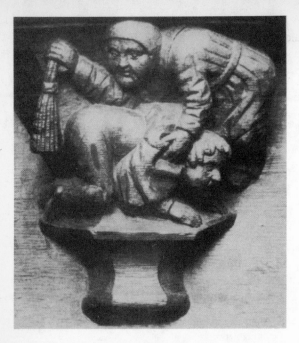

Figure 1.6. Mother birching her son. Misericord carving, sixteenth century. Eglise de Brou, Boug-en-Bresse.

missions.[5] Artists regularly provided preliminary drawings, and the overall design was developed with the patron's wishes in mind. The idea of placing a flagellation so prominently may have originated with an ecclesiastical official at S. Agostino's rather than with Gozzoli. This panel has negligible value with respect to St. Augustine's life, and whatever value it may have had for mid-fifteenth-century viewers is difficult to discern five centuries later.

Icons of flagellation are not confined to frescos on the walls of churches; one must look under the seats. Carvings on the bases of misericords exhibit an astonishing variety of scenes from everyday life, people at their quotidian occupations and amusements. Dorothy and Henry Kraus illustrate a sixteenth-century misericord from the choir stalls of the Eglise de Brou at Bourg-en-Bresse that shows a mother birching her son (fig. 1.6), the boy's shirt tucked up, his rump bared.[6]

Another at Rouen Cathedral portrays Aristotle and Phyllis; she sits sidesaddle on his loins and holds the bridle, but there is no whip, and both are fully clad. The genre was not confined to French churches; a similar scene is found on a misericord in Zamora Cathedral, the victim's legs being held down by a third party. The Reverend William Cooper illustrates his late-nineteenth-century text with a drawing from a stall at Sherborne Minster (ca. 1500) in which a schoolmaster birches a pupil before three other students who seem to be disregarding the proceedings.[7] Similar reliefs can be found in masonry among the decorative borders that adorn facades of late medieval or early Renaissance institutions of learning. Erotic suggestions are not found in these carvings; the anonymous artists were presenting a *tranche de vie*, a note on the variety of human behavior, not a moral or a message. The exposed *nates* have more of a humerous than a sensual character; they can be equated with a pratfall in vaudeville. The figures are, if one will permit the pun, a bit wooden.

After line engraving developed in the fifteenth century and woodblock printing a few decades later, a number of broadsides, *Flugblätter*, and other ephemera were produced, many of them as calculated erotica. They run the gamut of flagellatory situations and fall somewhere between art and pornography. A fair sample can be found scattered through the ponderous, pseudoscholarly compilations of *Sittengeschichte* by Central European writers that were published in the first third of this century.[8] With the advent of photography after the 1840s, nothing was left to the imagination, and a clandestine trade in such prints and pictures soon developed. That each generation preserves an almost atavistic interest in representations of "old-fashioned discipline" can be seen in the endpapers of Cheetham and Parfit's *Eton Microcosm*, which depict a flogging, purportedly at Eton, in the style of an early-sixteenth-century woodcut (fig. 1.7) but actually of modern execution.[9] The book was illustrated by Edward Pagram, who may have executed the woodcut himself, perhaps "inspired" by an earlier drawing or print.

It is a far cry from the homely carvings on seats designed to ease the tired rumps of plebeian choristers and the rude accoutrements of the schoolroom to the high art that decorated the public rooms in the sumptuous *palazzi* of Roman nobility, and the social distance required a different style and a change in tone. A painting titled *Cupid Chastised*,

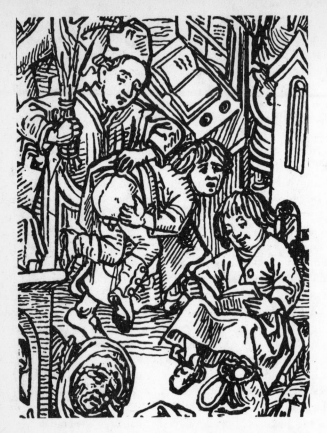

Figure 1.7. Birching at Eton. Twentieth-century woodcut imitating early-sixteenth-century style. *Eton Microcosm,* 1964.

attributed to Bartolemeo Manfredi (1580–1620/1), may have been commissioned by the Marchese Giustiniani or one of his circle in the first decade of the seventeenth century (fig. 1.8). Manfredi was an imitator of Caravaggio, as the bold curvilinear composition with its intersecting diagonals and the chiaroscuro indicate. It depicts an anecdote from classical mythology in which Mars punished Cupid for discharging his arrows at the wrong target. Mars is shown whipping Cupid with knotted cords as Venus tries to intercede for her mischievous son. Cupid is blindfolded and lies almost supine, squirming under the lash,

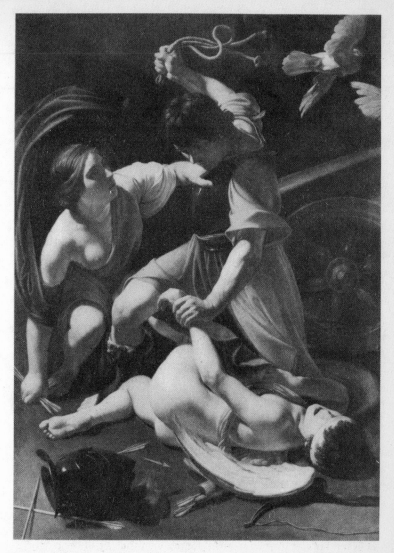

Figure 1.8. *Cupid Chastised*. Bartolomeo Manfredi, ca. 1605–10. Oil on wood. Courtesy of the Art Institute of Chicago.

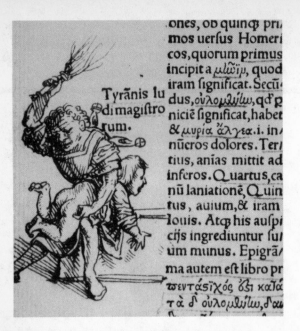

Figure 1.9. *The Schoolmaster's Tyrannical Game*. Hans Holbein, 1516–17. Marginal drawing in his personal copy of Erasmus' *Laus stultitiae*. Basel, 1516.

his quiver and arrows strewn untidily around him. Mars has grasped him by the left wrist, turning the youth's body so that his buttocks are exposed to the cords and the viewer's gaze. The artist was fully aware of the erotic implications of the scene and accentuated them. The source of light is from the upper left, and it highlights Venus' exposed breast, Mars' muscular forearm, and the boy's buttocks and thighs, which are sensuously modeled. It was a daring painting for its time. A generation earlier the Council of Trent, taking time from its weighty deliberations on church reform, had decreed that it was improper to paint an exposed female mamma except in the case of the Virgin and Child or of the legend of the Roman matron. Regarding exposure of the buttocks, the cardinals, bishops, and their learned advisers were silent. (Bottoms yes, bosoms no—*mes fesses!*)

Beating schoolboys' bottoms is a constant and recurring theme in both the literature and iconography of flagellation. Gozzoli's fresco of St. Augustine is an example from the Italian Renaissance, but it can be found in medieval art, and it persisted through the new humanism of the late fifteenth and early sixteenth centuries. When Hans Holbein the Younger (1497/8–1543) left his father's workshop at Augsburg in 1515, he settled in Basel, then a center of humanistic ideas. One of the young man's early acquisitions for his own library was a copy of Erasmus' *Laus stultitiae* (*The Praise of Folly*), the Lucianic satire written in England in 1509 in response to Sir Thomas More's stimulus, a work that had rapidly become the most popular and influential embodiment of the new spirit of intellectual inquiry that swept Western Europe during the first quarter of the sixteenth century. Young Holbein made marginal illustrations in his copy (the 1516 edition) and chose to adorn the section dealing with follies of the prevailing educational system with a drawing of a schoolmaster birching a pupil whom he has taken across his knee and who is naked from the waist down (fig. 1.9). He labels it "the master's tyrannical game," and perhaps it was a rueful recollection of his own schooldays of recent memory. A late-twentieth-century illustration of the same section of *The Praise of Folly* by Fritz Eichenberg shows an even more chaotic scene, a schoolroom with three sinister masters and a dozen terrified students (fig. 1.10). In the foreground, a schoolmaster dressed in early-sixteenth-century costume brandishes a birch in his left hand as he displays with his right hand a picture of Adam and Eve in their original sin to the students below him. Just behind him, a second master in monk's garb is beating the bared buttocks of a small boy bent over a bench. He is using a knotted cord, and the boy is kicking up his heels in pain. At the rear is the third master at his desk, twisting the ear of one boy and pulling the hair of another, while in front of the desk at a simulated altar a boy who has just been beaten is praying to an emblem of Christ crucified. The boy's hands are not in front of his face, as is customary when praying, but are massaging his *podex* for obvious reasons.

Holbein's drawing is not an isolated example of the period. Secular subjects found their way into the Books of Hours so popular among the French upper classes. A 1526 edition of *Les petites heures à l'usage de Chartres* depicts a more formal treatment of the subject (fig. 1.11). The elaborately robed schoolmaster is in his *sedia* and his victim is ensconced over a flogging block, his hands and feet held by two ushers while three of his schoolmates witness his punishment from the background. The motto in the scroll reads *Initium sapientie timor domini* (The beginning of wisdom is fear of the schoolmaster).

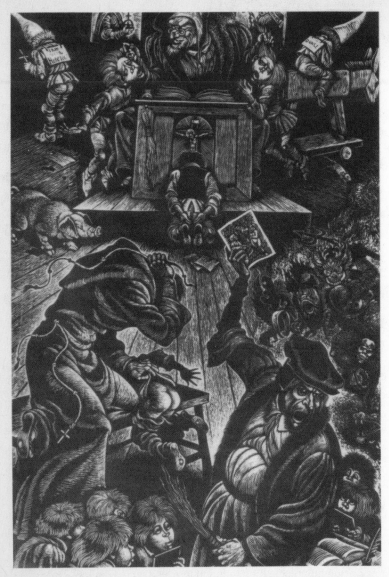

Figure 1.10. Illustration for Erasmus' *The Praise of Folly*. Fritz Eichenberg, woodcut. Baltimore: Aquarius Press, 1972.

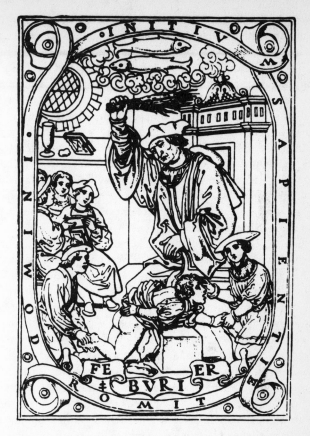

Figure 1.11. *Feburier: Initium sapientie timor domini.* Woodcut. From *Les petites heures à l'usage de Chartres.* Paris: Veuve de Thielman Kerver, 1526.

The uneasy symbiosis between art and flagellation reached its peak in England during the eighteenth century. That English society was prepared for it is evident even earlier. In act 3 of Thomas Shadwell's *The Virtuoso* (1676) there is an abortive flagellation scene between Snarl, a libertine, and Mrs. Figgup, a prostitute. Snarl proclaims, "I love castigation mightily. . . . I was so us'd to't at Westminster School that I could never leave it off since." But just as the rods are revealed under the carpet the action is interrupted by the arrival of Mrs. Figgup's brother.

The silent emblem of eighteenth-century flagellation in England is found in plate 3 of Hogarth's familiar series *The Harlot's Progress* (1731). We come upon her just as her decline is beginning, no longer in luxurious quarters "under the protection of a gentleman of quality," but set up in business for herself as a prostitute. She is just receiving a visit from Sir John Gonson, the magistrate who was determined to exterminate houses of ill repute. Hogarth has managed to fill his plate with any number of symbols that bear upon the meaning of the squalid scene, but the one item relevant here is the birch hanging on the wall just above the left side of the harlot's bed of transaction. No actual use of it is being made, nor is the engraving in any way indecorous; all personages are fully clad, and indeed the harlot herself is at breakfast. But the implication is that the birch is an instrument that no well-equipped prostitute would be without. Lichtenberg's famous commentaries are skittish about explaining it:

> At the head of the bed . . . there hovers between canopy and earth a comet with a terrific tail—the broom of education—the birch. We have been rather slow to mention it although among all the other inanimate objects on the plate this is usually the first, after the watch, to attract the eye of the spectator. We have called it terrible, but merely in accordance with linguistic custom; for these comets on the firmament of morals do just as little harm to that system as those in the sky to the system of the physical world. . . . If, however, we see them not as birches but merely as a bundle of faggots, then their use is really limitless; one might well ask, for example, what would become of the rushing stream of instruction and learning which in school pours through both our ears, if they were not in due course to build a dam at the other end of such faggots to prevent its escaping there helter-skelter. But how does the pedagogic faggot or rod of philanthropy come to be here, and just on the head-board of the bed? The problem, I must admit, is really not an easy one. I wish it were even more difficult. . . . Oh! that sort of problem makes the most wonderful material for authors who are paid by the page. . . . It is merely the point where morals themselves prohibit moralizing, and the most eloquent interpretation grows dumb or at least pretends to be dumb and makes only signs to passersby, or if it is compelled to speak, will say nothing more than I am dumb.[10]

Nowhere does Lichtenberg state frankly that the use to which the birch was put was, surely, a datum "that every schoolboy knows."

Hogarth's silent reminder that addresse with the birch was expected of prostitutes soon gave way to explicit representations. The 1766 edition of John Cleland's *Memoirs of a Woman of Pleasure* (usually known as *Fanny Hill*) is illustrated by a drawing showing Fanny about to apply the birch to Mr. Barville, who is shown lying prone on a couch, his trousers down, while Fanny, dressed in the latest French fashion, brandishes the birch behind him (see fig. 7.2, p. 164). The victim's haunches are raised to disclose his erection. A similar piece serves as the folding frontispiece for the first edition of *Madame Birchini's Dance*, a flagellation poem of some length.[11] The book sold for 3 shillings, but an advertisement in it informs us that proof impressions of the plate could be purchased from the publisher for 5 shillings and colored impressions (not proofs) at the same price. Then as now, there was a thriving trade in "soft" pornography in London. In this engraved plate the man's buttocks are exaggerated to steatopygia, but his genitals are not shown. The *mise-en-scène*, the chamber's furnishings and decorations as well as the woman's costume, is in the French style, a characteristically English use of displacement in which matters of sexual irregularity are ascribed to the French, as in French kiss, French letter, French pox, etc. But in general French flagellatory art was less direct than the English variety. For example, a copper engraving by Avril after J. F. Troy shows Venus punishing Psyche.[12] The scene takes place in an elegantly furnished neoclassical boudoir. Venus reclines imperiously on a four-poster bed while Psyche *en déshabielé* is shown falling backward in a swoon, her bosom and abdomen exposed, having been punished by three scantily clad attendants carrying birches. The emphasis seems to be on the display of undraped female flesh rather than on the flagellatory act.

The leading exponent of flagellation in English eighteenth-century art was the caricaturist James Gillray (1756–1815). Draper Hill estimates his total output during his active years (1782–1807) as slightly less than 1,000 prints, of which about two dozen display either an overt flagellatory act or something suggesting it: not an overwhelming percentage but disproportionate in comparison with the scant contributions by Rowlandson and Cruikshank to the genre.[13] According to Hill, much of Gillray's work before 1780 "had to do with brothel or privy," and this preoccupation never left him. The idea of using flagellation as a vehicle for satire came to him spontaneously, and he used the

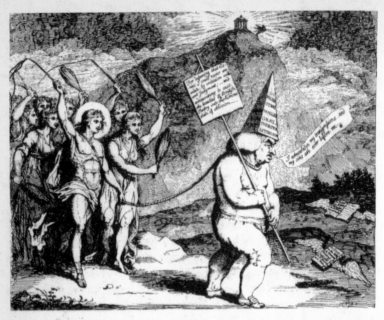

Figure 1.12. Samuel Johnson as Dr. Pomposo. James Gillray, 1783. Etching.

motif in a variety of contexts. As early in his "mature" career as 1782, four years after he entered the Royal Academy to study under Bartolozzi, his political satire *Evacuation before Resignation* depicts defecation, and his *Patience on a Monument* (1791) does the same. The droll transformation of the kettle's spout to a phallus in *The Kettle Hooting the Porridge Pot* (1782) is a bit more than outspoken. But later that year, when Judge Buller ruled that it was legal for a man to beat his wife with a stick provided it was no thicker than a thumb, the topic so exercised Gillray's fancy that he turned out an engraving showing the effect of "Judge Thumb's" opinion, namely, a man beating his wife with a stick.

Gillray used flagellation as an instrument of literary criticism. Though today we look back on Samuel Johnson's *Lives of the Poets* (1781) as one of the great monuments of English critical writing, its reception was by no means unanimous. Gillray shows Dr. Johnson as Dr. Pomposo, an epithet applied by Charles Churchill over twenty years earlier, being flogged out of Parnassus by Apollo and the Nine Muses (fig. 1.12).

The pyramidal dunce cap lists some of the poets in his *Lives*—Milton, Otway, Waller, Gray, Shenston[e], Lyttleton, Gay, Collins—and the placard over Johnson's shoulder reads, "For defaming that Genius I could never emulate by criticism without Judgment;—and endeavouring to cast the beauties of British Poetry into the hideous shade of oblivion." Johnson is shown as a penitent, a tear falling from his eye, and he is made to recant: "I acknowledge my transgressions, and my sins are ever before me." To Johnson's right two books take flight, one titled *An Essay on the Milk of Human Kindness dedicated to Dr. Johnson as a Man,* the other *An Essay on Envy dedicated to Dr. Johnson as an Author.* The verdict of literary history is somewhat different.

The give-and-take of politics sometimes made Gillray conceive of political satire in flagellatory images. His best-known plate in this form is titled *Westminster School* (1785) (fig. 1.13), an institution whose reputation for floggings went back a century when Dr. Busby was headmaster; recall Shadwell's *The Virtuoso* (1676). Gillray shows Charles James Fox applying the birch to William Pitt and his fellow Tories. The scene is a lofty hall with stone walls. Pitt lies across Fox's knees; marks of previous beatings are shown on his gluteal skin. Fox, playing the role of Dr. Busby, has already birched at least a score of Pitt's supporters, and a sea of birched bottoms proceeds *ad infinitum* to the right. In a niche over Fox's head is a statue of Justice, her scales in one hand, a birch in the other. Near his left foot is a large chamber pot filled with a supply of fresh birches. The details of the comments allude to minor political issues of the day, long forgotten. A decade later, Gillray's aquatint *Promis'd Horrors of the French Invasion* (1796) shows Pitt tied to a garlanded pole with a Liberty cap on its top, while Fox flogs him severely with a birch in each hand. Other acts of violence fill out the plate, the motive for which was Edmund Burke's *Reflections on a Regicide Peace,* in which he opposed Pitt's attempt to negotiate peace with the French government that had executed Louis XVI three years previously.

Burke was not exempt from Gillray's political flagellatory images. In *Crumbs of Comfort* (1782), Burke is shown being offered a scourge by a devil. In a double aquatint titled *Morning Preparation and Evening Consolation* (1785), Burke is shown in the latter attired as a Jesuit, stripped to the waist and holding a rosary, about to birch himself, presumably in penance for a political maneuver that had failed.

Other politically motivated plates by Gillray include *The Royal Joke* (1788), in which the Prince of Wales is shown spanking one Mrs.

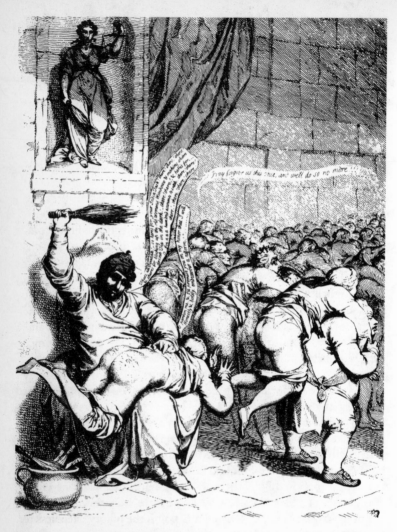

Figure 1.13. *Westminster School, or Dr. Busby settling accounts with Master Billy and his Playmates.* James Gillray, 1785. Etching.

Sawbridge; it was etched during the Regency crisis. Other examples are related to the French Revolution, such as *A Representation of the Horrible Barbarities Practised upon the Nuns by Fishwomen* (1792), in which the fishwives are shown scourging a group of nuns, and the gruesome *Petit Souper à la Parisienne* (1792), showing the sansculottes at a cannibal feast. Among the barbarities Gillray depicts is a bare-bottomed man seated on the amputated breast of a woman whose throat has been slit; he is chewing on a human arm. On the table lies a decapitated head, and another bare-bottomed wretch is about to eat an eye plucked from it. Three evil-looking women are also seated at the table, one eating a heart, another a pair of testicles, while the third looks on enviously. At the left rear, a hag is basting the body of a child on a spit in front of the fireplace. The spit has been inserted in the child's anus (cf. Taddeo di Bartolo), and he is suspended upside down (cf. the crucifixion of Peter), his thorax transfixed by a spike into which his arms are tied. However bloody-minded the French sansculottes were, they were not cannibals, and Gillray's excess piled upon excess satirizes both the coarseness of the French revolutionaries as well as the British purveyors of atrocity stories. Less bloodthirsty is his caricature of the Dutch Parliament (1796), in which he shows its members' heads distributed among the twigs of a birch. He etched this plate after an original drawing by a Swiss officer, David Hess, who later took up caricature semiprofessionally and signed himself as Gillray, Jr.

Gillray went beyond using flagellation as a vehicle of literary and political satire, employing it for contemporary scandals of the lesser sort. When Lady Buckinghamshire was forced to appear at the Marlborough Street police court on charges of maintaining a gambling house at her home in St. James's Square, he engraved *Discipline à la Kenyon* (1797), showing the judge, Lord Kenyon, flogging her with a scourge in one hand, a birch in the other, as she is paraded through the streets with her wrists tied to the back of a cart. Two of her wellborn colleagues in this floating faro game are shown in the pillory. Needless to say, no such punishment was ever carried out, and one suspects Gillray executed the plate to embarrass his pretentious neighbors. Another minor brouhaha occasioned his engraving *The Caneing in Conduit Street,* dedicated to the Flag Officers of the British Navy (1796).

Even less appropriate to the circumstances is *Lady Termagant Tinglebum: The Lovely Flagellation* (1795?), a print much altered by erasures and watercolor. On the print is inscribed "Vide [Covent Garden]

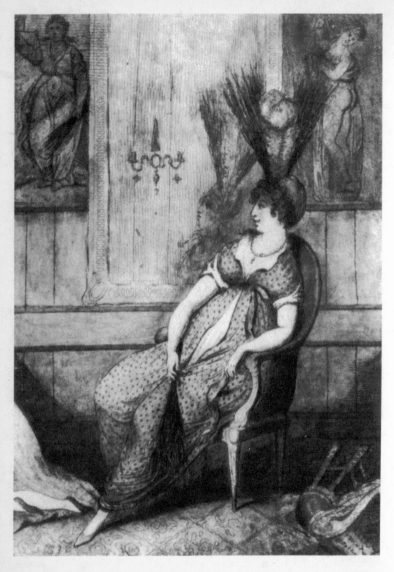

Figure 1.14. *Lady Termagant Tinglebum: The Lovely Flagellation*. James Gillray, 1795? Etching.

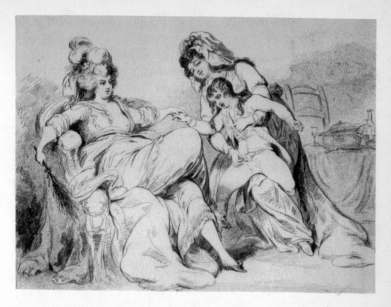

Figure 1.15. *Lady Termagant Flaybum going to give her Stepson a taste of her Desert After Dinner, etc.* James Gillray, 1786. Etching.

Monthly Recorder, June the 1st 1792. The Pupils of Birch, or the Severe Aunt, a Scholastic Scene Frequently Performed by Lady Eliza W******, the Beauty of Worcester upon her Juvenile Offenders, etc." (fig. 1.14). Gillray retouched the elaborate headdress of the lady flagellant, replacing three of the four feathers by two birch rods. Creeping away to the left is a young girl who evidently has just been flogged. An overturned stool suggests the girl has been birched upon it and struggled. Panels on the wall show Justice with her scales and a young lady disrobing. Although the act of flagellation is not shown, it is clearly a scene of lubricity. Precisely why Gillray was motivated in 1795 to take for his text a magazine article of the sort implied by its title is not known, but it is unmistakable evidence of his interest in flagellation and its literature. To be sure, the assigned date of 1795 is questioned, but there is no evidence that Gillray intended it as an illustration for the lurid story when it appeared.

Gillray's attraction to flagellation is even more visible in an earlier plate with the elaborate title *Lady Termagant Flaybum going to give her Stepson a Taste of her Desert after Dinner, a Scene performed every day near Grosvenor Square to the annoyance of the neighbourhood* (1786) (fig. 1.15).

The caricature took its origin from a local scandal when Lady Strathmore left her husband's home in Grosvenor Square and obtained a court order known as Articles of Peace against him. In point of fact, she had no stepson. Again we see the lady flagellant in fancy headdress, and though no actual flagellation is shown, the depiction of the lady's maid undoing the placket of the boy's trousers to prepare him for it is the sort of suggestive illustration designed to elicit fantasies in the minds of purchasers whose sensibilities were so oriented. It sold for 7s 6d., not a small sum in those days. Gillray's relationship to the domestic problems of the Strathmores is not known. Perhaps Lord Strathmore was an acquaintance or a customer, and Gillray took his side in the quarrel, but the engraving seems not only out of proportion to the event but also inaccurate.

Spencer Ashbee describes as a companion piece to the above engraving an untitled print which he describes as follows:

> Size 18 × 14½ inches. Interior. A lady in a high head-dress, with bosoms exposed, is seated on a long sofa, which extends across the picture, and is birching a lad stretched across her lap with his breeches down. A pretty girl, in a round hat, stands behind the sofa, and with her left hand holds the boy's left leg. To the right of the picture, in the foreground, a little girl is rubbing her naked bottom with her right hand and wiping her eyes with her left. . . . The design, which is very spirited, is in outline only.[14]

From the description there can be no doubt that Ashbee actually examined the print, but I have not been able to retrieve a copy. Ashbee left his books to the British Museum and his collection of paintings to the Victoria and Albert Museum, but this engraving is in neither collection, nor is it mentioned in any compendium or catalogue of Gillray's works. It is, of course, possible that Ashbee saw it in the collection of another connoisseur or that the attribution to Gillray is incorrect, the print being the work of a contemporary imitator. But more likely is the possibility that it was issued in a small edition and the extant copies destroyed. Nonetheless, sight unseen, it is a classcial pornographic icon of flagellation, designed to whet the prurience of those susceptible to such stimuli.

Perhaps some light can be shed on the lost print Ashbee describes by adding to the canon an as yet uncatalogued engraving by Gillray (fig. 1.16). It shows a middle-aged man sans breeches, still wearing stockings and slippers, horsed on the back of a madam while being birched

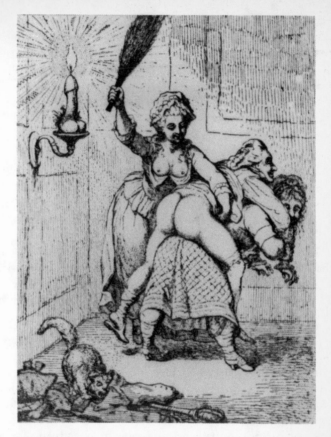

Figure 1.16. Flagellation scene in a brothel. James Gillray, 1780–85. Etching.

on his exposed buttocks by a fully dressed young woman whose bosom is exposed. At the bottom a cat rummages through the gentleman's discarded breeches, and his sword lying nearby on the floor attests that he is either a military or naval officer. The room seems unfurnished, and the priapic candle on the wall sconce completes the orgy in a flagellation brothel. Both Andrew Edmunds and Draper Hill have independently confirmed the attribution to Gillray and assign it an approximate date of 1780–85, somewhat early in his career. I suggest that Gillray ran a profitable sideline of making such plates and issuing the prints to a limited number of personally known collectors of "curiosa."

It would be an exaggeration to suggest that Gillray was obsessed with flagellation, but he seems to have more than a usual interest in it. Biographical details are scanty, but there are clues that suggest a possible background, granted the risk inherent in retrospective analysis based on incomplete evidence that is two centuries old. At the age of six, Gillray's strongly religious parents sent him to a Moravian boarding school in Bedford, an atmosphere scarcely designed to promote what we today would call mental health. A few lines from Hill's account indicate the tenor of the establishment:

> The rules forbade students to gather among themselves. No boy was supposed to be out of the immediate supervision of a master. Any fault of action, work or thought was severely rebuked as soon as it was suspected, and the practice of informing was generally encouraged. . . . The Moravians regarded the world with ill-concealed horror and worked to instill into their children a sense of the worthlessness of life. Four centuries of persecution had encouraged a view of death as a glorious release from earthly bondage. . . . They welcomed the thought of death, were delighted by funerals, and desired passionately *not* to recover from illness.[15]

Gillray's brother actually died at the school after a wasting disease, saying he "had fixed his mind on going over to the Saviour" and on his deathbed begging that his coffin might be brought nearby. That chilling, morbid event occurred in the first half of 1762, shortly after James Gillray had been entered as a pupil. Fortunately, the Moravians found it too expensive to maintain the school, and it was disbanded in 1764, at which point Gillray's formal education came to an end when he was eight and one-half years old.

There are no allegations of excessive corporal punishment at the Moravian school, but one may assume that the boys were punished in the manner then customary in all schools. Gillray returned home to Chelsea and lived with his parents. One item seems certain: he was not beaten by his father. That unfortunate man had lost his right arm at the battle of Fontenoy in 1745. We know almost nothing about Gillray's early adolescence except that it was passed in London. In his mid-teens he was apprenticed to an engraver, but after learning the rudiments of the craft he found apprenticeship irksome and deserted his master for a vagabond life with a group of strolling players. He returned to London in 1775 and slowly began his career as a caricaturist.

His early work was published by William Humphrey, and in the 1780s he worked for several different publishers, but after 1791 he worked exclusively for Hannah Humphrey, a woman a few years older than himself; she was the unmarried sister of his first publisher. He occupied lodgings over her shop successively in Old Bond Street, New Bond Street, and finally St. James's Square. According to Hill, their "friendship undoubtedly progressed beyond the stricter limits of professional cooperation."[16] The curtain of privacy drops upon what went on in the rooms above the shop, but in addition to this irregular liaison there is other evidence of emotional disturbance. Though in no sense an alcoholic—his consistent output from 1782 to 1807 negates such an idea—he did drink to excess on occasion, enough for one of his contemporaries to write that he was intemperate. He was also subject to wide fluctuations in mood: He "experienced soarings and plummetings of mood which a psychiatrist would nowadays regard as signs of a manic-depressive temperament."[17] Not overtly psychotic—far from it—he was nevertheless highly strung. Although he was generally described as morose and introverted, one correspondent described him as a "fountain overflowing with joke." Gillray's was a complex personality, and there is not enough information for a careful assessment, but there are enough clues in both his life and his work to indicate that he was emotionally labile and, on occasion, unbalanced. Osbert Lancaster's assessment is fair: "One thing alone Gillray lacked—compassion; had he possessed it, he would be, what he so nearly is, the equal of Daumier."[18] But the circumstances of his life were not so ordered that compassion played any role. More than any British caricaturist, his satires are severe and biting, even bitter and frequently cruel.

To contrast Gillray with Thomas Rowlandson (1756–1827) is an obvious device. Born the same year as Gillray, Rowlandson too studied briefly at the Royal Academy and became a caricaturist, equally well known for his individual prints and his series of illustrations for popular books. Like Gillray, he drew upon current events and fashions for inspiration, and even more than Gillray his life can be described as dissolute; gambling, drinking, and fornicating occupied the time he spent away from the drawing board and copper plate. Yet despite his knowing insistence on the animalism in human nature, few of his prints match Gillray's for savagery. Even in later life, when he felt his Kraft ebbing and turned out more than one hundred explicitly sexual drawings, he exhibited a good-humored randiness that amuses rather than titillates.

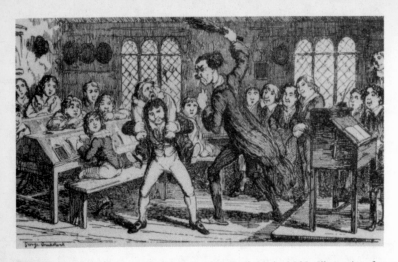

Figure 1.17. *Take Down his Breeches!* George Cruikshank, 1839. Illustration for Thackeray's "Cutting Weather." *The Comic Almanack,* February 1839. Facing p. 164.

In only one of these is there a suggestion of flagellation; a plate titled *The Fort* shows a bare-breasted woman prisoner, presumably a prostitute, being led downstairs in a prison while a potbellied, ithyphallic jailer looks on. Escorting the woman is a turnkey who carries a cat-o'-nine-tails, clearly indicating what will shortly take place downstairs but not actually denoting the act of flagellation.

Contemporary with Gillray and Rowlandson was the Marquis de Sade. Editions of his *La nouvelle Justine* and *L'histoire de Juliette* in the 1790s were illustrated by a number of prints portraying *à la manière française* any number and variety of flagellations, often with a number of participants. One, for example, shows four nude women stacked one on top of another while a nude man flagellates them seriatim as he is being masturbated by a fifth nude woman. Such illustrations are clearly pornographic in intent and outside the boundaries of art.

George Cruikshank (1792–1878), who followed Gillray and Rowlandson as England's leading caricaturist and book illustrator, seems to have depicted only one flagellation scene, a print titled *Take Down His Breeches!* The scene is a schoolroom with leaded lozenged windows, the schoolboys at their benches, and front and center the schoolmaster about to birch a student who is horsed upon another's back (fig. 1.17).

The illustration was for Thackeray's "Cutting Weather" in the *Comic Almanack* for February 1839. Though schoolboys were regularly flogged at the time, Cruikshank abided by the mid-Victorian distaste for displaying undraped gluteal flesh.

The two isolated examples by Rowlandson and Cruikshank can be taken as comment on the mores of their day, but not only the number but the quality of Gillray's prints exceed the usual conventions of his time. More in keeping with the almost jocular allusions to flagellation by Rowlandson and Cruikshank is an isolated etching by Goya (1746–1828). Many of his etchings portray human cruelty, notably *Caprichos* (1797–99) and *Desastres de la guerra* (1808–14), first published in 1863, thirty-five years after his death. It is not surprising that one of the *Caprichos* should show a spanking scene, albeit a temperate version (fig. 1.18). *Se quebro el cantaro* (The Broken Jug) shows a mother, who has been hanging laundry on the line, in the act of spanking her young son with a slipper. A broken clay water jug lies in the left foreground, and the boy's clumsiness has occasioned the maternal wrath. The mother holds up the boy's shirttails with her teeth, lowers his trousers with her left hand, and assails his bottom with the slipper in her right hand. Her face is contorted with anger, the boy's with anguish. It is unlike the calmly administered floggings by schoolmasters from Gozzoli on, but there is no intimation of excessive brutality beyond the anger of the moment and certainly no erotic intention. It seems reasonable to interpret the etching as Goya's comment on how children were treated circa 1800 in Spain (not much different from elsewhere) and, perhaps, on how not to rear them. It is the reality of "domestic discipline" rather than the fantasy.

Superficially similar to Goya's etching but different in purpose is Honoré Daumier's (1808–79) lithograph *Le toucher,* first published as one of the series *Les cinq sens* in *Caricature,* September 13, 1839, later in *Charivari,* January 15, 1843 (fig. 1.19). The similarity is that a very young child is being beaten, presumably for a domestic offense against good order, by a wrathful woman. The old crone is quite savage, her facial expression that of rage. The birched child, whose sex is indeterminate, is yelping, as one would expect. The scene is the kitchen of a lower-middle-class or working-class household. Daumier, even at the age of thirty-one, was a confirmed Republican, anti-Royalist, certainly anti-Bonapartist. Perhaps the picture of Napoleon on the wall suggests

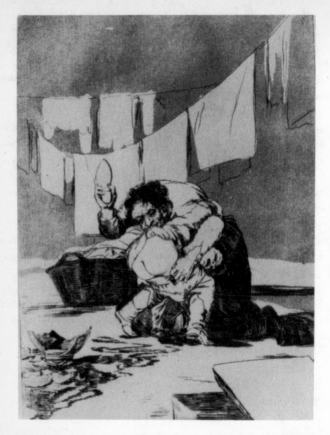

Figure 1.18. *Se quebro el cantaro* (The Broken Jug). From *Los caprichos*. Francisco Goya, 1799. Etching.

that Daumier may have been trying to equate Bonapartism among the lower orders with unbridled violence. It is easy enough to read ideology into a picture, but actually the lithograph was one of a series of five, each dealing with one of the five senses. This was a recognized form of demotic genre art. For example, in the Mauritshuis there is a comparable painting by Jan Molenaer (1610–68) titled *L'odorat* (The Sense of Smell), which shows a woman wiping the exposed bottom of an infant who has just defecated, while to her right her husband holds

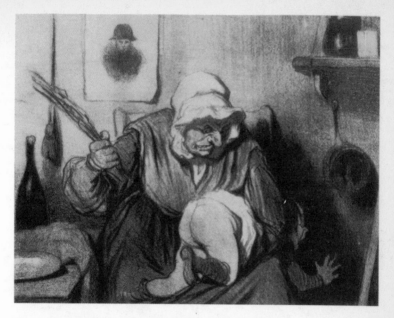

Figure 1.19. *Le toucher.* Honoré Daumier, 1839. Lithograph.

his nose and grimaces at the offensive odor, a scene of domestic intimacy that Daumier may have chosen to satirize (though he had a fair number of comparable French examples) instead of making a political statement. Whichever interpretation one chooses, the flagellation is a social comment with no hint of eroticism.

Continuing in Cruikshank's tradition across the Atlantic was True Williams, who provided the illustrations for *Peck's Bad Boy,* that Tyl Eulenspiegel of the Wisconsin frontier.[19] Young Henry's pranks may seem crude to modern readers, but they struck a responsive vein in the audience of the 1880s and 1890s, sufficiently so to propel their author and publisher George W. Peck into the governorship of Wisconsin from 1892 to 1894. Many of the "bad boy's" escapades were designed to expose the hypocrisy of the older generation, and his father carried out his reprisals in the woodshed or attic (fig. 1.20). As in Cruikshank's scene of schoolroom discipline the boy's buttocks are not exposed, and the American barrel stave has replaced the British birch. Also in Cruikshank's tradition are a few illustrations by Norman Rockwell, notably

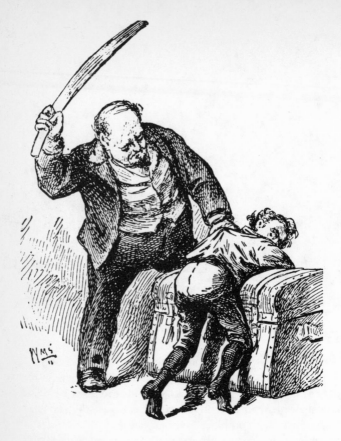

Figure 1.20. "Pa said, 'Now Hennery.'" Illustration from *Peck's Bad Boy,* True Williams, ca. 1883.

one for a 1935 edition of *Huckleberry Finn* showing the schoolteacher beating Tom Sawyer with a switch for having whispered to Huck in class.[20] Another from the same period, executed with deliberate archaism, is an advertisement for Interwoven Socks which makes the pun on "socks" by showing a man in late-eighteenth-century costume applying a slipper to a boy's upturned bottom; it is titled *Father's Day*. In both of these the man is standing, his knees slightly bent, and he is holding the boy off the ground, more or less against his thigh. This is a most awkward position in which to apply a series of smacks to a squirming

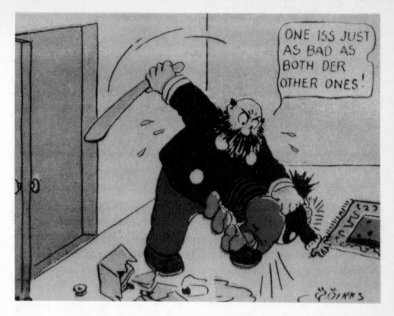

Figure 1.21. Hans and Fritz on a Sunday morning. From *The Katzenjammer Kids.* Rudolph Dirks, ca. 1906–7.

boy. A *Saturday Evening Post* cover for 1933 repeats the Goya theme; a mother is shown seated spanking a rather young child across her lap with a hairbrush; she is holding a book titled *Child Psychology* in her free hand.[21] The little boy seems to have broken seriatim a vase, a mirror, and a clock. Needless to say, all Rockwell's boys receive their punishment decorously with their trousers on.

Further dilution of the theme is seen in Rudolf Dirks' *The Katzenjammer Kids,* a comic strip that started in 1897 and continued in weekly appearances for over half a century under a succession of cartoonists.[22] The captain's drubbings were usually administered by hand, but occasionally with a barrel stave or bed slat (fig. 1.21); the panel selected for illustration shows a broken box camera, an echo of Goya's broken pitcher. The humor of the situation seems to have lost its public appeal by the middle of the twentieth century. In recent years it appears for popular consumption in the guise of sophisticated wit in which the actual beating is replaced by innuendo (fig. 1.22).

The long list of examples cited indicates that like the drama, opera,

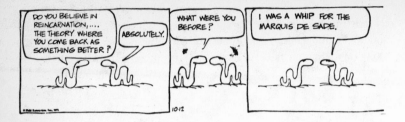

Figure 1.22. Remembrance of things past. From *B.C.* Johnny Hart, ca. 1971. Copyright © 1971 by King Features Syndicate. Reprinted with special permission of King Features Syndicate, Inc.

and ballet, flagellation and its icons developed from religious rituals. Originally the province of a priesthood, the act became demotic and even democratic. With reference to hedonism, John Stuart Mill pointed out that it required no *a priori* proof of its validity as a motive; the proof lay in mankind's conduct. In the same sense, one may infer that flagellation and its representation fulfill and satisfy a deep-seated human need. Not only do artists at many different levels of achievement take pleasure in executing such images, but viewers enjoy looking at them. From what we know about the artists cited, none seems to have had a reputation for cruelty. Only Rowlandson and to a lesser extent Gillray can be impeached for leading disorderly lives, but in that respect they were no worse than many of their contemporaries at the close of the eighteenth century in London.

With rare exceptions (Taddeo di Bartolo's fresco of the punishments of Hell), none of the flagellations depicted suggests the infliction of serious bodily harm. The erotic implications cannot be gainsaid; consider Leopold Bloom's comment in Joyce's *Ulysses:* "I meant only the spanking idea. A warm tingling glow without effusion. Refined birching to stimulate the circulation." This notion can be traced to Meibom, who argued that flagellation of the gluteal area stimulated circulation to the pelvic region in general, hence its erogenous effect.[23] Meibom's book was translated into English, French, and German, some editions with further amplifications by Bartholin. The theory was widely accepted in the seventeenth and eighteenth centuries and was given further credence by Abbé Boileau's *Historia flagellantium, de recto et perverso flagorum usū apud Christianos* (Paris, 1700).

It is evident from the exemplars given above that, pornography excepted (much of it of recent vintage), icons of flagellation more frequently exhibit males rather than females being beaten, adult males by women, adolescent and younger males by men. The homoerotic implications of beating schoolboys are obvious, best expressed in the verses Lytton Strachey wrote to Roger Senhouse in 1929:

> How odd the fate of pretty boys!
> Who, if they dare to taste the joys
> That so enchanted Classic minds,
> Get whipped upon their neat behinds;
> Yet should they fail to construe well
> The lines that of those raptures tell
> —It's very odd, you must confess—
> Their neat behinds get whipped no less.

2
Robert Musil: What Price Homosexual Sadism?

*I*n a recent article I commented that neither Somerset Maugham nor D. H. Lawrence nor James Joyce, each of whom wrote an autobiographical novel on the eve of World War I, proved in later life to have been successful in exorcising his personal devils by literary autocatharsis.[1] Their subsequent careers were characterized by a variety of neurotic maladjustments, and literary biographers have made capital of them ever since. To this list might be added the case of Robert Musil (1880–1942), the Austrian novelist, whose work is less familiar to English readers because it has been translated only in recent years and, even now, not completely.

His reputation, that of a German Proust manqué, rests chiefly upon his labyrinthine stream-of-consciousness novel *Der Mann ohne Eigenschaften* (*The Man without Qualities*), set in decadent Viennese society during the declining days of the Austro-Hungarian Empire. In that respect it resembles Proust's study of Parisian salons under the Troisième République before World War I, but unlike Proust's achievement Musil's novel was left unfinished at its author's death and has not yet been completely translated into English. But Musil's first novel, an experiment in autobiography, was finished and published in 1906, a few years before the public self-exposures of Maugham, Lawrence, and Joyce. It bears the title *Die Verwirrungen des Zöglings Törless,* that is, the perplexities (or confusions, or aberrations) of the military-school student Törless, and has been published in English translation under the simpler, but less accurate, less defining title, *Young Törless.*[2]

A writer who publishes an autobiographical novel in his twenties, when his career is just beginning, runs the risk of having the events of his earlier life reinterpreted in the light of his subsequent career. Such postmortem examinations are not carried out under the high bright spirit of young promise but in the chillier atmosphere of the dissecting room, where the most frequent questions are: What is the nature of the disease? How did it begin? What were the symptoms? What course did it pursue? What finally happened to the patient? In such circumstances, purely literary values are modified by historical and biographical ones, and the argument is less concerned with letters quā literature than the relation between letters and life.

Like so many novels of its genre, a few precursors but many more since, *Young Törless* deals with the sexual and intellectual awakening of an adolescent hero who is modeled on its author and recapitulates, how accurately one cannot be certain, many of its author's actual experiences. That these experiences include a complex episode of homosexual sadism is not, by the standards of 1987, a novelty. But by the standards of 1906 the subject was daring, not to say unconventional. That it should have been related in such explicit detail and yet not have been subjected to censorship is, in the light of American and British experience, quite surprising, all the more so because *Reigen* by Arthur Schnitzler, which deals with so banal a subject as heterosexual promiscuity, had been interdicted in 1900. *Young Törless* may have scandalized a few readers, but its erotic contents do not whet the reader's prurience nor, clearly, was it designed to. For a first novel it met with fair success, and the generally favorable notices decided Musil on adopting a writer's career.

Available biographical data about Musil, especially his childhood years, are scanty; the details of his life have not been subject to the businesslike scrutiny of American literary scholars. But the general outline is clear, and some specific anecdotes are telling. In his afterword to the American edition of *Young Törless,* John Simon tells us that Musil was born in 1880, the only son and surviving child of an engineer who rose to a high position in the Austro-Hungarian civil service, whose later career included a major teaching position, and who was eventually knighted. The father is described as "essentially scholarly, mild and pliable." Musil's mother, we are told, was "a tempestuous woman, presumably frustrated by marriage to the point of not even showing particular love for her son who, nonetheless, cared more for her than for the meek father who carefully softened the rod with which, at his wife's insistence, he would give the boy a caning." Given a family constellation with such a configuration of interpersonal relations, the question is not so much why the son developed psychopathic tendencies but what form they took. Added to this information is the datum that before Musil was born his parents had had a daughter who died before she was a year old. Simon concludes that the image of what this sister might have been, added to what the mother should have been, was to haunt his work and thought forever. The ambiguous figure of a sister, lost before his own birth, might well be part of the reason why Musil was never able to finish *The Man without Qualities,* unable to resolve the consummation of the love between two of its chief characters, Ulrich and his twin sister, Agathe, into either overt incest or into "some abstinent otherworldly rapture." The lack of a real sister, coupled with his mother's lack of affection, or overt rejection, may have been the unconscious motive for Musil's innocent "abduction" of a very young schoolgirl some time in early puberty. Shortly after this incident, his parents sent him to the military school in which the events of *Young Törless* are set.

Confronted by an autobiographical novel, the reader is faced with the problem stated by Coleridge when he tried to distinguish between poems of fancy and poems of imagination. Is it a rearrangement of experience rather than a transformation of it? We can never be sure of the historical accuracy of some of the incidents Musil relates or of the specific behavior of some of his characters, but there is no doubt that Musil attended a military school where upper-class Austrians sent their sons to prepare them for a career in the army, that he was a student there from circa 1893 to circa 1896, and that he did participate in an affair which involved homosexual behavior and sadism. Of equal importance is the fact that in these years his inquiring mind developed; he became proficient at physics and mathematics, and he developed an interest in metaphysics, epistemology, and psychology. The transition from a boy's home to boarding school marks the change from being exposed and subject to his parents' values and judgments, and the emotions they invest, to the values and judgments of society, in this case as in so many, a societal hierarchy based on command and status, coupled with the inevitable comparison to and by his peers. The rhetorical framework of such an environment, artificial and set apart from the real world outside, affords the novelist considerable advantage in setting his stage and controlling the movements of his characters. Many novelists have created such environments from imagination for the sake of their fiction, but in Musil's case it was real, and he drew on direct personal experience.

The action in *Young Törless* centers around four boys: Törless, modeled after Musil himself; two slightly older boys, Beineberg, who represents a mystical view of life, and Reiting, who embodies ruthless activism and an aptitude for intrigue; and Basini, of an age with Törless, the victim. John Simon conjectures that Reiting may represent a transformation of the name Reiter, a constant companion of Musil's parents, a man Musil hated because he suspected him, rightly or wrongly, of being his mother's lover. Whether Musil's belief had a foundation in fact or was a fantasied projection of an unresolved oedipal situation is not clear; what was decisive, however, was that his belief in his mother's unchastity determined his conduct.

The novel opens with a scene in which Törless, still homesick after three years at the military school, says goodbye to his parents at the railway station. They have paid him a two-day visit and entertained his friends Beineberg and Reiting, who are also at the station to bid them adieu. After the train leaves, Törless, somewhat disconsolate, walks back to the school with his two friends. They stop off at a cake shop or tavern where a rather coarse barmaid named Božena, apparently sexually available to some of the military cadets, teases Törless unpleasantly and makes crude innuendos about his mother's sexual promiscuity, claiming to have been in service with the boy's aunt. In this scene we are introduced indirectly to Basini; Božena describes him as a youngster who boasts of love affairs he pretends to have had at home but whose advances she, with the intuition of her class and occupation, readily identifies as those of a lad who is with a woman for the first time.

An abrupt transition from this shabby scene initiates the plot. Reiting has identified Basini as the person who has been stealing from other cadets' lockers. He and Beineberg lay plans to deal with Basini according to their whim, and they persuade Törless to join the fun. Previously, Reiting and Beineberg have found a "secret chamber," a small room under the eaves in the attic of an unused wing of the school building. They have furnished it with a variety of juvenile mementos and accoutrements. One senses that Törless is privy to the arrangement and has been there before. In this chamber Reiting and Beineberg subject Basini to a series of humiliations including conventional beatings, tying up, and sexual abuse. This continues for a period of several weeks.

At first, Törless is merely an onlooker. Musil interposes a number of metaphysical and psychological digressions but finally makes the point that during one of these séances Törless experiences sexual excitement.

Another abrupt transition, and we are confronted with the device Musil uses to symbolize Törless' *Verwirrungen,* his adolescent perplexities, confusions, and doubts. He falls afoul of the mathematical convention of irrational numbers. At first he discusses the problem with Beineberg: "But that's just it, I mean, there's no such thing . . . there can't be any real number that could be the square root of a minus quantity." Beineberg cannot help him resolve his doubts, so he takes them up with the mathematics master, an equally unproductive discussion, but the master lends Törless a volume of Kant. That Kantian metaphysics and epistemology may prove more dangerous to a confused adolescent than hard-core pornography appears never to have occurred to German schoolmasters. Törless' perplexities increase.

The consolations of philosophy lead easily into psychopathology. Törless has a nightmare, a scene involving Beineberg and the mathematics master. The master, who is carrying the book, says, "If that is really so, we shall find the right answer on page twelve, page twelve refers us then to page fifty-two, but then we must bear in mind what is pointed out on page thirty-one, and on this supposition. . . ." The dream sequence rapidly switches to the sensation of sexual excitement Törless had felt when he watched Basini being used sadistically, and intermingled with this is a recollection from early childhood of his feeling himself to be a girl. He wakes up. Later that day he has hallucinatory experiences in which Basini figures prominently.

A two-day public holiday occurs, and the school is almost emptied of cadets and masters. Törless and Basini are left more or less alone together. That night the inevitable occurs: Törless consummates a homosexual act on Basini, who has, in effect, solicited it. Musil describes Basini's body as "lacking almost any sign of male development . . . chaste, slender willowyness, like that of a young girl." To a medical eye this suggests a form of hypogonadism without obesity. In a note dating from 1906, the year the novel was published and ten years after the events took place, Musil wrote that Basini could just as easily have been replaced by a woman and that instead of "bisexuality" there could have been any other perversion. Musil's abduction of a little girl a few years before might indicate that he had not yet fixed on a sexual object-choice, but given the deliberate setting of the novel in a military school, his later comment appears like a hasty attempt at rationalization by displacement and sex reversal. By endowing Basini with a female habitus, Musil fuses both male and female object-choices into one partner, his own literary pseudohermaphrodite. Following this epicene epiphany of ephebic eroticism, Törless experiences a profound guilt reaction. The sense of guilt is made explicit in the next few paragraphs when he abruptly rejects further sexual advances from Basini.

The denouement follows swiftly. The other students return from their brief holiday. Another episode is presented in which Reiting and Beineberg torture Basini by sticking pins into his naked body while Törless watches, unhappy and lacking in grace. Basini finally becomes terrified and seeks Törless' advice. Törless advises him to confess what has been going on to the masters. Guilt and anxiety press so heavily on him that he makes only a feeble effort to exculpate himself. Reiting and Beineberg manage to put most of the blame on Basini, who is so thoroughly frightened that he is almost mute. Their task is made easier because Törless has made a maladroit effort to run away. "In short, it was a well-rehearsed farce, brilliantly stage-managed by Reiting, and the highest possible moral tone was assumed in putting forward excuses that would find favor in the masters' eyes. . . . Then Törless was brought in. He had been picked up, dead tired and very hungry, in the next town."

When interrogated in the headmaster's chambers, Törless is agitated, unintelligible, and unable to give a coherent account. He mumbles something about imaginary numbers, then delivers himself of the following speech:

> No, I wasn't wrong when I talked about things having a second, secret life that nobody takes any notice of . . . ! It was more as if I had a sort of second sight and saw all this not with the eyes of reason. Just as I can feel an idea coming to life in my mind, in the same way I feel something alive in me when I look at things and stop thinking. There's something dark in me, deep under all my thought, something I can't measure out with thoughts, a sort of life which can't be expressed in words and which is my life, all the same. . . . The silent life oppressed me, harassed me. . . . I was tormented by the fear that our whole life might be like that and that I was only finding it out here and there in bits and pieces. . . . Oh, I was dreadfully afraid! I was out of my

mind. . . . Now it's all over. I know I was wrong after all. I'm not afraid of anything any more. I know that things are just things and will probably always be so. And I shall probably go on forever seeing them sometimes this way and sometimes that, sometimes with the eyes of reason, sometimes with those other eyes. . . . And I shan't ever try to compare one with the other. . . .

Musil has put into the mouth of his fictive alter ego the speech of a person recovering from a psychotic episode, but it was his own self divided. Basini, of course, is expelled; Reiting and Beineberg stay on. Törless withdraws from the school by mutual consent. His mother comes to fetch him. She expects to find an overwrought and desperately perplexed boy but is astonished by his cool composure. The last lines of the novel are:

"What is it, my dear boy?"
"Nothing, Mama, I was just thinking." And, drawing a deep breath, he considered the faint whiff of scent that rose from his mother's corseted waist.

In real life Musil never received more than vicarious affection from his punitive, dominating mother.

But Musil tipped his hand long before that. Just after describing the homosexual scene between Törless and Basini he interpolates a sententious passage:

Later, when he had got over his adolescent experiences, Törless became a young man whose mind was both subtle and sensitive. By that time he was one of those aesthetically inclined intellectuals who find there is something soothing in a regard for law and indeed . . . for public morals too, since it frees them from the necessity of ever thinking about anything coarse. . . . For the only real interest they feel is concentrated on the growth of their own soul, or personality, or whatever one may call the thing within us that every now and then increases by the addition of some idea picked up between the lines of a book, or which speaks to us in the silent language of a painting—the thing that every now and then awakes when some solitary, wayward tune floats past us and away, away into the distance, whence with alien movements tugs at the thin scarlet thread of our blood—the thing that is never there when we are writing minutes, building machines, or following any of hundreds of other similar occupations.

Gauchely written though the passage is, it merely represents a form of retreat from reality, a retreat into a solipsistic world in which illumination or growth occur only intermittently, and then in response to random aesthetic stimuli. However, this is Musil's image of himself as of 1906, after he had purged himself of guilt.

It appears to be time to return from Musil's ramblings, first as the guilt-stricken Törless, later as the novelist trying to relieve that guilt. What actually happened in the ten years between 1896 when he left the military academy and 1906 when *Young Törless* was published? The decade covers Musil's years from sixteen to twenty-six, a decisive period in most men's lives. The objective record tells us that he floundered a bit. At first, possibly spurred by the scent of his mother's corseted waist, he considered following in his father's footsteps, and he studied civil engineering. His nimble mind served him well; he even invented a chromatometer which was known by his name. But engineering did not satisfy him, so he went off to the University of Berlin to study philosophy and experimental psychology. It was probably at this time that he became aware that his intrapsychic conflict still persisted, partly digested but unresolved. Accordingly, concomitant with his work toward his degree, he began writing *Young Törless*. When it was published, he felt a sense of relief for a time, but he had yet to establish a firm, mature, heterosexual relationship.

In 1907 Musil met Martha Marcovaldi, whom John Simon describes as "a Jewish woman seven years older than himself, estranged from her husband, mother of two children, unattractive, free-thinking, highly intelligent, and a talented painter." Viewed in terms of the standards of the outside world, his parents' world, this was just another example of a neurotic young man making an unsuitable choice of mate. From Musil's point of view, unconscious though it may have been, she combined the attributes of mother-sister-friend and fellow artist. Unable to elicit an affectionate response from his mother, Musil found a substitute in an older, experienced woman. His marriage rather than his novel appeared to resolve some but not all of his problems. Simon informs us that when they were able to marry a few years later, Martha gave up painting to become a "dedicated helpmate-hand-maiden to the impractical genius she had married, and the two remained happy with each other to the end." Probably not a bad compromise for both of them, but what about the objective record?

Musil received his doctorate from the University of Berlin in 1908. Presumably backed up by Martha Marcovaldi, he decided not to pursue an academic career. He took a position as librarian at the Technische Hochschule in Vienna. In 1913 he returned to Berlin to become one of the editors of *Die neue Rundschau,* an avant-garde literary magazine. During World War I he served as an officer in the Austrian army. After the war he worked as a liaison official in the War Ministry of the newly formed Austrian republic. From 1922 on he supported himself as a free-lance writer that he might have time to work on *The Man without Qualities.* He left Germany in 1933 for obvious reasons and returned to Vienna where a "Musil society" was formed to provide him with financial support. After the Anschluss of 1938 he moved to Switzerland, where he died four years later. During these years attempts to interest American organizations to sponsor his emigration to the United States failed, despite support by men of such reputation as Albert Einstein and Thomas Mann.

Apart from *Young Törless* (1906) and *The Man without Qualities* (unfinished at his death, 1942) Robert Musil's publications, excluding journalistic ephemera, include two longish short stories or contes, "The Perfecting of a Love" and "The Temptation of Quiet Veronica," published together as *Unions* in 1913; three comparable stories, "Grigia," "Tonka," and "The Lady from Portugal," published as *Three Women* in 1924; an expressionist drama, *Die Schwärmer* (*The Enthusiasts*), performed once only in 1921 and published that year; and a farce, *Vinzens* (1924). The short stories have in common what Kermode calls "a nervous obliquity, a mystique of the erotic, a deep interest in the borders of the human mind, those uneasy frontiers with the human body and with inhuman reality."[3] This sensibility is more fully explored and exploited in *The Man without Qualities,* which numbers among its themes nymphomania, incest, and sex murder, "not at all for their prurient interest but as indices of the reaches of consciousness." To these works, most of which are available in English, one must add the amusing sketches called *Posthumous Papers of a Living Man* and the light-textured, quasi-satirical fictions called *Stories Which Aren't Stories,* neither of which, so far as I can determine, has appeared in English translation. It is not exactly a voluminous output for a writing career of four decades.

One begins to question whether Musil suffered from neurotic work inhibition. If so, it might well be interpreted as the expression in later life of the same forces which determined his indecision regarding a choice of career during the decade after leaving school. He began *The Man without Qualities* in 1922 and left 2,000 pages of it twenty years later at his death in 1942, a production rate of 100 pages a year. Granted that during this period he wrote many ephemeral pieces merely to earn a living, granted that he took enormous pains, polishing and rewriting continually, it is not surprising that even a critic disposed in his favor such as John Simon should write, "Though these works contributed to making him famous among a small elite, they achieved scarcely more than a succès d'éstime, and the larger public has remained to this day, even in his own Vienna, ignorant of Musil." Small wonder! He had but little to say to that "larger public." Kermode epitomizes Musil as "the interesting limiting case" and decides that *The Man without Qualities* as a novel "turns into something else: a metaphysician's miscellany, interspersed with subtle exempla."[4]

Musil's doctoral thesis was an analysis of the ideas of Ernst Mach (1838–1916), the physicist-psychologist-philosopher who developed the epistemological notion that knowledge is based primarily on experience and that the individual is united with the external world only through sensory impressions. Musil puts much of this ideation into the mouth of Ulrich, the hero of *The Man without Qualities,* another fictive alter ego. Immobilized and impotent, torn like Musil by conflicts between his intellect and emotions, Ulrich can only maintain his facade of being in complete control of his life situation by withdrawing from the crises engendered by irrational elements (Törless' anxiety over irrational numbers) both in his own psyche and in society. In terms of Musil's relation to his parents, it is significant that Ulrich rejects the values of his father, a character who bears a partial resemblance to Musil's own father, and there is no mention of Ulrich's mother at all. In Elliott's apt phrase, "Like Schoenberg's Moses, he is condemned to know the word of God but to be unable to communicate it."[5]

Other evidence of neurotic maladjustment can be found. We learn that Musil was an effective editor of military newspapers during World War I, that he was demobilized as a captain with many citations and decorations, and that "something military remained in him, consolidating an anterior aristocratic-snobbish streak," hardly surprising in view of his family's status and his own education at military school. But then, "However poor the Musils were . . . [his] clothes had to be expensive and immaculate . . . the sight of an unpolished pair of shoes hurt him physically." That is not merely an aristocratic-snobbish streak; it is overt narcissism, prefigured in the passage from *Young Törless* in which Musil preens himself on the subtlety and sensitivity of his mind. Musil chose this image of himself to defend his ego and keep it from crumbling. In effect, he suppressed his homosexual and sadistic tendencies, substituting a private cult of self-adoration for them.

Perhaps nothing became him so fittingly as his death. Always vain of his slim, athletic figure and fine physical condition, he kept in trim by strenuous gymnastic exercises, continuing them even after his physicians had warned him that his heart was weak. He died of a heart attack incurred at his daily calisthenics, carrying his body beautiful with him to the grave. Writing *Young Törless* did not resolve his underlying psychopathologic characteristics; it merely drove his idiosyncratic sexual drives into narcissism, work inhibition, a marriage tailor-made for his convenience, and a role of dependency on his wife and their friends not only for the psychological energy to carry on but for the basic necessities of life. In return he offered desultory work on a novel which he could not bring himself to complete, for had he done so, his raison d'être would have been extinguished. All the more so because Ulrich, the man without any definable qualities, was another projection of Musil's own character into a fictional setting. The perplexities of the youthful Törless matured into the indecisions of Ulrich in parallel with Musil's own development.

Had Musil concentrated his self-analysis not on the incident of his military school career, in which his effort at self-understanding was equivocal and his self-dramatization ignominious, but on the intrafamilial polarities which preceded it and were in large measure its cause, he might have become better adjusted and more productive. As matters developed, having deceived himself into thinking he had solved his problems by writing about them in *Young Törless,* having propitiated his private Eumenides by exposing his guilt publicly, he had to devote the major portion of his psychological energies into maintaining the facade he had created. He managed this role with fair success for a number of years, and doubtless his wife's sympathetic support was of inestimable value, but one speculates whether at the end of his career he came to recognize that the chief victim of his aborted homosexual sadism was himself.

3

Carlo Gesualdo, Prince of Venosa: Murder, Madrigals, and Masochism

Music may be less explicit than literature in denoting the details of emotional experience, and in many instances the listener's response may reflect as much of his or her own emotions as the composer's. A special case occurs when words are set to music. Not only the selection of the text but also the means of musical expression inform the listener of the intended emotion and delimits the response. An illuminating example can be found in the life and work of Carlo Gesualdo (1560–1613), who is best known for his madrigals, which appeared between 1594 and 1626.

Gesualdo's music has been studied extensively by musicologists, and the known facts of his life have been recorded, but the relation between his psychic ailment and his music has not been explored. Admittedly, anamnestic data are sketchy. The passage of time has effaced many documents, and there is no account of his early formative years. Nonetheless, a distinctive pattern emerges when the outline of the important events of his life is taken in conjunction with his musical practices. Serious lacunae in the case history render interpretation of many problems conjectural, but the known facts and an examination of texts almost speak for themselves.

Gesualdo was the second son of Don Fabrizio, prince of Venosa, duke of Caggiano, marquis of Laino, and count of Cossa. His father's brother, Cardinal Alfonso Gesualdo, was at one time a contender for the papacy. His mother's brother, St. Carlo Borromeo, was one of the most influential leaders of the Counter-Reformation. Gesualdo passed his youth on the family estates in southern Italy and in Naples, but there is no information about his youthful experiences or his musical training. He first came to notice when he fell heir to the family titles and estates in 1585 on the death of his elder brother Luigi. We are told that up to this time he cared for nothing but music.[1]

Dynastic considerations compelled his marriage in 1586 to his first cousin, Donna Maria d'Avalos, then a young lady of twenty-one years who had been married twice before and had two children by her first husband. Gesualdo was twenty-six at the time. Cecil Gray comments that "the idea of marriage was uncongenial to his temperament, for . . . the nobility were accustomed to marry at an extremely early age."[2] Donna Maria was what one might euphemistically call ardent. She was first married, at the age of fifteen, to Federico Carafa, son of the marquis of San Lucido. Rumor credits his early death to excessive marital exercise (*"forse per aver troppo reiterare con quella i congiungimenti carnali"*).[3] Two years later she married Alfonso di Guiliano, also the son of a marquis. According to Gray, he "seems to have had a stronger constitution or at least greater moderation and prudence."[4] A papal dispensation for divorce was granted in 1586, and her marriage to Gesualdo followed almost immediately.

The marital happiness of the couple was short-lived. She bore him a son, Don Emmanuele, but at some time in 1589/90 Donna Maria took as her lover Fabrizio Carafa, third duke of Andria and seventh count of Ruovo. It was not a casual affair but a liaison that continued for some time. Whether Donna Maria was a woman of insatiable lust or Gesualdo was below average as a sexual partner cannot be ascertained; however, he was inadequate for her. Precisely how and when Gesualdo became aware of his wife's infidelity is not clear, nor is there any evidence regarding the precipitating cause for his rather extreme solution of the domestic problem.

According to the recorded testimony, Gesualdo told his wife that he was going out on an overnight hunting expedition. Actually he merely went a few blocks away to the home of a friend, giving the lovers time to get together. At midnight he returned to his home, the Palazzo Sansevero in Naples, accompanied by three armed followers. He found his wife and her lover in bed together and proceeded to have them killed, participating in the deed himself. Whether his conduct constitutes entrapment is a nicety of Anglo-Saxon law which would not have applied in southern Italy of the sixteenth century or even today. What is significant is the brutality with which the two victims were dispatched. According to Gray, "The lady's wounds were all in the belly, and more particularly in those parts which she ought to have kept honest; and the duke was wounded even more grievously."[5] Verbatim accounts of the proceedings at the Gran Corte della Vicaria confirm that Donna Maria died of multiple stab wounds by sword and dagger, but the official record mentions only that her throat was cut and that she had received additional stab wounds in the head, face, right arm, and breast as well as two sword thrusts in the flank. Duke Fabrizio had been shot through the head with an arquebus and was also wounded in the head, face, neck, chest, stomach, arms, hands, shoulders, and flanks by multiple sword thrusts which passed through his body from front to back. A somewhat discordant note is struck by the unexplained statement that Duke Fabrizio, when slain, was wearing one of Donna Maria's night dresses. This might pose a problem for the costume designer of this opera but not for the librettist.

Gray comments on Gesualdo's dexterity as a murderer:

> [He] handles the firearms with commendable restraint but with enormous effect. Not one shot does he waste, as we see from the coroner's inquest. On the other hand, the figuration of the steel weapons is exceedingly elaborate and complex. Wooden instruments he neglects entirely; this is perhaps the only conspicuous defect of the work. A few judicious blows with a bludgeon impart a variety, expressiveness, and much charm, which cannot be attained in any other way. On the whole he perhaps tends to use too many instruments; his work is a trifle thickly scored here and there.[6]

So speaks the music critic. But one element of style was lacking: Gesualdo had violated a local canon of the unwritten law. The approved procedure in his social circle would have been for him to murder his wife and her lover himself, unassisted. The use of hired hands in such matters was beneath the dignity of the occasion. It is evident from the testimony that Gesualdo's *sbirri* struck the first blows; he added the final thrusts after both victims were either helpless or dead. Though the *vicaria* exonerated him of any criminal act, his lapse in etiquette provoked the wrath and vengeance of the victims' families, and Gesualdo left Naples for Ferrara soon after his acquittal.

At an indeterminate time after the murders Gesualdo allegedly killed a child born to Donna Maria after the birth of Don Emmanuele; he believed it to be the fruit of her adultery. Gesualdo's father died in 1591, the year following the domestic tragedy, and Don Carlo succeeded him as prince of Venosa. After a while he made his peace with Donna Maria's family, and he continued to devote his time to music.

Gesualdo's journey to Ferrara was leisurely. He was accompanied by Count Fontanelli, a Calabrian nobleman, whose letters record that Gesualdo suffered from asthma. We are not informed whether his attacks were mild or severe, frequent or occasional, nor whether his respiratory difficulty dated from childhood. The travelers stopped in Rome and Florence, participating in many musical activities in both cities. Fontanelli informs us that when Gesualdo arrived at Ferrara he had with him in manuscript the first two of his six books of madrigals. These were his entrée to the court of the Este family, which had made Ferrara a center of late Renaissance learning: "Ferrara was the most cultured, enlightened, and splendid city in the whole of Italy. Indeed, one might say that Ferrara dominated the closing period of the Renaissance in Italy, as Florence [had] dominated its early stages; the Medici were the wet-nurses; the Estensi were the undertakers."[7]

In addition to eminence in scholarship and the visual arts, Ferrara had a distinguished tradition of music and music making. Such names as Josquin dePrès, Luzzasco Luzzaschi, Adrian Willaert, Giovanni Palestrina, and John Dowland are associated in one way or another with the musical interests of the Estensi, evidence not only of Ferrara's achievement in Italy but also of its international importance. Members of the ruling family as well as their courtiers were adept as singers and instrumentalists. It was not unusual for several concerts a day to be performed in the castellated palazzo in the city's center, designed by Bartolino Ploti in 1385 and completed in 1472. Gesualdo found Ferrara congenial to his musical tastes, and he published there his first two books of madrigals in 1594, his third in 1595. The Estensi did not hold his Neapolitan marital scrape against him, for in 1594 he took as his second wife Donna Eleanora d'Este, a sister of the reigning duke. The marriage proved reasonably successful; it was blessed by a son and two daughters. Unfortunately the son died in childhood and, following Don Carlo's death in 1613, the Gesualdo male line became extinct.

Extinction of the male line also afflicted the Estensi. When Alfonso II died in 1597 he was without male issue despite three marriages, and the duchy passed to Pope Clement VIII, thereby bringing to a close the reign of the house of Este, which had held Ferrara and the Duchy of Modena in fief since 1240. Since there was no reason for Gesualdo to remain after the luster of the court had dimmed, he soon returned to southern Italy with his new family, living both in Naples and at his family seat at Gesualdo.

During the last two decades of his life Gesualdo developed profound feelings of guilt and remorse for his crime of 1590. In an effort to expiate his guilt he endowed the construction of a monastery, the Convento dei Cappucini at Gesualdo, and commissioned a remarkable altarpiece for it. Although devoid of artistic merit, it possesses great iconographic value. It depicts Christ the Redeemer sitting in judgment and pardoning repentant sinners. Disposed around him are the Virgin Mary, the archangel Michael, St. Francis of Assisi, and St. Dominic invoking mercy for a particular sinner. Mary Magdalen and St. Catherine of Siena are shown in postures which suggest that they are instructing the sinner to trust in God and in their intercession. In the lower left corner of the panel kneels Carlo Gesualdo, prince of Venosa, bare-headed and wearing a large white ruff. Stretching a protective arm around this crouching creature is none other than the late Carlo Borromeo, cardinal archbishop of Milan, who had died in 1584 and was canonized in 1610, and who was, among other things, Gesualdo's uncle. Below the center of the painting is an attractive bambino to represent the murdered infant; below him are two souls burning in hell's fire, Donna Maria and Duke Fabrizio. Just how efficacious this painting was in saving Gesualdo from damnation will be known only on the Day of Reckoning; let us hope there are no art critics on the jury.

Gray has commented on Gesualdo's likeness in the picture:

> It is not necessary to know anything of his life to detect in these long, narrow, slanting eyes . . . in the small, puckered, and sensual mouth, aquiline nose, and slightly receding forehead and chin, a character of the utmost perversity, cruelty, and vindictiveness. . . . [I]t is a weak rather than a strong face—almost feminine, in fact. Physically, he is the very type of degenerate descendant of a long aristocratic line.[8]

These lines, published in 1926, seem curiously dated now that the Lombroso's idea of correlating physiognomy with character has been discarded, and Gray's reasoning seems post hoc. Nonetheless, Gesualdo is a singularly unappetizing character (fig. 3.1).

Gesualdo's contrition did not stop with erecting a monastery and commissioning a painting. During the last decade of his life he was tormented by demons, and he developed a penchant for being beaten. He

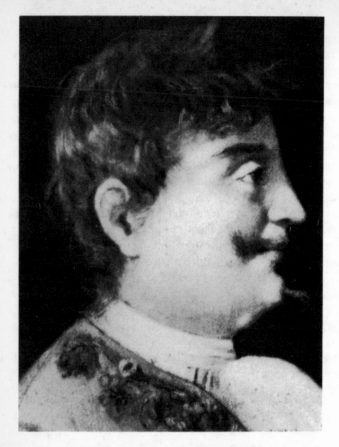

Figure 3.1. Carlo Gesualdo, Prince of Venosa.

maintained a troupe of ten or a dozen young men whose duty it was to flagellate him three times daily, "during which operation he was wont to smile joyfully."[9] Masochism may have kept the demons at bay for a while, but Gesualdo soon developed the unusual symptom of being unable to move his bowels unless he was whipped—"Princeps Venusae musica clarissimus nostro tempore cacare non potest, nisi verberatus a servo ad id adscito."[10] In the absence of specific information which only Gesualdo could supply, it is difficult to ascertain the psychodynamic significance of this idiosyncratic fusion of masochism and anal retention. But through it all he kept on writing madrigals until his death in 1613.

Gesualdo's fame as a composer rests upon his 140-odd madrigals, most of which were published in six books between 1594 and 1611. All but three of these are for five voices; a posthumous book of madrigals for six voices was published in 1626 (the quinto part alone survives). His other extant compositions include two books of sacrae cantiones and responsoria. All his known music is a capella; not a scrap of instrumental music survives, though Vatielli informs us that he was a virtuoso on the lute.[11] Gesualdo's harmonic vocabulary sounds extreme, even to twentieth-century ears. By its chromaticism, it differs considerably from the typical modal or diatonic progressions of his time, leading the listener to remote tonal regions seemingly unrelated to each other. In the background, however, the basic tonal language of the period is present. More than any composer of his period, he found inspiration in the texts he chose to set, and his music is closely wedded to the words. Philip Heseltine, better known as Peter Warlock, the composer, offers the perceptive comment:

> The form of Gesualdo's madrigals is almost invariably conditioned by verbal antitheses. The harmonic and contrapuntal styles seem to have been sharply differentiated in his mind, quite apart from any consideration of the notes . . . employed in either; he pits one style against the other according as the sentiment of the text provides him with opportunities for sudden change.[12]

Gesualdo's expressive effects are achieved by slow progressions of chromatic chords and short, piercing cries of melody, which express pain, suffering, and thoughts of death—they alternate with brilliant contrapuntal passages to match words of joy, love, or any sort of active movement. He concentrated his imagination upon the darker aspects of life: the tragic, the grisly, and the bizarre; as a consequence his joyful moods and passages seem perfunctory, almost negative. The words upon which he seems to focus his most profound emotion are *duolo* and *dolore, martire* and *morire,* all to the accompaniment of *sospiri* and *lagrime.* It is the vocabulary of a masochist, and it permeates almost every single madrigal he wrote. The actual words are not unique to Gesualdo. Other contemporary poets and madrigalists, not known to be masochists, wrote of sighs and tears, pain and suffering. What distinguishes Gesualdo from them is a difference of degree, not of kind; he carried the expression of these feelings to extremes, using such subjects almost to the exclusion of others, almost obsessively. For a literary equivalent one must go beyond John Webster, who was "much possessed by death," and on to Thomas Lovell Beddoes' *Death's Jest Book*. In Gesualdo's madrigals the particular emotion that determines the relation between words and music, between feeling and expression, is epitomized in the second strophe of "Luci serene," a madrigal from Book 4 (1596):

> Dolci parol' e care,
> Vio mi ferite, voi;
> Ma prov' il petto
> Non dolor nella piaga, ma diletto.

Englished, this antedates the romantic agony by two centuries:

> Words, sweet and dear,
> You make me suffer;
> But the wound in my heart
> Feels not pain but only delight.

Gesualdo's vocabulary was not unique. Many composers set Tasso; it is a question which verses they set and what emphasis was placed on the words relating to the vocabulary of masochism. Gesualdo adapted his harmonic technique to enhance his emotional expression. Unlike his predecessors Cipriano and Monteverdi, who expressed themselves within received harmonic traditions, Gesualdo broke the system by employing violently juxtaposed chords, indefinite cadences, and shifting harmonic patterns to express his grief and pain.

Nonverbal and nonpictorial as the expressive powers of music are, affinities with literature and the visual arts suggest themselves almost automatically. Rowland explores comparable literary reverberations in John Donne and finds common aesthetic ground between Gesualdo and such Mannerist painters as Jacopo da Pontormo and Salvatore Rosa, though perhaps the violence in the life and work of Caravaggio, his contemporary, might be a more apposite choice.[13] Aldous Huxley reminds us that Ernest Walker, the Oxford musicologist, remarked that the madrigal "Moro lasso" sounded like "Wagner gone wrong," and Wagner was another case of harmonic experimentation for musicoliterary effect.[14] But the most unexpected conjunction is that of Gesualdo with John Milton. Milton bought at least one book of Gesualdo's madrigals during his travels in Italy (1638–39) and shipped it home from Venice. We can assume only that he sang them with friends at informal soirees in England on the eve of the Civil War. Milton was much concerned with the question of sin and redemption, to say nothing of suffering eternal punishment in hell everlasting. One can speculate whether Milton was acquainted with the events in Gesualdo's life, but almost surely he did not know that the composer's uncle was St. Carlo Borromeo. Milton would have ducked from under the cardinal's protective arm, and no one has ever hinted that its reach was ecumenical enough to embrace Cromwell's Latin secretary. But one cannot escape the intuition that Milton sensed a feeling in Gesualdo's suffering which was akin to his own.

Texts for Italian madrigals are almost exclusively nonstrophic vernacular verses. Gesualdo selected his texts from a wide variety of contemporary sources, most of them now forgotten. It is the specific type of text he most frequently chose that marks the relation between his psychic disease and his musical expression. As early as book 1 (1594) he set verses by Torquato Tasso:

> Se da il nobil mano
> Debbon venir le fasce a le mie piaghe,
> Amor, che non m'impiaghe
> Il sen con mille colpi?
> Ne fia ch'io te n'incolpi,
> Perche nulla ferita
> Sarebbe al cor si grave
> Come fora soava
> De la man bella, la cortese aita.

Here we find wordplay based on such antitheses as *piaghe-impiaghe* and *colpi-incolpi*, and a free translation reads: "If from so noble a hand should come the rod which wounds me, Love, why not inflict a thousand blows upon my breast? Feel no blame, for nothing wounds the heart so deeply as the mild wrath of a beautiful hand." A majority of Gesualdo's madrigals deal with this theme and variations upon it. Gesualdo cast himself in the role of the victim of a *belle dame sans merci*. Many poets and composers have used this theme on one occasion or another; the difference between them and Gesualdo is that he was obsessed by it.

Many of Gesualdo's dramatic effects were achieved by a concentration of expression. Heseltine has described him as "the perfect master of the short, poignant phrase."[15] A characteristic example is his treatment of the line "Debbon venir le fasce a le mie piaghe" in Tasso's verse. Its first exposition requires a mere two measures in the lower voices, and the phrase is repeated, using a different strain, in another two measures for the higher voices—four measures in all devoted to the instrument of his suffering. The key word is not *fasce:* Gesualdo did not worship the rod; he simply enjoyed its pain. *Piaghe*—his wound, the received stigma—is given emphasis by assigning its first syllable to a half note, and on its first appearance the leading voice is given a short turn upon it which terminates upon another half note. Additional weight upon the word is achieved by giving its second syllable a half note on its first exposition; then, on its second appearance, only a quarter note placed strategically a whole tone lower. All this in four measures—a short phrase indeed. One might wonder whether Gesualdo's predilection for the short, concentrated phrase might be related to the difficult expiratory phase of breathing in bronchial asthma. Yet every composer has employed short phrases for dramatic expression, and it seems unlikely that a quantitative analysis of phrase length in asthmatic versus nonasthmatic composers of vocal music would merit subvention. It is difficult to resolve the question posed by Alfred Einstein on examining "Io pur respiro in cosi gran dolore" from Book 6 (1611): "Where are we to draw the line between stark naturalism and highest expression, between symbolism and self-confession? The laborious 'breathing,' the 'pain,' the agitated invocation of Death—everything is depicted. . . ."[16] And a few lines farther in the text the phrase *un colpo solo* is concealed as a single measure in the next to lowest voice, a phrase not taken up and developed in other voices. This has "an uncanny effect when it is declaimed by a murderer who is haunted by his victims' wounds."[17] It is in passages like these that Gesualdo's medical history, psychological pattern, and his reaction to both become fused into a single musical expression, content synthesized with form, emotion identical with its expression.

Gesualdo had other devices at his command and used them skillfully to heighten the values of the text. In "Tu m'uccidi, o crudele" from Book 5 (1611) the opening words are set to an ascending chromatic progression in half notes, another example of "the short, poignant phrase," and this rhetorical device is repeated in the phrase *al mio morir*. He set the rhyming words of the closing couplet in different styles: *gri-*

dando (screaming with pain) is set to a florid melismatic figure of eighth notes and sixteenth notes, terminating with an ictus on a quarter note. Another device is the judicious use of dissonance: lest the *do* syllable of *gridando* seem too euphonious with its G-major triadic harmony (G-B-D), Gesualdo locked into the vertical line the first syllable of the next phrase, the *Oi-* in *Oima,* and assigned it to B-flat, thereby achieving both textual concentration as well as a musical equivalent for the cry of the suffering victim.

Similar tropes are found in his madrigal "Moro lasso" from book 6 (1611). The two opening words are set to a descending chromatic progression of whole notes and these are contrasted with the figurations of eighth notes and sixteenth notes on the word *vita* in the next line of text. The last line of the madrigal, "Chi dar vita mi puo, mi da morte" (She who could give me life, is my death) is given its "dying fall" by a series of dissonant suspensions in slow tempo which are not resolved until the final chord.

Having examined Gesualdo's life and glanced into his workshop, can we now construct an explanation? Perforce, any attempt at psychobiography at a remove of three and one-half centuries has severe limitations. Important details are lacking, and a sequential reconstruction of events cannot be attempted. Nor is a review of such data as are known and an examination of musical materials any sort of substitute for a doctor-patient confrontation during which so much material information is exchanged, when events can be put into perspective and nuances of emotional valence attached to them, then reexamined and corrected in the light of further discussion. Any schema we construct will be merely a broad outline, a framework upon which to rest the case. But, like any other form of scientific hypothesis, its validity can be tested in terms of how well it fits the known facts and its internal consistency.

Gesualdo did not begin to act out in overt form his masochistic impulses until after 1597, when he was thirty-seven years old. There is evidence of covert masochism in the texts chosen for his first two books of madrigals, which appeared in 1594. Coventional feelings of guilt for the murders in 1590 could have been neutralized by such recognized acts of penitence as confession, building a chapel, commissioning a painting. It seems reasonable to infer that the roots of Gesualdo's masochism were set in his personality before that time, possibly established in youth or childhood. One may conjecture that his inadequacy as a sexual partner for Donna Maria may have been the result of an unexpressed masochistic passivity. One may even speculate that his interest in flagellation might have been initiated by witnessing a religious procession in which flagellation was a prominent feature, an institutionalized, socially acceptable manifestation of masochistic submission. Such scenes were not uncommon at that time in southern Europe, and their history goes back to many of the forms of primitive religion long before the advent of Christianity. But this is mere surmise; other causes for marital inadequacy can be proposed. Gesualdo's choice of a male flagellant in later life at least suggests homosexual impulses which were presumably repressed. That he might have had such impulses is by no means rebutted by his apparently adequate sexual performance with his second wife. Masochistic and homosexual impulses often coexist and, acting singly or in concert, could have set the background for the domestic tragedy.

From all accounts the murder of his wife seems to have been excessively brutal even by the standards of his time and place, and the murder of the infant child can be described as *un acte gratuit*. The crime bears the hallmarks of sadistic murder, and the presence of an anal-sadistic component in Gesualdo is in part confirmed by the later development of anal-retentive behavior. Anal fixation at an early age could account for displacement of sexual impulses from the genital organs to the anogluteal region, a common clinical observation in both homosexual and masochistic personalities. We lack information to fill out the framework with evidence of such frequently associated traits as a parsimonious attitude toward money, the continuous wearing of shabby clothes, infrequent changing of linens, even frequent enemas. Available biographical data do not permit so close a scrutiny. If the above hypothesis fits the facts, some of which we shall never surely know, we can infer that during his youth and young manhood Gesualdo maintained his personality intact and conformed to the dictates of society and religion by repressing unacceptable sexual impulses, convincing himself that he was heterosexually competent and "normal." His first wife's infidelity destroyed this carefully developed self-image and, in one hideous act of destruction, he tried to restore its integrity. During that climactic scene the sadistic element of his anal fixation was dominant.

Murder was neither a satisfactory catharsis nor a permanent solution. The sadistic component may have subsided, but not the masochistic personality structure. Composing madrigals provided an outlet for temporary relief, especially because in so doing Gesualdo could identify his role as the punished victim, suffering and dying at the hands of a cruel, denying woman. But in the long run composition proved insufficient, and his needs could be satisfied only by his submitting to actual flagellation by a man. It is not difficult to trace the effects of his life experience in his music, but the music itself transcends the psychic disturbance from which it developed. It contains an emotion which is so universal that it encompasses all forms of human suffering. Like Philoctetes, Gesualdo suffered from an incurable wound. His personal tragedy was that he inflicted it on others, with a show of violence. His redemption lies not in the whim of *la belle dame sans merci* nor even *per fasces* but in a later age with its own martyrdom and pain, for which his music is singularly fitting.

4

The Sticky End of
František Koczwara,
Composer of
The Battle of Prague

The New Grove Dictionary of Music and Musicians informs us that František Koczwara (ca. 1750–91) "gained special notoriety by the manner of his death. . . . He was reputed to have unusual taste in his vices and was accidentally hanged while conducting an experiment in a house of ill repute." Little more stimulus is required for the medical detective and sometime musicographer to scurry into the library in search of the anonymous pamphlet titled *Modern propensities . . . with Memoirs of Susannah Hill and a Summary of her Trial . . . on the Charge of Hanging Francis Kotzwara, &c.*[1]

Koczwara is known to music history as the composer of *The Battle of Prague,* a piece of battle music popular from circa 1790 to circa 1820, when the vogue for such music was high. Battle music is not to be confused with military music. Military music is written for the troops—marches, quicksteps, and somewhat rowdy songs. Battle music is written for the folks at home, a semipopular genre designed for the salon or concert hall that enables listeners to participate vicariously in the pain and glory. An early example is Heinrich von Biber's *Battalia* (1673), which tries to recreate the sounds of battle by various means. In the first movement the violinists strike their instruments *col legno,* with the wood of their bows instead of the hairs. Armed conflict is suggested in the second movement by the cacophony of eight different folk songs played simultaneously, a device later imitated by Charles Ives' father, a Connecticut bandmaster who experimented by having two military bands play different marches as their paths intersected during a parade. Other movements of von Biber's *Battalia* include a solo violin and drum, *pizzicati,* to represent bombardment by cannons, followed by an antiphonal lament for the wounded.

Battle music was an agreeable art form for the eighteenth-century audience. Handel's *Royal Fireworks Music* celebrated the Treaty of Aix-la-Chapelle in 1748. Even Mozart composed a contradanse (K. 587) to honor Prince Friedrich Josias of Saxe-Coburg-Saalfeld for his victory over the Turks at Martinestie in 1789. Composers of lesser renown, such as Jean François Dandrieu (1682–1738) and Franz Christoph Neubauer (1760–95), also composed battle symphonies. Dandrieu's *Les caractères de la guerre* (1718) is a glorification of military life with movements labeled "Charge," "Retraite," and "Boutte-selle" (Boots and Saddle), all written relentlessly in D major. Neubauer's *Sinfonie,* op. 11 ("La Bataille"), composed in 1789, also celebrates the victory at Martinestie; it is a full four-movement symphony with a strain from "La Marseillaise" in the third movement and a "Celebration de la victoire" as the finale. Beethoven's *Battle Symphony* of 1813 (properly titled *Wellingtons Sieg, oder die Schlacht bei Vittoria,* op. 91), a potboiler he turned out for Mälzel's mechanical organ and which proved to be his best seller, is still heard on recordings, albeit rarely in the concert hall. Tchaikovsky's *1812 Overture* must be rated the smashing success of the battle music genre, perhaps the only one to hold its place in the standard orchestral repertoire.

The foregoing pieces are all orchestral, and perhaps the big bang of a big band is necessary to give the full flavor of a battle. Less familiar to twentieth-century ears is battle music written for the keyboard. Perhaps the earliest specimen is a short piece for harpsichord titled "The Battel" in *My Lady Nevell's Book* (1591), ascribed to William Byrd. Compositions of this type became more popular in the latter half of the eighteenth century when the fortepiano replaced the harpsichord. Arthur Loesser remarks that

> pianistic battle pieces came into great general favor and were
> dished up in large quantity, if not variety, by publishers, compos-
> ers, virtuosos, and of course young ladies—the ultimate retailers.
> These compositions were, indeed, extraordinarily conventional in
> conception; they all show a remarkable family resemblance, not
> always short of actual plagiarism: all are rigorously provided with
> approach marches, bugle calls, cannon shots, cavalry charges, fog

of battle, cries of the wounded, national anthems, and victory balls. These items were always carefully ticketed in the printed notes, and we wonder whether players generally announced the captions orally to their hearers in the course of the performance.[2]

One reason for this vogue was the invention of the so-called janissary pedal as an attachment to the fortepiano. It was supposed to supply "Turkish music," a Levantine effect derived in some peculiar fashion from the many contacts, military and nonmilitary, that Central Europe had with the Ottoman Turks from 1453 on. A twentieth-century listener is surely familiar with the "Turkish" section in the finale of Mozart's A-major Violin Concerto K. 219, and what boy or girl has not struggled through the "Turkish March" that is really the rondo of Mozart's A-major Piano Sonata K. 331. More apposite for the venue are the "Turkish" effects in Mozart's *Die Entführung aus dem Serail* (1782), where the action takes place in the Pasha's palazzo. The vogue even crossed the Atlantic, where James Hewitt's *Battle of Trenton*—following which Washington crossed the Delaware—was a popular piano piece in the early days of the republic.

But the all-time favorite piece of battle music from around 1790 to 1820, at least in England, was Koczwara's *The Battle of Prague*. It was the sort of piece Jane Austen's heroines could have (and would have) played in the drawing rooms of country gentry. Born in or near Prague circa 1750, Koczwara could not have had firsthand experience with the actual battle there in 1756, but doubtless he heard story after story about it during his boyhood, and when he came to write a battle piece, that was the natural name for him to affix. Unlike his fellow Bohemian Smetana's *Aus meinem Leben,* Koczwara's *The Battle of Prague* is not youthful emotion recollected in tranquility. The music is generic rather than specific for time and place. In point of historical fact, the Battle of Prague, which was fought on May 5, 1756, was an early engagement in the Seven Years' War and a famous victory for Frederick the Great's Prussian soldiers over Maria Theresa's Austrian troops commanded by Feldmarschal Doun. For almost two centuries textbooks on military tactics devoted long sections to Frederick's masterful disposition of his men and his ability to take advantage of terrain.

As is so often the case with minor eighteenth-century composers, biographical details about Koczwara are scanty, and what little we know can only be inferred from publications of music bearing his name plus occasional scraps in memoirs of the period. The entry in *New Grove* describes him as a "Bohemian composer and instrumentalist." His education and musical training are unknown, but he must have moved to London before he was twenty-five, because his compositions were published there from 1775 on. In the early 1780s he lived in Bath, and he lived in Ireland during the late 1780s. The itinerant returned to London for the Handel Commemoration in May 1791, and it was only a few months later that he met his unhappy end in a Soho bordello. At the time of his death he had a job playing double bass at the King's Theatre. Koczwara's instrumental skills were varied; he was professionally competent on the violin, viola, cello, double bass, flute, oboe, bassoon, fortepiano, and cithern. *The Battle of Prague* was first published in 1788 while he was in Dublin. It met with phenomenal success and was widely reprinted (and pirated) in London, America, and continental Europe. Almost forty issues have been traced, and in Federalist Boston it was considered the indispensable climax to every concert, much as Arthur Fiedler's performance of "The Stars and Stripes Forever" was for a later generation.

The earliest editions of *The Battle of Prague* provide accompanying parts for violin, bass, trumpet, and drum so that not even the most unimaginative listener could miss the point. Later versions were printed for solo piano, and in such performances the janissary pedal helped. The music does not pose technical or intellectual problems; patrons of the Assembly Rooms at Turnham Green in 1792 heard it performed by a Miss Hoffman at the keyboard accompanied by her brother on the drum, the young lady being six years old, her brother three and one-half. It opens with a slow march, then cannon bursts followed by bugle and trumpet calls. Then we have the attack, the cries of the wounded, and the trumpet of victory which leads to "God Save the King." The last three movements are Turkish music, finale: allegro, and "Go to Bed Home." Perhaps the sequence of the last two sections could be reversed depending on whether the player wanted a rousing bravura finish or a gentle close at the end of an evening's music.

The Battle of Prague had such flexible musical lines that the versatile musicians of the period adapted it for any plausible combination of instruments. In September 1791, just after Koczwara's death, Michael Sharp played it at his benefit concert in Norwich for a full complement of strings plus oboes, clarinets, bassoons, French horn, bugle horn, trumpets, fifes, side drum, bass drum, kettledrum, and Abbey double drums.³ The decibels ran high in the Assembly Rooms that evening.

Koczwara's unusual death did not pass without comment in London's musical circles. The last entry in Haydn's first notebook recording the events of his first visit to London is the cryptic note, "Kozwarra."⁴ H. C. Robbins Landon, in *Haydn: Chronicle and Works,* goes on to quote from W. T. Parke's *Musical Memoirs,* published in 1830:

> Kotzwara was a great imitative composer and was engaged by certain music-sellers to compose trios, quartets &c. in the style of the popular writers of the [C]ontinent, [H]aydn, [P]leyel, and others; and his productions displayed so accurately the taste and science of his prototypes, that, like the admirable copies of the old masters by Reinagle, the best judges considered them to be originals. He had been found hanging in a house of ill fame. . . . As it was proved that he was suspended by his own desire, and that neither he nor the parties implicated in the transaction ever contemplated death, [the whores] were acquitted.⁵

Modern Propensities &c. is what a bookseller might describe as "curiosa." It runs to some forty-six pages, the first twenty-nine being devoted to an archly written preamble discussing the putative effects of hanging on the body's "physiology." Only the last seven pages deal with the trial of Susannah Hill, who assisted Koczwara in the fatal event. Broadsides and pamphlets describing capital crimes were frequently published in eighteenth-century London for the mass market, and this one offered the added cachet of a lurid death with sexual overtones. Richard Wolfe conjectures that the pamphlet may have been written by Martin Vanbutchell, a Mount Street quack who had developed spring bands and elastic garters that were presumably used in autoerotic practices and the sale of which he wished to promote.⁶

The anonymous pamphleteer leads us from Dr. Graham's celestial electric bed to the theory that "if . . . the most robust and youthful require certain *aids* to ascend the upper sphere of conjunctive transports, what must be the situation of those *elderly* and *antiquated* PEERS AND COMMONERS?" He cites the example of General S——, who suffered from "a certain corporeal debility which prevented him from *regular* enjoyments," and presents a circumlocutory account, perhaps fictitious, of the attempt by Parson Manacle, who attended prisoners at Newgate, to regain his potency by undergoing a brief hanging by Mrs.

Birdlime. Next comes a brief digression on flagellation as a sexual stimulant, and finally we are let in on the secret that it was the notorious Jonathan Wild who first discovered, while examining the pockets of hanged felons, that "they evinced *certain emotions* and *commotions,* which . . . proved that all flesh must die to live again."

In the section "Memoirs of Susannah Hill," we learn that Hill was a country girl abandoned by her lover, that she came to London, where she found "protection" from "a certain pale-faced Quaker, of the most primitive order, a Lombard-street discounter" who soon tired of her, and that she decided "to depend upon the events of the evening for support." She found "lodging in a place not subject to the curious and prying observations of the World"—namely, the front parlor at 5 Vine Street, Soho (a location obliterated in 1810 by urban improvements, when Nash designed and built what is now Regent Street).

The pamphlet summarizes the evidence given at the trial on September 16, 1791, two weeks after the event:

> That in the afternoon of 2nd of September, between one and two o'clock, a man whom she had never seen before, and who was the deceased, came past the house where she lived—That he came into the house, the street door being open (as usual, it was observed by the counsel) and asked her if she would have anything to drink. That she replied, if she chose anything, it should be a little porter. The deceased said he should like some brandy and water; and gave her money to buy porter and brandy—with two shillings for some ham and beef, which she accordingly bought. Some time after this, they went into a back room, where several acts of the grossest indecency passed; in particular he pressed her to cut off the means of generation, and expressly wished to have it cut in two. But this she refused. He then said he should like to be hanged for five minutes; and while he gave her money to buy a cord, observed that hanging would raise his passions—that it would produce all he wanted. But as a cord large enough could not be immediately procured, she bought two small ones, and put them round his neck. He then tied himself up to the back parlour door, a place where he hung very low, and bending down on his knees. . . . After hanging five minutes, she cut him down; he immediately fell to the ground: she thought he was in a fit,

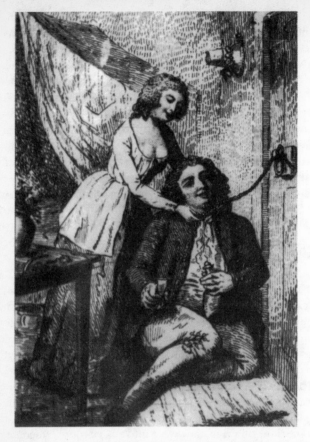

Figure 4.1. Frontispiece from *Modern Propensities, & c.* (1791), purporting to show how Susannah Hill slipped the noose around Koczwara's neck.

and called to an opposite neighbour for help. She then went to a publican, ... and he ran for a surgeon, who came and attempted to bleed him.

The prosecution had charged Susannah Hill with manslaughter on the ground that she had assisted Koczwara to commit suicide, but Judge Gould dismissed the case.

The pamphlet's frontispiece is a woodcut (fig. 4.1) that purports to reconstruct the scene. Susannah Hill is shown placing the cord around

Koczwara's neck. Both participants are fully and decorously clad, which seems improbable if "acts of the grossest indecency" had just transpired in the back parlor. Koczwara wears a simpering smile, again improbable if he was intent on summoning his faltering flesh. His right hand holds a glass, and his left hand grasps the neck of a brandy bottle. The shape of the bottle and its stopper as well as the position of his hand suggest masturbation. It is reasonable to infer that he was no stranger to the practice of using suspension to induce sexual excitation; the evidence indicates it was done at his suggestion. However, he seems to have been seriously disturbed, anxious about his potency and filled with guilt about its loss, if we can credit his request for dismemberment. The immediate cause of death was asphyxia, the result of compressing the trachea with a ligature.

The notion that hanging can produce erection and ejaculation persists in literature and art as well as in life. Contemporary with Koczwara's fiasco is de Sade's *Justine* (1791), in which Thérèse helps Roland achieve orgasm by hanging him briefly. Whether Koczwara had access to that novel, published anonymously in Paris earlier that year, is not known. A similar scene takes place in *Gamiani, ou Deux nuits d'excès* (1833), a novel filled with sadism and bestiality, often attributed to Alfred de Musset. In *Ulysses* (1922) James Joyce describes the aftermath of the hanging of the Croppy Boy: "He gives up the ghost. A violent erection of the hanged sends gouts of sperm spouting through his dead clothes on to the cobblestones. Mrs. Bellingham, Mrs. Yelverton Barry, and the Honorable Mrs. Mervyn Talboys rush forward with their handkerchiefs to sop it up." In recent years William Burroughs has offered similar scenes in *Naked Lunch* (1959) and *Cities of the Red Night* (1980). Representation of the supposed effects of hanging are uncommon in the visual arts, but Phillipe Mohlitz's etching *Le pendu* (fig. 4.2) displays the phenomenon.

Sexual hanging, better labeled autoerotic asphyxia when it proves fatal, is predicated on the belief that when the carotid arteries and jugular veins are compressed, the effects on cerebral circulation elicit sexual stimulation.[7] Compressing the carotid arteries decreases the supply of oxygen to the brain (hypoxia), and compressing the jugular veins increases the blood carbon dioxide level (hypercapnia); in addition, the cerebral veins become congested. Shutting off the carotid circulation for a short time (transient ischemia) does produce a sensation of light-headedness and often a tingling sensation in the extremities. If carotid

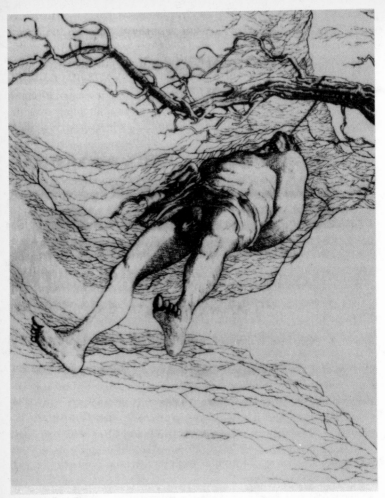

Figure 4.2. Detail of *Le pendu*. Phillipe Mohlitz. Etching.

flow is reduced for a somewhat longer time, consciousness may be altered, but there is no physiological mechanism by which it can produce an erection in psychologically normal males. The prevailing notion that criminals executed by hanging ejaculate as they gasp their last is a canard. It is difficult to imagine that a man with a noose around his neck, about to be "jerked into eternity," can develop an erection and have a pulsatile ejaculation of semen. That the clothing of hanged criminals is often stained with urine, feces, or semen merely reflects the passive emptying of the bladder, rectum, and seminal vesicles when the cervical spinal cord and autonomic nervous system are disrupted and the usual controls abolished. Individuals who come to medicolegal attention as the result of autoerotic asphyxia are the victims of a psychosexual disorder. Unfortunately, they do not come to medical attention until too late, after the noose has slipped and compressed the trachea, producing asphyxia as well as hypoxia. It takes about five pounds of external pressure to compress the jugulars, about eleven pounds to compress the carotids, but about thirty pounds to compress the trachea. The victims of tracheal compression in autoerotic hanging do not come to the psychiatrist's office but wind up on the medical examiner's slab. Park Dietz has proposed the term *hypoxyphilia* or *Kotzwarraism* to describe individuals who produce sexual excitation by mechanical or chemical asphyxia or intentionally induce cerebral hypoxia to the point where consciousness or perception is altered.[8]

It is important to distinguish between erection, which is physiological, and priapism, which is pathological. Priapism is more often idiopathic than a complication of systemic or local disease, such as sickle cell anemia, leukemic or other neoplastic infiltration, trauma and thrombosis, inflammatory processes, or a variety of uncommon neurological disorders involving the spinal cord.[9] As long ago as 1897, Hughlings Jackson described priapism as an occasional sequel to cervical fracture-dislocation, assigning the mechanism to release of an inhibitory center in the medulla or higher upon the *nervi erigentes,* the parasympathetic fibers that arise from the third and fourth sacral segments and stimulate the penis to physiological tumescence.[10] This mechanism accounts for the occasional instance of ithyphallism following judicial hanging, but it plays no part in autoerotic asphyxia.

The results of judicial hanging depend upon the placement of the knot. Frederic Wood-Jones demonstrated that if the knot is placed beneath the chin, the resulting hyperextension of the neck will produce a fracture dislocation of the first and second cervical vertebrae with compression, if not actually division, of the spinal cord at that level, whereas a knot placed at the angle of the jaw beneath the ear produces a fracture of the base of the skull.[11] With a submental knot, death is instantaneous; with a subaural knot, death is slower and probably due to strangulation. Priapism can occur when the submental knot is used, but in the eighteenth century the knot was placed at the angle of the jaw; thus, the observations attributed to Jonathan Wild are apocryphal. In my own hospital experience, a twenty-three-year-old man who sustained a fracture of the first and second cervical vertebrae with damage to the spinal cord did develop priapism that lasted for three years. He at last succumbed to the side effects of paraplegia, but such priapisms do not persist very long after death.

Autoerotic asphyxia is a problem in forensic rather than clinical medicine. Even as a patient's medical history is essential for the clinician, so is the "scene" for a medical examiner. The body is usually that of a young man, often an adolescent. In a recent study of 132 cases of autoerotic asphyxia, the researchers identified only 5 women and only 16 men over the age of forty.[12] In addition to the fatal noose, there is often evidence that the victim has been using bondage as a psychosexual stimulus. Joseph Rupp catalogues the major variations:

> [T]here may be binding of the head with a gag, mask, or blindfold; binding of the trunk and extremities with ropes, ligatures, tape, or chains; pinioning of the extremities with handcuffs, shackles, leg irons, belts, or leather thongs; binding of the genitals or suspension of heavy weights from [them]; or insertion of foreign bodies into the rectum. In many cases the binding of the body is elaborate and intricate; however, detailed investigation always reveals that the restraints were self-applied. . . . Not infrequently one finds pictures of nude females, bondage literature, or drawings surrounding the body where they may be easily viewed. In other cases the act has been performed in front of a mirror.[13]

It is not uncommon to find protective padding or towels underneath the rope or belt used for suspension, applied in order to protect the neck from abrasions. Some degree of cross-dressing may be an added feature, not necessarily a complete female costume but such items as panties, tights, girdles, garter belts, nylon stockings, brassieres. Articles suggesting fetishism are occasionally found: leather goods, high-heeled boots, and the like. The act is almost always performed in a location where privacy is assured; Koczwara was unusual in having an assistant to place the noose around his neck. Investigation of the past history usually indicates that few of the victims had consulted psychiatrists, but questioning of their families and friends will often elicit accounts of unusual sexual preoccupations or practices. Most of the victims are single men who have had only heterosexual contacts; only a few are overtly homosexual.

Except in prepubescent boys, the genitals are usually exposed, and in older individuals exposure may extend to complete nudity. Young boys excepted again, there is almost always evidence of masturbation, which seems to be the point of the exercise. Rupp traces a sequence of development in the complexity of the associated psychosexual paraphernalia, a systematic progression of the embellishments and the fantasies they represent, but this has not been confirmed. There is considerable variation from case to case, and it is often evident from examining the equipment, especially in older individuals, that the act was not improvised but had been practiced many times. If the body is found by a family member, the clothing may be readjusted before the authorities are notified; detailed questioning may be necessary to exclude suicide.

Until recent years there was little salacious literature describing this variety of sexual behavior, and it does not seem to be the sort of activity into which one is initiated by an older practitioner. With few exceptions it is a solitary act that each individual seems to have developed to satisfy the needs of a personal sexual fantasy. If we consider that the act comes to notice only when accidental asphyxia occurs and that accidents do happen to men who have practiced it on many occasions, it is reasonable to infer that a considerable number have practiced it successfully and without accident, perhaps for most of their sexually active lives.

The evidence from forensic pathology provides us only with an end point to a complex of psychodynamic processes. The dead bodies and the circumstances under which they are found tell us only what has happened, not why; successful practitioners of autoerotic hanging do not come to a psychiatrist to discuss it and be treated. We lack a body of case histories that tell us why they began the practice, how it evolved, and the fantasies accompanying the act. It can be described as masturbation "with all the trimmings"—that is, with masochism, bondage, cross-dressing, and fetishism as integral parts of the act. To this must be added the extra thrill provided by the risk. Except for the most inexperienced boy, anyone who chooses this technique for self-gratification must surely be aware of the risk of death by misadventure. That hanging is the common denominator and some degree of bondage extremely frequent suggests that expiation of feelings of guilt for sexual activity must play an important role in initiating the behavior. The individual may be acting out on himself what he fantasizes doing to others. There is even a suggestion that by assuming the posture of a hanged man the actor is paying in advance for his pleasure, and the added elements of masochism, bondage, and even self-mutilation form a constellation of reactions to that guilt.

While we remain ignorant of what can produce such a disturbed state of mind, we can only recall the couplet from Hugh Kingsmill's parody of A. E. Housman's pessimistic style:

> But bacon's not the only thing
> That's cured by hanging from a string.

Part Two

The Iconography of Death, Disease, and Dirty Books

5

Weighing the Heart against the Feather of Truth

*M*ost physicians accept with complacent pride the descent of the medical profession from Apollo's son Aesculapius and the high priests of his cult. With less complacency we trace our lineage to the medicine men and shamans of primitive tribes, but the relation between magical spells and rites and the evolution of modern medical practices cannot be gainsaid. One specialty in particular, pathology, can trace its roots to the Roman *haruspex,* who prophesied future events by examining the entrails of sacrificed animals. Indeed, much of the discipline of today's experimental pathology consists of precisely that. Archaeological retrieval of clay and metal representations of the liver in Babylonian and Etruscan remains (fig. 5.1) testifies to the remote origin of the *haruspices* and to the principal organ upon which their divinations focused, but the Romans never accorded them official status. There was no Royal College of Haruspices. For official divination the Romans relied on the guidance of *auspices,* who drew their inferences from the flight of birds and such melodramatic effects as flashes of lightning and crashes of thunder. The rules of practice for *auspices* were well codified and their nomenclature well standardized. But one contribution of magic to medicine has been largely overlooked, namely, the ancient Egyptian idea of weighing the heart after death.

To be sure, the Egyptians weighed the heart for eschatological purposes rather than for prophecy or application to medical judgments. The ancient Egyptians were far more concerned with the afterlife than the transitory and ephemeral concerns of life on earth. Orientation of their thought toward the hereafter probably accounts for such latter-day judgments as, "One might imagine that the widespread practice of

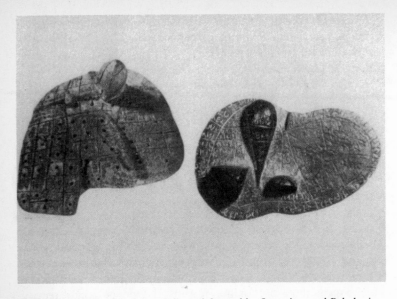

Figure 5.1. Clay model of sheep's liver (*left*) used by Sumerians and Babylonians for divination, ca. 1830–1530 B.C. Courtesy of the British Museum. Bronze model of sheep's liver (*right*) used by Etruscans for divination, ca. 1000–800 B.C. Courtesy of the Piacenza Museum. It is conjectured that using the liver of a sacrificed animal for divination originated in Mesopotamia and was transmitted to northern Italy. Putatively, *haruspex* is derived from the Chaldean *har*, meaning liver.

embalming the dead body would have stimulated the study of human anatomy, but it was not the case."[1] Nonetheless, even as weighing the heart was an integral part of Egyptian religion, an essential element in the judgment of the dead, so at the autopsy table pathologists of today weigh the heart religiously and form judgments based upon that datum.

The Egyptian embalmer is the precursor of the anatomist, but it would be a mistake to regard him as one. He was a sacerdotal technician concerned only with preventing decomposition of the body, and his procedures were ritual in origin and purpose—in fact, utilitarian. That anatomic knowledge accrued was incidental, even accidental. Nonetheless, this knowledge was unrivaled elsewhere in the ancient world, a body of information denied to cultures that inhumed or cremated their dead. It led to speculation regarding physiological functions, and, imperfect as that was, it provided the basis upon which later, more scientific insights could be erected.

Egyptian religion was based on a solar monotheism appropriate for official and ceremonial purposes, supplemented by a polytheistic pantheon of gods and goddesses of varying degrees of importance and influence. The latter ranged from an "executive cabinet" of major deities charged with specific departmental functions down to a host of regional or local deities serving demotic needs. Such familiar names as Osiris, Isis, Horus, Amon, Set, Geb, Nut, Ptah, Maat, Thoth, and Anubis were important figures in the "cabinet" and were the prototypes of the Greek deities of Olympus. They were usually considered to be the children or grandchildren of the sun god, Re (Ra). The cult of Osiris was one of the most important, largely because Osiris was god of the Underworld.

Osiris began his career as a vegetation-fertility god, one of many such. He was killed in a quarrel with his brother Set, who cut his body into pieces and threw them into the Nile. After a long search his sister-wife Isis (cf. later Ptolemaic marriages between siblings) recovered the pieces—except for the genitals, which had been eaten by fish—sewed them together, and restored Osiris to life. The idea of a mutilated and resurrected god ought not seem strange to Christians. In *Areopagitica* Milton compared Isis' quest to the search for truth:

> Truth indeed came once into the world . . . then straight arose a wicked race of deceivers, who . . . dealt with Osiris, took the virgin Truth, hewed her lovely form into a thousand pieces, and scattered them to the four winds. From that time ever since, the sad friends of Truth, such as durst appear, imitating the careful march that Isis made for the mangled body of Osiris, went up and down gathering up limb by limb still as they could find them. We have not found them all, Lords and Commons, nor ever shall do so, till her Master's second coming [when] he shall bring together every joint and member, and shall mould them into an immortal feature of loveliness and perfection.[2]

One may also construe the metaphor as a statement of the scientific method, collecting the data and assembling them to form a faultless statement.

Because he had once died, Osiris was charged with supervision of the Underworld, and it was to his realm that the king and later the nobility and priesthood were translated. After a few generations had passed, it became the goal of every Egyptian to join Osiris and the blessed company of the honored dead in paradise. For the ancient

Egyptian, life after death was a real physical resurrection with sensory and motor functions restored. It was considered his duty to cultivate the domains of Osiris and keep the dikes and irrigation canals in good order; the kingdom of the dead was a replica of the Egyptian state. Food and utensils stored in tombs indicate their expectation of normal gastrointestinal function despite the fact that the stomach and entrails were removed prior to mummification and stored in canopic jars. That normal sexual function was anticipated in paradise is indicated by a coffin text that reads in part, "For any man who shall know this spell, he shall copulate in this land by night and day, and desire shall come to the woman beneath him whenever he copulates."[3] Life in the Underworld was business as usual, and, as befits most African religions, its gods and inhabitants were apperceived at a level of reality corresponding to Marc Connelly's *Green Pastures*.

The cult of Osiris survived for over two millennia and was one of the dominant themes in Egyptian faith. Much of our knowledge about its eschatology comes from the so-called *Book of the Dead* (literally, *The Book of Coming Forth by Day*), papyrus scrolls recovered from mummy wrappings containing a variety of texts, and an even more varied assortment of illustrative vignettes. The earliest versions of the *Book of the Dead* date from the Eighteenth Dynasty (1567–1320 B.C.), and they continued to be written until the fourth century A.D. The text was not codified until the Ptolemaic period some time in the third century B.C. Until then the scribes who prepared the scrolls used whatever texts were at hand and suited their customers. Some passages can be traced back to the Pyramid Texts, spells and incantations incised in the stone walls of burial chambers dating back to the Fifth Dynasty under Wenis (Unas) circa 2360 B.C. At that time translation into the company of the gods was reserved for the king, who was their descendant and enjoyed the prerogative by right of birth. One such text proclaims that the king was pure of heart. It may seem anomalous that magical spells should be used to ensure the king's safe passage into the afterlife; in theory he required no such assistance.

Over the next few centuries the privilege of joining Osiris and the king was extended to courtiers, the nobility, and the priesthood. Their bodies were mummified and buried in coffins, hence the development of Coffin Texts, elaborations from the incantations of the Pyramid Texts, written on the sides of the coffins. Needless to say, mummification, an expensive and time-consuming process, was beyond the reach of commoners. The bodies of the ordinary Egyptian and his family were consigned unceremoniously to the desert sands where they decomposed anonymously, even as do the bodies of their descendants today.

What elevates the *Book of the Dead* above the level of primitive magic is its incorporation of a moral code and the idea of a judgment of the dead. These are embodied in the famous chapter 125 as the so-called Negative Confession and the rich iconography of the judgment scene in which the heart is weighed against the feather of truth. A contemporary example of the use of a scroll containing a religious text as protection against an evil fate can be seen in the *mezuzah* that Jews fasten to their gateposts.

After the *ba* (or soul) of the deceased had entered the Underworld, it was led into the Hall of Maat, the goddess of truth, justice, and cosmic order, whose symbol was a feather. The hall is sometimes referred to as the Hall of Two Truths, perhaps because a statue of Maat was placed at either end. Seated in the hall were the forty-two assessors (or judges), their number corresponding to the number of nomes (administrative districts) of ancient Egypt. It was to this panel that the deceased recited the Negative Confession, not truly a confession of sins in the modern sense but rather a blanket denial of wrongdoing supplemented by claims of virtue, charity, and purity of heart. The confession consisted of forty-two separate declarations, one addressed to each assessor, with considerable duplication among the postulations of innocence. The scribes were rather unimaginative at constructing a litany of evil. The deceased denied having committed murder, acts of violence, a variety of forms of theft and fraud, perjury, blasphemy, and sexual misconduct, as well as offenses specific for an agrarian society, namely, "I have not laid waste the lands which have been ploughed"; "I have not made light the bushel" (i.e., given short weight); and "I have not fouled running water," nor presumably the footpath. The sins denied seem to include most of those listed in the Ten Commandments and some of the forms of misconduct proscribed in Leviticus. The only significant item added in the Decalogue is the matter of graven images, a prohibition that may explain why Judaism was noted for its exegetical textual criticism but impoverished in representational fine arts such as painting and sculpture. It is notable that in Judaica the "arts" largely feature such decorative *Kleinkunst* as elaborate finials for Torah scrolls and fancy spice boxes. Not until the twentieth century was there a Jewish painter or sculptor of first rank. A communal form of confession, albeit in a positive sense, is found in the Yom Kippur service, when Jews assembled for prayer ask forgiveness for a comparable catalogue of sins, but this liturgy dates from Rabbinic times.

The exodus of the Israelites from Egypt is said to have taken place during the Nineteenth Dynasty, circa 1280 B.C., in the reign of Rameses II, known as the Pharaoh of the Oppression. Like other newly developed religions, Judaism combined both innovation and imitation. With their happy faculty for oversimplification, the Israelites adopted monotheism as their innovation and buttressed it with the catchy slogan *adonai echod*. Their imitation, the continuation of tradition, was the moral element found in the Negative Confession. What we so proudly hail as Mosaic Law and Judaeo-Christian ethics seems to be a transcription, redaction, and recension of an idealized code of conduct for Nilotic noblemen. Perhaps Shelley underestimated the influence of Ozymandias.

Once the deceased had enunciated the Negative Confession and proclaimed his acts of charity, he was ready to have his heart weighed. This was feasible because in the embalming process preceding mummification, "the heart was purposely left *in situ,* to allow the future survival of the deceased. If by accident, it was detached, it was imperative to replace it inside the body, either free or attached by a ligature."[4] Parenthetically, the kidneys were also left behind, probably because their retroperitoneal location made access difficult and it was not essential that they be bathed in embalming fluid. There is no hieroglyph for the kidneys; they were unknown to Egyptian vocabulary. One recalls that prior to Richard Bright's study of renal disease in the first half of the nineteenth century the kidneys were not routinely examined at autopsy.

Scrolls of the *Book of the Dead* often depict this weighing of the heart, and additional representations are found as wall paintings in tombs, on mummy cases, and on the cerements used to shroud the cadaver. Seeber's comprehensive monograph classifies these vignettes with respect to period, location, content, and other features.[5] Considerable iconographic variation is evident. The artist was allowed considerable latitude in selecting and composing the representation, provided the essential elements were shown. Comparable tensions between freedom and restraint confronted Renaissance artists commissioned to paint such scenes of Christian symbolism as the many annunciations, nativities, crucifixions, and resurrections that adorn books of hours, missals, chapels, altars, and latterly museum walls.

The central element was the beam balance with the heart placed in one pan and balanced against Maat in the other. Maat was often represented symbolically by her hieroglyph, the feather, but sometimes a statuette of the goddess wearing her feather was used. The actual weighing was conducted by the jackal-headed Anubis; sometimes he was assisted by the falcon-headed Horus, and in a few examples Horus alone conducted the weighing. The result was recorded by the ibis-headed Thoth, chief secretary to the Egyptian pantheon; in many representations Thoth's cynomolgus monkey sits on top of the center post, probably to indicate how scrupulously the scales of justice were watched. If the deceased's heart were pure and balanced evenly with Maat or the feather of truth, he was considered "justified," and after a few ceremonial allocutions was admitted to the company of Osiris and the blessed. If his heart was heavy and laden with sin, it was cast to the devouring beast Ammit, depicted as a chimera with the head and jaws of a crocodile, the body of a lion, and the rump and tail of a hippopotamus. The idea is echoed in the handwriting on the wall at Belshazzar's feast (ca. 540 B.C.), in which *TEKEL* is translated as, "Thou hast been weighed in the balances and found wanting."

Portrayals of the judgment scene vary widely in complexity and detail. Most familiar is the frequently reproduced panel from the Nineteenth Dynasty papyrus of Ani (ca. 1250 B.C.), which displays all the elements cited above. By contrast, the Twenty-first Dynasty papyrus of Queen Nedjemt (ca. 1000 B.C.) merely exhibits a balance, with her heart balancing a statuette of Maat and no god present to conduct the weighing or record the result. Almost as simplified is the Eighteenth Dynasty wall painting from the tomb of the Noble Menna (ca. 1412 B.C.) showing Horus rather than Anubis weighing the heart against Maat (fig. 5.2). More detailed, including the hieroglyphic text of an appropriate prayer, is the Twenty-first Dynasty papyrus of Princess Entiu-ny (ca. 1025 B.C.) in which Anubis controls the balance, although Thoth is not shown as recording (fig. 5.3). In this papyrus an offering of food is placed before the seated figure of Osiris, the haunch of an ungulate, perhaps a lamb or a goat. This was the choicest cut of flesh, and perhaps the Talmudic interdiction against eating the hindquarters of even those animals that chew the cud can be traced to a rejection of what was thought fit for an Egyptian god. In such Ramesside papyri as those of Nesi-pa-ku-shuty and Ta-udja-re the food offerings are more sumptuous; included are a heart and lung, cuts of rib, loaves of bread, onions, leeks, and assorted vegetables, a basket of

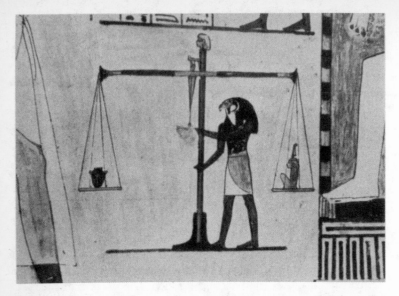

Figure 5.2. Horus weighing the heart against a statuette of Maat. Wall painting from the tomb of the Noble Menna at Thebes, Eighteenth Dynasty, ca. 1412 B.C.

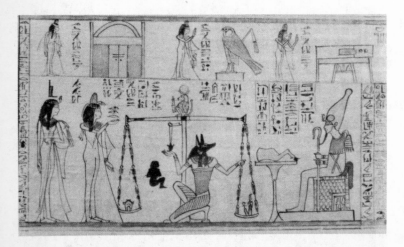

Figure 5.3. Judgment scene from the funerary papyrus of the Princess Entiuny, daughter of King Pay-nudjem. From the tomb of Queen Meryet-Amun at Deir el Bahri, Thebes, ca. 1025. B.C. Courtesy of the Metropolitan Museum of Art, Museum Excavations, 1928–29, and Rogers Fund, 1930.

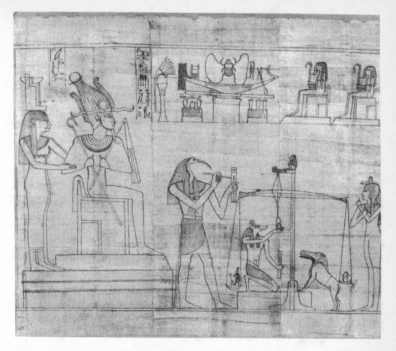

Figure 5.4. Judgment scene from the papyrus of Nestanebtashru. Thebes, Twenty-first Dynasty, ca. 1000 B.C. Courtesy of the Trustees of the British Museum.

fruit, even lotus flowers—clearly a more balanced diet. One of the simplest representations is the monochrome line drawing resembling a draftsman's outline in the Twenty-first Dynasty papyrus of Nestanebtashru (ca. 1000 B.C.), wherein Osiris closely supervises the scene in which Anubis weighs, his hand on the plummet, Thoth stands ready to record, and Ammit looks hungry, anxious to receive and eat the heart if it proves unjustified (fig. 5.4).

As in any other survey of the iconography of a set religious subject, one can find individual details of interest. The Twentieth Dynasty papyrus of Anhai (ca. 1150 B.C.) shows her just after justification, her body liberally decorated with the feathers of truth, resembling that of St. Sebastian pierced by arrows. The Twenty-first Dynasty papyrus of Tameniu (ca. 1000 B.C.) exhibits a curious juxtaposition. Just to the left of a conventional judgment scene and without intervening explanatory text is a vignette of the creation myth, the sky goddess Nut be-

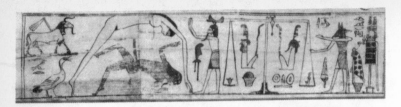

Figure 5.5. *Left*, sky goddess Nut being torn from ithyphallic earth god Geb; *right*, judgment scene. From the papyrus of Tameniu. Twenty-first Dynasty, ca. 1000 B.C. Courtesy of the Trustees of the British Museum.

ing torn from an ithyphallic earth-god Geb, who seems to be falling through space (fig. 5.5). The colorful Ptolemaic papyrus of Ker'asher (first century B.C.), a relatively late example, shows both Horus and Anubis weighing the heart beneath a frieze of the forty-two assessors. Earlier papyri showed fewer witnesses, sometimes a representation of the Theban Enniad, sometimes a miscellany of major and minor deities. A prominent feature of the judgment scenes—well displayed in the papyrus of Entiu-ny (fig. 5.3), occupying the space between Anubis' right hand and the pan with the princess's heart—is the dark figure of the birth child symbolizing resurrection. The papyrus of Hor-Netzi-Atef-Ef, a third- to second-century B.C. priest at Thebes, is notable for showing all forty-two assessors sitting in judgment above the weighing scene.[6]

Relics to indicate that weighing was an important aspect of life in the classical world are rarely encountered outside the Egyptian judgment scene. The Archaeological Museum at Athens has a set of gold scales recovered by Schliemann from a child's grave at Mycenae. The precious metal and small size suggest that the scales served no practical purpose, nor can a correlative be found for them in any Greek religious idea. A marble sculpture in the Museum of Fine Arts at Boston shows two women with an Eros poised between them.[7] Though parts of the sculpture, notably the scales, are missing, the presence of weights at the base and the disposition of the figures suggest a weighing scene. One of the women wears a happy expression, the other a sad one; perhaps it represents the result of a beauty contest. But the provenance and purpose of the group remain debatable. A fifth-century B.C. Attic black-figure *lekythos* shows Hermes weighing two winged *eidola* in a balance, presumably the scale of destiny, recalling the duel between Achilles and Memnon, but the scales symbolized the outcome of the contest rather than a judgment on the soul.[8] A sixth-century B.C. black-figure amphora by Taleides depicts two men weighing bales or cartons of merchandise in a balance, but its implication is commercial rather than otherworldly.[9] Balances for commercial use have been retrieved from Pompeii. Late medieval representations of Famine, the third horseman of the Apocalypse, often show him on a black horse with an empty balance in his hand.[10]

In Egypt, Coptic Christianity gradually replaced the old Egyptian gods. That the transition was gradual, even peaceful, can best be seen in the second-century Kom al-Shugafa catacombs at Alexandria, where Egyptian and Christian iconography are inextricably intermixed. By the fifth century only the faintest traces of Egyptian religion remained, and there are no examples of the *Book of the Dead* after this period.

The idea of a Last Judgment is, of course, explicit in the Revelation of St. John the Divine, but Christianity emphasizes the spiritual rather than the somatic aspect of resurrection. Exegesis of the parable of the valley of dry bones in Ezekiel 37 includes the notion of physical resurrection, but it is not generally taken as doctrinal. In the 1950s a painting by Sir Stanley Spencer of his friends and neighbors climbing awkwardly out of their coffins in the local churchyard at Cookham created some dismay, most of which centered around the feeling that Judgment Day couldn't be quite like that. Spencer was painting in a well-established tradition. The Guild Chapel at Stratford-on-Avon was decorated with a fresco showing the Last Judgment and Resurrection in which persons of both sexes and various ranks were shown rising from their tombs and graves. It was painted in the fifteenth century but was whitewashed over in Shakespeare's youth because of its papist imagery.[11]

The early Middle Ages provide no iconography of the soul actually being weighed and judged. But given the exigencies of artistic representation, it is not surprising that after a few centuries scenes depicting physical resurrection began to appear in painting, sculpture, and mosaics. In large measure the fine arts of the era existed to supply visual reification of spiritual ideas; the word was made flesh, or at least so depicted. Consider the common sentiment, "I shall see my Maker face to face," and, from Handel's *Messiah,* "In my flesh I shall see God." Related to the belief in physical resurrection is the observation that heretics and traitors were hanged, drawn, and quartered so that they could not be resurrected in the flesh.

By tradition the archangel Michael was given the role of psychopomp. The precise origin of that role remains obscure, but a fifth-century Coptic papyrus refers to him as a weigher, linking Egyptian and Christian traditions.[12] He was the only angel with a liturgical observance prior to the ninth century. He replaces the Greek Hermes and the Roman Mercury and is often depicted as youthful, agile, bare-legged, and wearing sandals. Emile Mâle informs us that

> anxious to divert to St. Michael the worship which the still pagan inhabitants of Roman Gaul paid to Mercury, the Church early endowed the archangel with almost all the attributes of the god. On the ruins of ancient temples of Mercury . . . rose chapels dedicated to St. Michael; a hill in La Vendée even today bears the significant name of Saint Michel-Mont-Mercure. St. Michael, already the messenger of heaven, became like Mercury the guide of the dead. . . . [He] is the angel of death, and it is in virtue of this that he presides at the Last Judgment.[13]

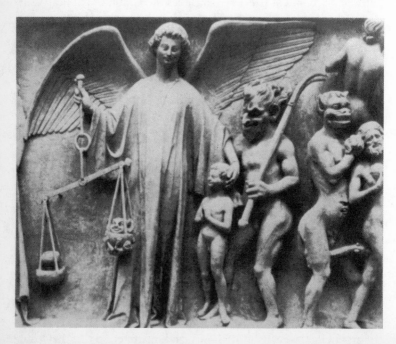

Figure 5.6. St. Michael weighing a soul in a balance. From a tympanum at Bourges, ca. 1280–90.

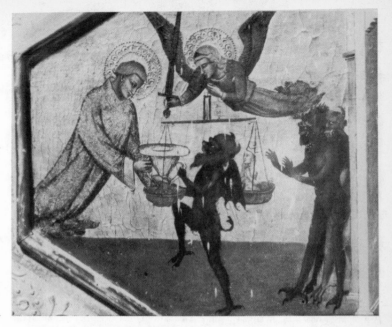

Figure 5.7. St. Michael weighing the soul of Emperor Henry II. Predella panel from S. Maria Novella, Florence. Orcagna, fourteenth century.

St. Michael is portrayed in a number of roles and guises, not only as a bare-legged, sandaled youth but also as a young knight in armor wearing a sword; he is sometimes shown in flowing robes. Like other saints, angels, and archangels he had many offices and duties to perform: God's messenger, the guide of souls, binding Satan with chains, killing a dragon. To these Pius XII added in 1941 his role as patron saint of radiologists and in 1950 of policemen.

The scales of judgment are a frequent attribute of St. Michael. Boase cites and illustrates a thirteenth-century Catalan altar frontal in which he is shown weighing a naked and supplicant soul in a balance.[14] The reliefs of the Last Judgment in the tympanums of the late medieval cathedrals at Autun, Bourges (fig. 5.6), and Notre Dame in Paris all show him weighing souls, with the added detail of mischievous devils trying to tilt the balance in their favor. These portrayals date from the twelfth and thirteenth centuries; in the next century a predella panel to a polyptych of the Virgin and Saints by Orcagna, executed for S. Maria

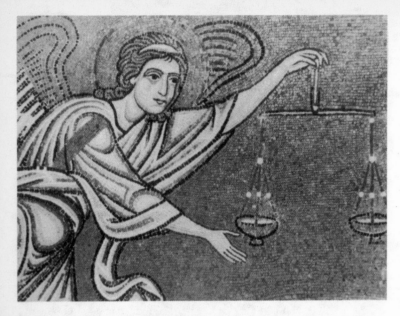

Figure 5.8. Angel with an empty balance. Detail from the Doomsday mosaic in the Cathedral at Torcello, thirteenth century.

Novella at Florence, shows him weighing the soul of Emperor Henry II against a golden ewer while a demon, encouraged by Satan himself, is trying to push the balance with the ewer upward so that the Emperor's soul will fall (fig. 5.7). In quite a different mode is the serenely floating angel with empty balances at equipoise in the Doomsday mosaic in the deserted cathedral at Torcello (fig. 5.8).

St. Michael's militant vigor is well captured in a panel now in the Portland (Oregon) Art Museum by the fifteenth-century Florentine Domenico Ghirlandaio. St. Michael is shown set in a shallow space in front of a garden wall, a sword in one hand and a balance in the other (fig. 5.9). A felicitous painting by a pupil of Leonardo, titled *La vierge aux balances* (ca. 1510) and now at the Louvre, shows the Madonna and Child with St. Anne and the infant St. John; at their left is an ephebic, epicene St. Michael playing with his balance and the Christ child (fig. 5.10). The museum at Le Bar-sur-Loup in Provence has an anonymous fifteenth-century wood panel with a *danse macabre* occupying the upper quarter. St. Michael is shown with scales at the left of a

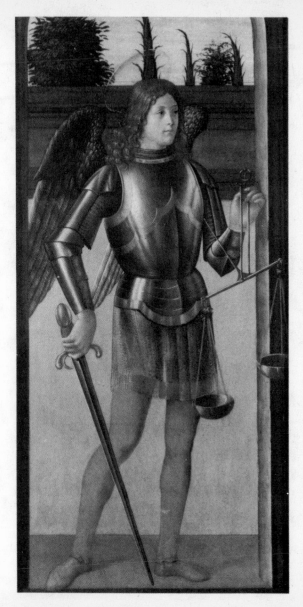

Figure 5.9. St. Michael. Follower of Domenico Ghirlandaio, ca. 1500. Portland (Oregon) Art Museum.

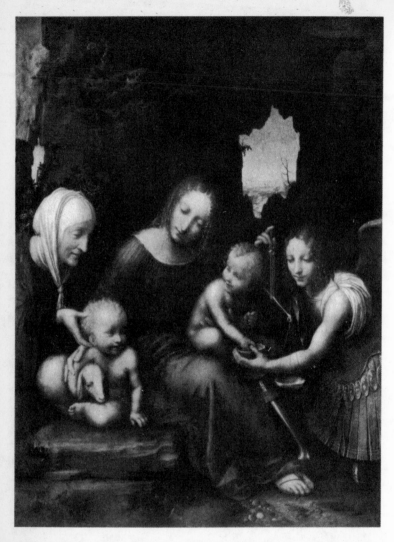

Figure 5.10. *La vierge aux balances*. Pupil of Leonardo da Vinci, ca. 1510. Photo Alinari.

circle of sinners dancing to their perdition; beneath is a monitory and hortatory text intended to remind the beholder of his certain fate should he die uncontrite and unshriven. Perhaps of a somewhat later date is the statue of St. Michael with his balances surmounting the portal to the cemetery bearing his name in Venice. Many legends have accumulated about St. Michael's role as an intercessor, but representations of him with a balance for weighing souls seem to have largely disappeared after the middle of the sixteenth century. An exception is a carved wooden *bulto* by an anonymous ninteenth-century *santero,* now in the Museum of New Mexico at Santa Fe.[15]

Also depicted with balances is the figure of Christ as an apothecary, a subject related to his healing mission that became popular in Germany and Austria between the sixteenth and eighteenth centuries, appearing in oil paintings, copper engravings, woodcuts, stained glass windows, and other media. Hein has located almost one hundred such representations.[16] Many show Christ in an apothecary's shop, surrounded by the jars and other appurtenances of the trade. A majority show him with a set of balances, often in the act of weighing out ingredients. The one at the Deutsches Apotheken-Museum at Heidelberg, an early-eighteenth-century oil painting by an anonymous artist, shows a vignette in the background of Christ healing the leper. But in this genre the balances are for weighing material substances, not truth.

In the Middle Ages the heart itself was not weighed, but on occasion it was accorded special treatment. Robert Bruce's heart was placed in a silver casket and dispatched by messenger for burial in the Holy Land. A crypt in the Church of St. Augustine in Vienna contains the hearts of fifty-four members of the royal house of Habsburg dating from 1618 to 1878. During the Middle Ages, postmortem dissection and embalming were carried out much less frequently than in Egypt. As in Egypt, it was reserved for royalty and a few members of the nobility and ecclesiastical hierachy, usually to refute a suspicion of death by poisoning; however, given the state of gross anatomic knowledge at the time, it is difficult to excogitate what anatomic experience might have served as a basis for a confident judgment. The effigies (ca. 1515) of Louis XII and his wife, Anne of Brittany, on the tomb in the abbey church of St. Denis recall evisceration and the embalming procedure to visual memory (fig. 5.11). On a happier occasion, that of their marriage, it was for these two monarchs that the celebrated and festive unicorn tapestries were woven. But with only sporadic exceptions the idea

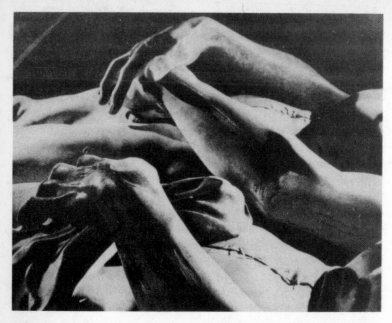

Figure 5.11. Detail of the tomb effigies of Louis XII and his queen, showing the incisions and sutures after evisceration and embalming. Abbey church of St. Denis, ca. 1515.

of weighing the heart for either religious or medical purposes was unimportant in Western Europe until the seventeenth and eighteenth centuries.

Weighing the heart for medical purposes is a post-Harveian idea, motivated by the need to estimate cardiac volume. The first record of this form of weighing is the observation by Theodore Kerkring in 1670 that the heart weighed seven ounces.[17] Eighteenth-century anatomists added the idea of linear measurements, namely, the circumference of cardiac valves, thickness of ventricular walls, and other measures of length and breadth. Yet Morgagni, who described so many examples of cardiac disease so well, never recorded the actual weight of the organ. Elaborating the clinicopathological concepts of Bichat, Laennec, and Corvisart, French anatomists and pathologists began to weigh hearts. Bouillaud, for example, gave the average weight of the heart as 8 oz., 3 gr., but his observations, as well as previous ones by Senac and Cruveilhier, did not distinguish between male and female hearts, nor did they take into account the effects of age.[18] Developing the concept of cardiac hypertrophy, Cruveilhier stated that weight was preferable to linear measurements to resolve the point, but it was a statement of principle rather than the result of systematic observations.[19]

Lobstein contributed a few observations on heart weight, but it remained for Clendinning to publish the first tabulation of the weight of the heart and other organs taking age and sex into account; these and the tabulations by Reid and Peacock are the basis for our modern ideas of heart weight.[20] But the idea of weighing the heart at the autopsy table was slow to take root. Rokitansky seems to have confined his observations to linear measurements, and Virchow's manual of post-mortem technique, written as late as 1875, does not instruct prosecutors to weigh the heart or any other organ.[21] Yet only a few years later, in 1883, Müller published his monograph dealing in a highly sophisticated fashion with partitioning the heart and weighing its anatomical subdivisions.[22]

The feather of truth has changed its colors as the paramount values of society have shifted. From the moral code of the ancient Egyptians through the spiritual values of medieval Christianity we have arrived at a modern society that prizes quantifiable information as its *summum bonum*. Today's youth are more familiar with baseball statistics than their catechism, and adults are more likely to have stock-market quotations and the cost of automobiles and their miles per gallon of gasoline at ready recall than to be able to quote chapter and verse of scripture. Homage to numbers permeates all walks of life, from Professor Max Gottlieb's commitment to the quantitative method in Sinclair Lewis' *Arrowsmith* to the fact that the simplest demotic game of chance, one requiring almost no cerebration or active participation by its players, is known as "the numbers game." For pathologists, the descendants of the jackal-headed Anubis, automated laboratory equipment churns out a daily quota of computerized printouts, and certainly the medical segment of today's society seems obsessed with numbers. It should be noted that it took longer for quantitative data to be applied to biological and medical problems than to other disciplines. Early in the history of science astronomers made quite accurate measurements of sidereal phenomena, and for cogent commercial reasons measurements of land were precise.

Without denying the usefulness of replicable and verifiable empirical data as one of the bases upon which science rests, there is more to science and medicine than coefficients of variance and standard deviation curves. Perhaps we ought to consider carefully Thomas Huxley's caution that although all science is measurement, not all measurement is science. In his presidential address to the American Society for Clinical Investigation, delivered in 1944 just at the time endocrinology was emerging as a scientific discipline, Fuller Albright spoke of the "dos and don'ts." One of his "dos" dealt with quantifying one's data, but he qualified it with a gentle reminder:

> Do measure something. I need not remind you gentlemen that science is based on measurements. Indeed this is so well understood today that at times one wonders whether the pendulum has not swung too far from the state of affairs in the Middle Ages. Then it was all metaphysics and no measurements; now it is all measurements and no metaphysics. Perhaps a dash of the latter would be a useful condiment.[23]

Carrying through the metaphor, if measurements and numbers can be taken to represent truth, then metaphysics is their feather.

6

Can the Leper Change His Spots? The Iconography of Leprosy

*W*e first learn about leprosy from Leviticus 13, the familiar chapter that describes "a rising, a scab, or bright spot . . . in the skin." The text is easily taken as an early statement of public health policy and procedure. It provides for isolation of suspected cases and it instructs priests charged with responsibility for diagnosis about the appearance of lesions as well as local spread and distant dissemination. Additional clinical features of the disease are mentioned, and various measures, including segregation of victims, are prescribed to control contagion. There is no suggestion in Leviticus 13 that leprosy, as the early Israelites understood it, was a visitation from God as a punishment for sin. That came later, and the punitive God of the Old Testament was not slow in making his appearance.

In Numbers 12 we learn that Miriam and Aaron expostulated with Moses because he had married an Ethiopian woman. Whether she was black or white we are not told, but clearly Moses had married outside the tribe. Aaron and Miriam are prototypical of opposition to intermarriage, a position taken by both the rabbinate and the Jewish matriarchy, the former for fear of decreasing the numerical strength of its flock, the latter out of sexual jealousy. Jehovah presumably took a more tolerant attitude toward intermarriage because he punished Miriam with leprosy for her strident objections. But Aaron interceded for his sister: "Lay not the sin upon us, wherein we have done foolishly. . . . Let her not be as one dead, of whom the flesh is half consumed. . . ." The good Lord remitted her affliction to a skin eruption that lasted only a week, after which she was readmitted to the Israelites' camp.

Leprosy of seven days' duration is not medically convincing, nor does the incident illustrate any concept that would be important for

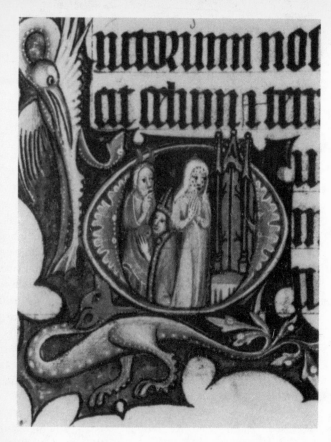

Figure 6.1. The leprosy of Miriam. English, before 1373. Oxford: Exeter College MS. 47, fol. 91v.

Christian ideology. Perhaps for these reasons Miriam's leprosy was rarely depicted by medieval or Renaissance artists. One such illumination in a late fourteenth-century English psalter (fig. 6.1) shows Miriam clad in white with only her hands and face exposed, her "leprosy" denoted by a few small violaceous spots on her face. Her folded hands suggest an attitude of prayer as she stands in front of a Gothic version of a tabernacle. To her right, also facing the tabernacle, is Moses, identifiable by his two horns. In the foreground, facing the other way, is Aaron, whose rank as high priest of Israel is indicated by a bishop's miter. Anomalous as that may seem to a non-Christian observer, it places him on equal footing with three of the Church Fathers, Saints Ambrose, Augustine, and Pope Gregory the Great, who were consecrated bishops of their own sees. Artistic convention awards the fourth Church Father, Saint Jerome, a cardinal's hat; although he antedates the College of Cardinals, it is generously assumed that had there been cardinals in his day, he would have been among them.

Miriam's leprosy is also illustrated in stained glass at the Ste. Chapelle in Paris (window N, bay 3), an early thirteenth-century miracle of light and color, as well as in a fourteenth-century *Biblia pauperum* in the Rosgarten Museum at Constance (fol. 6), to say nothing of several manuscripts of the *Bible moralisée* dating from the twelfth to the fifteenth centuries.[1]

Even before Miriam was afflicted, Moses himself was visited briefly by leprosy. When Jehovah commanded him to lead the Israelites out of Egypt, Moses asked for a sign lest his divine mission be challenged (Exodus 4:1–7). Turning Moses' rod into a serpent was one such sign; the next was the command that he put his hand in his bosom. When Moses withdrew his hand, it was white, "leprous as snow," and when he reinserted it and withdrew it a second time, it was healed. This transient, magically given, "presto-changeo" leprosy found no place in Christian art, but it is illustrated in two fourteenth-century Spanish *haggadot* (British Museum Add. MS. 27210; John Rylands Library MS. 6).[2]

The next Old Testament anecdote involving leprosy is in 2 Kings 5, Elisha's cure of Naaman, the captain of the Syrian army. The cure consisted of his dipping himself a magical seven times in the waters of Jordan. The rivers of Damascus whence he came, he was told, would not be efficacious. Cure by magical means suggests a supernatural origin for the disease, but we are not told what Naaman had done to incur God's displeasure. Elisha, being a holy man, had advised and cured Naaman without fee, but his servant Gehazi rode after Naaman surreptitiously and tried to extract money and clothing. Naaman generously gave him two talents and a change of garments, but Elisha punished Gehazi's cupidity by transferring Naaman's leprosy to him: "The leprosy of Naaman shall cleave unto thee and thy seed forever." Jehovah's prophets were endowed with uncanny epidemiological powers, even to the point of making an infectious disease inheritable.

Representations of Naaman's miraculous cure are more frequently

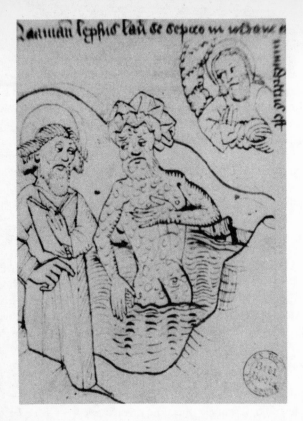

Figure 6.2. Naaman in Jordan about to be cured of leprosy by Elisha. English, fifteenth century. Oxford: Bodleian Library MS. Douce, f. 4, fol. 7.

encountered than ones of Miriam, but they are not numerous. Both an early-fifteenth-century *Speculum humanae salvationis* (C.C.C. Oxford MS. 161.5, fol. 48) and a Spanish manuscript of circa 1440 (Bodleian MS. Douce 204, fol. 12v) contain line drawings of Naaman standing in water up to his waist, his leprosy depicted by small spots or streaks over his chest, abdomen, and arms, Standing on the riverbank are his servants, who hold his cloak as he purifies himself. A slightly different version in a mid-fifteenth-century English *Speculum humanae salvationis* shows Naaman, nude except for a turban, mid-thigh-deep in running water, his torso and face covered with lesions drawn as open or closed

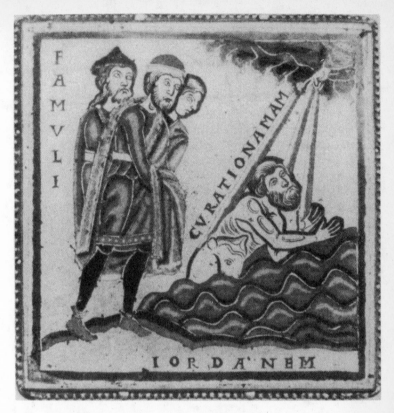

Figure 6.3. Naaman cured of leprosy by the hand of God. French Mosan enamel plaque, mid-twelfth century. British Museum, MLA 84, 6-6, 3. Courtesy of the Trustees of the British Museum.

circles (fig. 6.2). Elisha stands on the riverbank holding an open book while God looks down from a separate vantage point in the upper-right-hand corner. Primacy of quality in this late medieval tradition must be accorded a mid-twelfth-century Mosan enamel plaque showing the Syrian captain swimming in Jordan's waters (fig. 6.3). Divine cure is shown by rays emanating from God's hand in the upper right, and presumably they have done their work, for Naaman is unspotted. His three servants (*famuli*) stand on the left holding his cloak. That the bodies of the three servants arise from one pair of legs is an idiom of the workshop, not a prefiguration of the Trinity. The enamel plaque

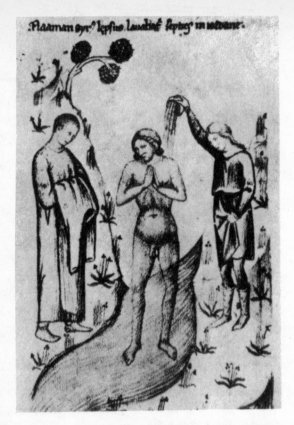

Figure 6.4. Naaman being washed in Jordan. Florentine, late fourteenth century. Riches MS. *Speculum humanae salvationis*.

and its equally striking companion piece showing Samson are probably parts of a larger altarpiece or cross. The late-fourteenth-century "Florentine" Riches manuscript *Speculum humanae salvationis* contains a drawing of Naaman being washed in the river Jordan that resembles pictures of Christ being baptized. Naaman stands naked in the river, his servants holding his cloak while Elisha pours the healing waters over his left shoulder; the cutaneous lesions of leprosy have vanished (fig. 6.4).[3]

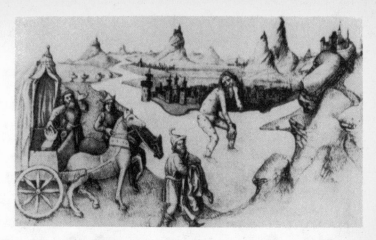

Figure 6.5. Naaman wading in Jordan. German, fifteenth century. Woodcut. Bettmann Archiv.

In contrast to the linear stylized images of the medieval illuminators, the humanistic artists of the Northern Renaissance provide an image different both in scale and in an attempt to depict the miracle as if it happened among people with real flesh and blood. An anonymous fifteenth-century German engraving (fig. 6.5) shows Naaman wading ankle-deep in shallow waters, his torso spotted with randomly distributed black dots. One servant holds his cloak; two others are in charge of a bathing machine that recalls Brighton in the 1880s. On a larger scale is the panel (ca. 1510–20) in the Kunsthistorisches Museum at Vienna by Cornelis Englebrechtsz (1468–1533), a Dutch artist (fig. 6.6). In the central panel, Naaman stands in the river to cleanse himself of his disease. *Mis à nu,* his pose resembles that taken four centuries later by "September Morn"; the waters have worked their magic, for his skin is immaculate. His three retainers stand on the bank behind him, and an opulently robed Elisha is on the near bank in the right foreground. In the background is the city of Samaria complete with a Dutch windmill. Disguised as citizens of Samaria going about their quotidian tasks are other elements of the story that fill in this sprawling composition. The wagon in the upper left shows Gehazi soliciting gifts from the departing Naaman; the two laden figures on the bridge have been interpreted as Gehazi and a helper returning with their ill-gotten

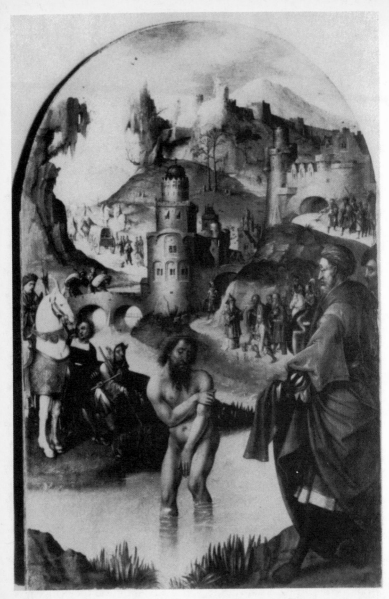

Figure 6.6. The prophet Elisha curing Naaman. Cornelis Englebrechtsz, ca. 1520. Central panel (folding wings not shown). Vienna: Kunsthistorisches Museum.

reward, though they seem to be traveling in the wrong direction. The left wing shows one of Elisha's aides, perhaps Gehazi, whispering in the ear of a man whose face is asymmetrical with left maxillofacial swelling and distortion of the left orbit, perhaps a leper being told of possible cure.

Earlier illuminations also show Gehazi's punishment. A late-twelfth-century Spanish bible at S. Millan de la Cogolla (fol. 210r) shows Elisha with a pearled nimbus seated on a cushioned bench, his right hand raised and extended toward Gehazi. A similar arrangement of the two figures occurs in the mid-fourteenth-century manuscript of Ulrich von Lilienfeld's *Concordantiae caritas* (fol. 145v). In an 1197 bible and Lives of the Saints at Amiens, Elisha is shown holding a *tau* staff in his right hand, pointing it at Gehazi, whose arms and hands are also extended (fol. 128v). None of these vignettes, however, shows Gehazi with spots denoting leprosy. Perhaps Elisha's curse has not yet taken effect; as we know, the disease does have a long incubation period.

Dutch narrative painting changed its style during the sixteenth century; the Italianate influence seen in Englebrechtsz's painting gives way to Mannerism in *Elisha Refuses Naaman's Gift* by Ferdinand Bol (1616–80). Now in the Rijksmuseum, it was painted in 1661 for the regents of the lazarette in Amsterdam. Naaman, clad in armor, is shown offering a decorated gold beaker to Elisha, who is decorously robed and wears a Levantine turban. Other gifts are in the background. At the extreme right Gehazi stands pensively in the doorway, presumably planning his next move. The river Jordan and its curative powers are not shown, and Naaman, having been healed, shows none of the lesions of leprosy. Perhaps the regents commissioned the painting as a cautionary tale for their employees, but the narrative element is uncanonical; nowhere in 2 Kings is there a hint that Naaman made such an offering. Such an attempt to inculcate acceptable moral values in an institution's staff is doomed to failure if the staff reads the Scripture carefully.

The remaining Old Testament legend dealing with leprosy is in 2 Chronicles 26, which relates the sad fate of Uzziah, the successful warrior-king of Israel who haughtily entered the temple and obstreperously attempted to burn incense as an offering to God. That particular act of devotion was the prerogative only of the high priests descended from Aaron. Uzziah, the reigning monarch, was clearly violating the separation between church and state; he was also guilty of Pride, the

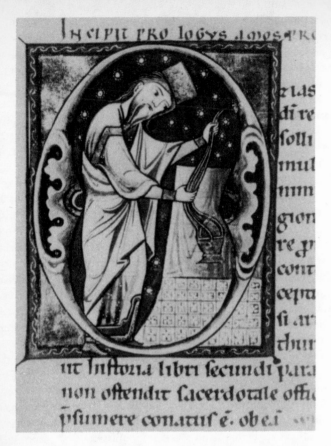

Figure 6.7. Uzziah swinging a censer. French, fourteenth century. Lyons: Bibliothèque de la Ville MS. 410–11, II, fol. 160vc.

chief of the deadly sins. The priests tried to stop him, and an altercation ensued. For such hubris God punished Uzziah with leprosy, and he was forced to abdicate in favor of his son Jotham.

Separation of powers between church and state was not an idea that found favor with patrons of art in the Middle Ages; it was an idea better left unvoiced or unlimned. As a result, iconographic representation of Uzziah is extremely rare. A fourteenth-century bible at Lyons shows him holding a censer, about to commit his act of impiety, but not yet smitten with leprosy (fig. 6.7). Among the scarce representations of Uzziah is an illumination in the ninth-century manuscript of the *Sacra parallela* of John of Damascus showing Azzahiah and another priest addressing Uzziah, who is crowned, holding an incense box, and about to enter the temple (Bibliothèque Nationale MS. Gr. 923, fol. 213v). A fourteenth-century bible at the Library of Congress contains an illuminated initial *O;* it is foliated and shows Uzziah in front of a curtain censing an altar (fol. 179r), but Uzziah's leprous lesions are not indicated.

Somewhat less lurid are the incidents involving leprosy in the New Testament. The account of Christ healing the leper appears in Matthew 8:2–4, Mark 1:40–44, and Luke 5:12–14. Healing was effected by touch, and Christ enjoined the patient to make a suitable thank offering to the priest rather than to himself. More consonant with the state of medicine today is the incident in Luke 17:12–19, where Christ healed ten lepers, only one of whom returned to thank him. Physicians who complain that few of their patients are grateful may find comfort in noting that Christ's rate of return was also low. The passage in Luke sets the stage for later faith healers: "Thy faith hath made thee whole." But in the absence of effective medical treatment, what other choice did patients have? These incidents in Christ's healing mission were frequent subjects for illustration; they lent themselves to pictorial and didactic aims, and only a sample can be discussed and illustrated.

Leprosy in the biblical, medieval and Renaissance eras was not diagnosed with accuracy. The criteria for diagnosis were imprecise; a few of the individuals so diagnosed may have had leprosy, but most of them did not. Many skin diseases, notably psoriasis, eczema, leukoderma, and other noninfectious dermatoses, were labeled leprosy, and the victims were doomed to a life of isolation, outcasts from society. The word *tzara'ath,* translated as leprosy in the Authorized Version, was used to denote the afflictions of Miriam, Naaman, Uzziah, and the beneficiaries of Christ's healing gift. It is a generic term denoting ritual uncleanliness rather than a specific skin disease. It includes a number of spots and blemishes, for it was used to describe cloth, leather, and even marks on damp walls of buildings. Alexandrian scholars who translated the scriptures into Greek rendered *tzara'ath* by *lepra,* using the word then employed to denote skin diseases characterized by scaling. First-century commentators used the synonymous term *elephantiasis graecorum,* which they distinguished from *elephantiasis arabum,* the equivalent of Bancroftian filariasis of today. To confuse vocabulary still further, *lepra arabum* was occasionally used to denote leprosy.

Aretaeus described the signs and symptoms of true leprosy toward

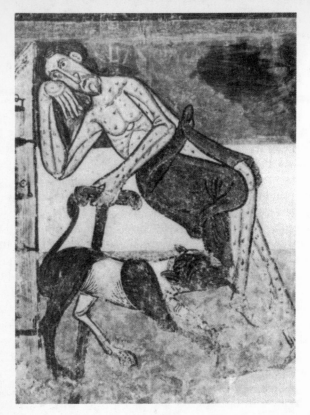

Figure 6.8. Lazarus at the rich man's door, his sores licked by a dog. Spanish, eleventh century. Fresco from the Abbey of St. Mary, Ripoll. Barcelona: Catalonia Museum.

the end of the second century; authorities concur that the disease was then diagnosed with some accuracy, but overdiagnosis was common. However, the ancients were able to distinguish between acute suppurative skin lesions and chronic granulomatous processes. *Tzara'ath* was quite distinct from *schechin,* the term for Job's boils, and *avabuah* (plural *avabuot*), the term for Lazarus' sores (Luke 16:20–21). The Vulgate follows the Septuagint closely; *schechin* became *pustulae ardentes,* occasionally *ulcus inflammatum,* and *avabuot* are simply *pustulae.* Curiously, the Lazarus whom Christ raised from the dead did not suffer from leprosy. The term *lazarette* for a building in which lepers were isolated conventionally alludes to Lazarus at the rich man's door, his sores licked by dogs (fig. 6.8), but one might cast a minority vote for an alternative allusion to Lazarus dead and resurrected, for in the Middle Ages a leper was considered as one dead (cf. Aaron's plea in behalf of Miriam), a person stripped of all human and civil rights.

The proscription against graven images largely precluded representation of the disease or its sufferers in Judaic culture, except for the *hiddur mitzvah* which permitted embellishment of holy books and objects, as in illuminated *haggadot* for the Passover service, and the same prohibition was later largely effective in Islam. I have not been able to identify leprosy in Christian art or artifacts in the early Middle Ages; its iconography does not seem to begin until the ninth century. Leprosy was certainly endemic in territories dominated by the Eastern Church, but Byzantine (later Greek, Turkish, and Russian) icons have not been catalogued to the same extent as the art forms of Western Christianity and are relatively inaccessible. The only example of leprosy I have been able to identify in Islamic art is the isolated figure of a leper in the mosaics decorating the fourteenth-century Kahrie Mosque in Istanbul. Clad only in a loincloth, the figure stands with his hands outstretched in a pleading gesture. His entire skin surface is covered with evenly distributed, prominent reddish spots. However, the style is more closely related to Byzantine Christian models than to figure representation in the Islamic tradition. Of related interest is an illustration in a manuscript titled *Chirurgia imperiale,* a translation into Turkish from a treatise probably composed in Persia circa 1300 by Abulcasis, now in the Bibliothèque Nationale at Paris.[4] The illumination (fig. 6.9) shows the points where cauterization was to be applied in treating lepromata. It shows rear and frontal views of a nude man wearing a turban; on the right is the seated figure of a physician holding the cautery iron in his right hand. The points for cauterization are indicated by round black spots, somewhat in the same fashion as sites for venipuncture or acupuncture might be demonstrated.

Though leprosy is supposed to have originated in the Indian subcontinent, the disease is not represented in Indian painting or sculpture.[5] A popular legend tells that King Simhavarman of the Pallava dynasty suffered from leprosy and was cured by the grace of the Lord Nataraja, in whose honor he erected a temple at Chidamvaram. Likewise, King Narasimhanarman of the Eastern Ganga dynasty of Orissa was cured

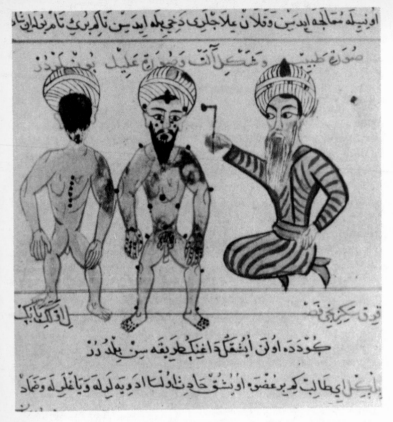

Figure 6.9. Cauterization points for treating leprosy. Turkish, ca. 1300. From *Chirurgia imperiale*. Paris: Bibliothèque Nationale.

by worshipping Surya; he later built a temple of the sun god at Konarak. But in none of the sculptures preserved in the National Museum at New Delhi is either king depicted with the stigmata of leprosy.[6]

A mid-nineteenth-century painting from Lahore showing considerable Western influence illustrates the charitable acts of Bhai Veer Singh. The small canvas contains more than one hundred figures, none executed in minute detail, but one figure in the lower right is that of an elderly man with a white beard wearing a turban. He is on crutches because his left leg is amputated, and there is a suggestion of a saddle nose. The amputation, however, is above the knee, suggesting either trauma or arteriosclerosis, and there are no indications of deformity in the digits of the three remaining extremities, nor are any cutaneous lesions painted. A confident diagnosis of leprosy cannot be made.

Many of the earlier studies on the iconography of leprosy have been unselectively inclusive rather than critically rigorous. Examples of lesions that are clearly not leprosy have been so labeled, and leprosy has been imputed when alternative diagnoses were equally possible, if not even more probable. For example, the legend of St. Martin informs us that he gave his cloak to a beggar, but there is no statement that the beggar was a leper. Although almost all lepers were beggars, only a minority of beggars were lepers. In many paintings and engravings of St. Martin the beggar is shown as a cripple, but physical deformity and a crutch are not sufficient for a diagnosis of leprosy. The distinction can be seen plainly in an illumination from Vincent de Beauvais' *Miroir historial* (fig. 6.10) which shows Jehosophat at the gate of Jerusalem welcoming a leper and a cripple. On the far right is the cripple, whose musculoskeletal deformity and crutches are explicit. The leper has a

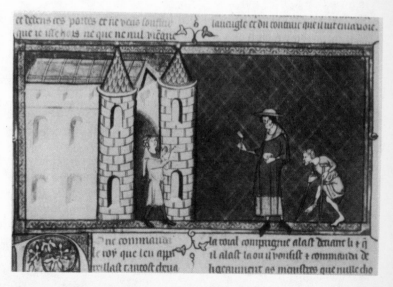

Figure 6.10. Jehosophat greeting a leper and a cripple at the gate of Jerusalem. French, thirteenth century. Vincent de Beauvais, *Miroir historial*. Paris: Bibliothèque de l'Arsenal.

normal body build, but he is carrying both a clapper and an ointment box, equally explicit. The *Perikopenbuch* of St. Erentrud, dating from circa 1150 (Bayerische Staatsbibliothek CML 15903, fol. 24), shows a leper supporting himself on a small crutch that reaches only waist high, but that leprosy has caused his deformity is indicated by the characteristic red spots randomly distributed over all exposed surfaces of his body.

The presence of a written tradition and availability of documentation make certain criteria obligatory. The emphasis must be on the artist's intentions insofar as we can ascertain them. Unmistakable illustration of an identifiable legend is, of course, optimal evidence. Presence of cutaneous lesions and facial or limb deformities designed to denote leprosy are equally valuable, but their representation will frequently conform more to the stylistic or symbolic conventions of the artist's period than to clinical perceptions. Identification of a leper in a painting or engraving may be legitimately claimed if the figure, almost always male, carries the attribute of either a leper's warning horn or clapper. Reasonable latitude in interpretation is permissible but one viewer's latitude may be another's longitude.

An occasional icon must be judged from its context rather than its content. The seal of Holy Innocents Hospital in Lincolnshire, founded as a leprosarium before 1135, depicts a man on crutches with an atrophic right forearm and possible atrophy of the left leg. Were it not the seal of a lazar house, one would consider the figure a cripple rather than a leper (Harleian MS. Ch. 44.A.29).

A common source of error is the oral tradition that may have accumulated about a given work of art, making the diagnosis of leprosy a received legend. A fine Rembrandt painting at Chatsworth, a half-length of a middle-aged man in Levantine costume wearing a white turban, is often reproduced with the title "Uzziah," but he exhibits none of the facial lesions associated with leprosy, nor is there any historical evidence that Rembrandt intended it as a picture of that bully. Also, it is sometimes labeled "Aaron" or occasionally "The Rabbi." But Uzziah it is surely not.

Goldman and Sawyer sound a useful caution in their study of Peruvian ceramics:

> One must be aware of certain distinct limitations before attempting diagnosis by the hazardous, though intriguing, technique of inspection. Differential diagnosis must take into account our in-

complete knowledge. . . . We must keep in mind that the ancient craftsmen expressed what is to us a bewildering complexity of mythological and religious concepts. What they intended to represent as a demon may look to us like dipsomania.[7]

Parenthetically, Vérut's statement that leprosy did not exist in pre-Columbian Mexico can be taken to exclude all mesoamerican artifacts from this essay.[8]

Artists do not work in a social vacuum, nor can the way they view disease be considered outside a social context. The intellectual tradition of Western Christianity interpreted leprosy as a mark of moral corruption—in Saul Brody's words, "a disease of the soul."[9] A few literary citations may serve to mark the late medieval attitude toward leprosy. Hartmann von Aue's poem *Der Arme Heinrich* (ca. 1195) tells the moral fable of a "parfit knight" stricken with leprosy because he chose material and secular goals over spiritual ones. Denying God's grace, he went to Montpellier and Salerno in quest of a medical cure, but the secular physicians offered him no hope. Resigned to becoming a leper, he distributed his wealth and retired to an isolated farm. He became aware of his sinfulness when a farmer's unspoiled daughter announced her willingness to sacrifice her heart's blood for his cure. Recognizing that her physical purity and beauty symbolized her spiritual immaculacy and perceiving his physical state as a symbol of his moral guilt, Heinrich rejected the proposed sacrifice as unnecessary because he required spiritual rather than physical purification. The homiletic point is that given such awareness, he was then cured, and more wealth and honor accrued to him than before. Implicit in the farmer's daughter's offer to sacrifice herself is the notion that a disease of supernatural origin can be cured by shedding blood.

Three centuries later, Robery Henryson's *Testament of Cresseid* (ca. 1500), a sequel to Chaucer's *Troilus and Criseyde,* describes the high-born wanton as "with fleschelie lust sa maculait," spotted with leprosy because of her promiscuity. The image is most unclassical; the Greeks and Trojans did not punish concupiscence with skin diseases, but Henryson was a Scot. Nonetheless, to the medieval mind a disfiguring disease was a fitting punishment for the sins of the flesh, and in that sense leprosy was considered a venereal disease. Cresseid finally admitted the justice of her punishment and accepted moral responsibility for her pride and lust.

Lepers, or sufferers from diseases resembling leprosy, are also found in the eighth circle of Dante's *Inferno* (canto 29:73–84). In Malebolge, where perjurers are punished, two alchemists are described as covered with scabs from head to foot ("Dal capo al pie di schianze macolati") which they scrape in the same way fish are scaled ("Come le coltel di scardova le scaglie"). But their skin lesions are pruritic, intractably so (". . . per la gran rabbia/Del pizzicor, che non ha piu soccorso"), and leprosy characteristically does not itch. Yet a few stanzas later (29:124) we are told ("Onde l'altro lebbroso") that they are both lepers, at least moral lepers to Dante.

The attitude of medieval and Renaissance writers and artists to leprosy can be traced to ideas promulgated in the early Middle Ages, which in turn can be traced back to Old Testament sources. Typical of these is the comment by Rabanus Maurus (780–856), Archbishop of Mainz, who wrote that "sickness is a disease caused by vice. . . . Fever is a fleshly desire burning insatiably. . . . Swelling leprosy is puffed-up pride. . . . He has scabs on his body whose mind is ruined by the lusts of the flesh."[10] Three centuries later, Richard of St. Victor (d. 1173), the great theologian of the century preceding Aquinas, wrote:

> Omnes enim immundi fornicarii, concubinarii, incestuosi, adulteri, avari, feneratores, falsi testes, perjuri, qui etiam dicunt fratri, fatue, et qui vidunt mulierum ad concupiscendam eam, etso non opere, tamen mali sunt voluntate, inquam . . . judicantur esse leprosi.[11]

> (In fact all filthy fornicators, concubines, the incestuous, adulterers, the avaricious, usurers, false witnesses, perjurers, those who call a brother fool, and who look upon a woman with lust in their hearts, who though not evil in deed are wicked in inclination: all these, I say . . . are judged to be leprous.)

A few years later, Maurice of Sully (d. 1195), the redoubtable Bishop of Paris, took the passage almost verbatim for one of his famous homilies: "Le lepre signifie les granz pechez dampnables, si cum est fornicacions, avoutire, usure, roberie, laroncine, glotonie, ivresce, fausetez, tricherie, homocide, clamer son prosme fou ou musart . . . esgarder femme pur lie coveiter."[12] Rabanus Maurus' reasoning is not far removed from doctrines of twentieth-century Christian Science that equate sin with "error," and disease its consequence. One is reminded, perhaps irreverently, of the dialogue between master and schoolboy.

"Are you troubled by impure thoughts?" To which the schoolboy replies, "Why no, I rather enjoy them."

In keeping with theological ideas about leprosy, medieval artists depicted the disease typologically. They presented a formalized, even a universal, image of leprosy rather than a picture of an individual suffering from it, and there was certainly no intention to produce a clinically accurate likeness. Lepers were to be avoided, and it is unlikely that any medieval illuminator stayed near one long enough to look closely at him. Precisely when the artistic tradition and the conventions associ-

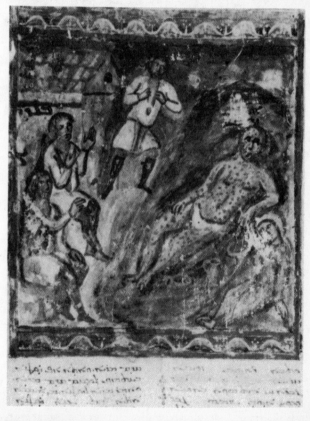

Figure 6.11. Job and his comforters. Syriac bible, seventh century. Paris: Bibliothèque Nationale.

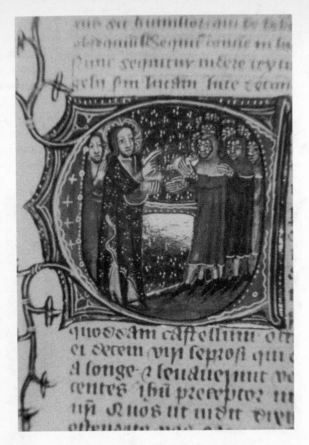

Figure 6.12. Christ healing ten lepers. English, ca. 1397. Oxford: Bodleian Library MS. Laud Misc. 165, fol. 363.

ated with it began is not certain, a process lost in the mists of antiquity, but a seventh-century Syriac bible in the Bibliothèque Nationale contains an illumination showing Job and his comforters. Job is reclining, nude except for a loincloth, and his entire body is covered with symmetrically distributed bright reddish-orange spots (fig. 6.11) to indicate he is covered with boils. Analyzing the transition from roll to codex, Kurt Weitzmann develops the idea that for the scenes with which they embellished their texts, medieval artists sought simple standardized representations available from model books in the studio.[13] The use of red spots to depict the lesions of leprosy continued for several centuries. In general, the spots used for Job's boils were a bit larger than those used to denote leprosy, but exceptions exist. Attempts to portray the leonine facies of nodular leprosy, as in an English commentary of about 1397 showing Christ healing ten lepers (fig. 6.12), were a great rarity. For the most part artists relied on the tried but untrue formula, as the less imaginative treatment of Christ healing the single leper in the same 1397 Gospel indicates (fig. 6.13).

The artist's problem was to compose and execute a scene in which

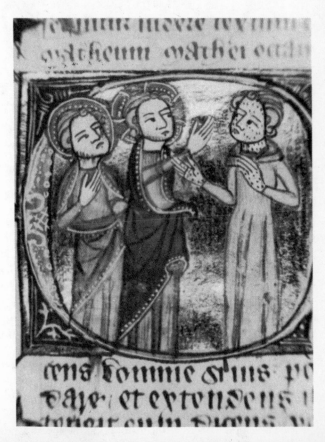

Figure 6.13. Christ healing a leper. English, ca. 1397. Oxford: Bodleian Library MS. Laud Misc. 165, fol. 186.

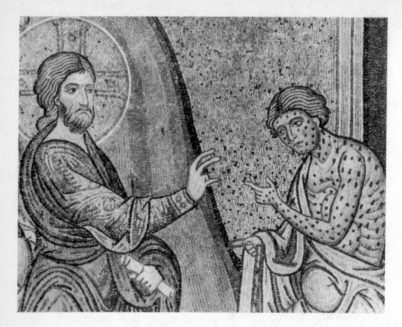

Figure 6.14. Christ healing a leper. Norman Sicilian, twelfth century. Mosaic from Monreale Cathedral, near Palermo. Courtesy of the Wellcome Trustees.

the leper would be plainly identifiable at a glance, and the "red spot" convention was uniformly observed in Western Europe from the ninth through the fifteenth centuries. In a late manuscript of Bishop Theodoric's *Cyrurgia* (1498/99) we see a leper with his clapper; the disease is denoted by small red spots on his face. Theodoric's original text dates from 1266; whether this was deliberate archaism or mere persistence of an antique style is not certain; perhaps it was an artist's tribute to an authority over two centuries removed. That the use of an immediately recognizable convention would make communication direct and simple is self-evident when we look at a mosaic high above eye level in the twelfth-century Norman cathedral at Monreale near Palermo, executed in a modified Byzantine style with one tessera equal to one leprous nodule (fig. 6.14). But a twentieth-century observer may question why the convention persisted in manuscripts designed for close reading by a more literate audience for whom more precise depiction might be meaningful. One reply might be that the medieval readership was not particularly interested in leprosy as a disease or in lepers as individuals.

A few medieval manuscripts exhibit the beginning of sequential narrative technique. The ninth-century *Sacra parallela* of John of Damascus, probably executed in Palestine under the Abassid Caliphate and now in the Bibliothèque Nationale, tells the story of Naaman in four vignettes, each depicting a different episode. Examples of the two-part sequence are common in the Rhineland school that flourished from the ninth through twelfth centuries.[14] The earliest example is from a ninth-

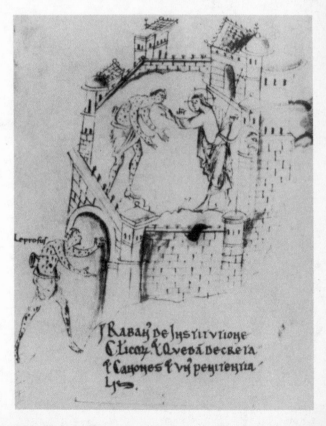

Figure 6.15. Christ healing a leper. Rhineland, latter half of the ninth century. Gospel from Essen Abbey, originally from Coblenz (Monastery of St. Florinus?). Dusseldorf: Landesbildstelle Rheinland MS. Cod. B, 113, fol. 5r.

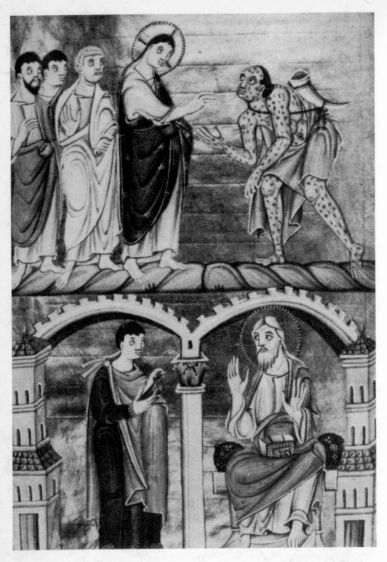

Figure 6.16. Christ healing a leper (*upper panel*) and the leper giving thanks (*lower panel*). German, ca. 1000. Evangelarium of Otto III. Munich: Staatsbibliothek MS. Lat. 4453, fol. 97v.

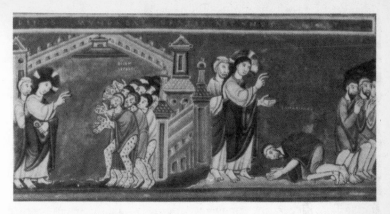

Figure 6.17. Christ healing ten lepers, only one of whom returns to thank him. German, 1020–30. Echternach Gospel. Nuremberg: Germanisches National-museum MS. 156142, fol. 55.

century Gospel probably executed at Coblenz, now in Düsseldorf, showing the spotted leper entering the gate of Christ's castle, then in the forecourt receiving Christ's blessing (fig. 6.15). More sophisticated than the line drawing of that vignette is an illumination from the Evan-gelarium of Otto III executed circa 1000 at Reichenau, now at Munich. The upper panel shows the leper clad in rags, wearing his horn and covered with spots from head to foot as he receives Christ's blessing; the lower panel shows him cured of his cutaneous lesions, now in new raiment, making a thank offering of two doves to God (fig. 6.16). It is one of the most striking "before and after" pictures of the epoch. Al-most equally attractive, though not formally divided, is the Echternach Gospel version of Christ healing ten lepers, an early eleventh-century illumination, now at Nuremberg, in which the lepers' spots are slightly larger than average for the period (fig. 6.17). The same technique was used to paint the skin lesions of Lazarus at the rich man's door in that Gospel. Though the scriptures distinguished between *tzara'ath* and *avabua,* the eleventh-century illuminator did not.

Legends of Christ's healing mission were popular with medieval il-luminators because their message was direct and lent itself to a design within a small compass as well as in a variety of media. The gold relief binding of the *Codex aureus* of St. Emeran from Regensburg (Baye-rische Staatsbibliothek Lat. 14000) shows Christ in the center flanked by two apostles on one side and a leper receiving his blessing on the other side. The leper's spots are shown in raised relief. A different technique was usually used for ivory; a ninth-century Carolingian carving of the scene shows the leper's spots as depressed, carved out of the material. An illuminator's imagination occasionally outran the text; the depiction of a leper being cured by the emperor Tiberius' worshipping Christ (Bodleian MS. Canon Ital. 280, fol. 218) is unhistorical and uncanonical.

An occasional icon indicates that Christ's healing skills were thought to be passed on to his disciples. The lower range of figures in a silver-gilt altar frontal (ca. 1300) in the treasury of the Basilica San Marco at Venice shows fifteen scenes from the saint's life, one of which shows him healing a leper. The arrangement of the two figures resembles that of Christ and the leper; the stigmata of the disease are indicated by rounded punch marks on the exposed surfaces of the arms and legs.

Two special legends require separate mention: those of the emperor Constantine and of St. Thomas Becket. Constantine's leprosy is seen in a fresco in the Church of the Santi Quattro Coronati in Rome (fig. 6.18).

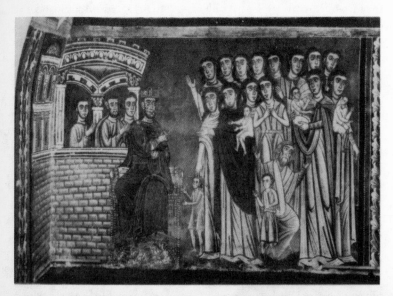

Figure 6.18. The emperor Constantine stricken with leprosy. Italian, thirteenth century. Fresco from Chiesa di Santi Quattro Coronati, Rome. Photo Alinari.

The present thirteenth-century church replaces one erected soon after Constantine's conversion to Christianity in the fourth century. The frescos in the chapel of St. Sylvester date from circa 1248 and are an example of the late Italo-Byzantine style that immediately preceded the Giottesque revolution. Among the miracles credited to that saint is his cure of Constantine's leprosy, in gratitude for which the emperor converted. The painting shows him seated on a throne before his castle giving audience to a group of sorrowful women accompanied by a few children. His leprosy is indicated by the conventional red spots. The women are indeed sorrowful, for they have heard that they and their children are to be sacrificed on the advice of non-Christian physicians so that the emperor will be cured—the primitive notion of cure by spilling blood.

However, there is no fourth-century evidence that Constantine ever had leprosy; on the contrary, he seems to have been vigorous and healthy to the end of his reign. The legend that he contracted leprosy and was cured by St. Sylvester seems to have arisen some time after the tenth or eleventh century, and his conversion to Christianity seems to have been prompted by political expediency, the need for imperial unity, which in turn required religious unity. The Christians, whose numbers had increased steadily over three centuries, formed the most unified sect in the heterogeneous, polyglot territories that made up the fourth-century Roman empire. As Penniman points out, "The union of Church and State made heresy and civil dissension the same. Freedom of thought was dead." [15] For that reason the legend of Uzziah was not popular in later centuries, hence its sparse iconographic representation. Like the famous forged decretals upon which the Church based its claim to temporal authority, Constantine's spurious leprosy was a necessary fiction for the medieval church. However, the first hospital for the care of lepers was founded circa 320 at Rome during Constantine's reign, and St. Basil established a leper colony at Caesarea in 372. Illustrations of Constantine's legend were not confined to Rome. A fifteenth-century English manuscript of John Gower's *The Lover's Complaint* shows children being brought to Constantine to cure him with their blood (Bodleian MS. New College 26, fol. 53).

St. Thomas Becket was martyred in 1170 at Canterbury, where a leper colony had been in existence since 1096, and he surely must be accounted a victim of the conflict between church and state. The famous "miracle windows" at the east end of the choir at Canterbury

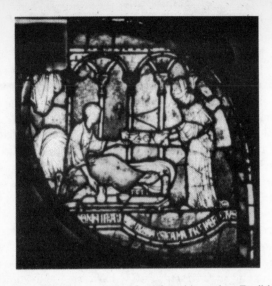

Figure 6.19. Richard Sunieve receiving food from his mother. English, ca. 1220. Stained glass from Canterbury Cathedral. From Canterbury Cathedral Chronicle, no. 28, October 1937, pp. 4–8. Courtesy of the Dean and Chapter of Canterbury Cathedral.

Cathedral date from about 1220, by which time the martyred archbishop's tomb had become a place of pilgrimage. One set of roundels tells the story of Richard Sunieve, a herdsman, who contracted leprosy by sleeping outdoors. His history was written by the monks William and Benedict, who relate his eight years of suffering while the disease spread so that his entire body was covered with purulent, putrefying ulcers. He became so loathsome that only his mother could approach him, bringing him food placed at the end of a long-handled shovel-like tray (fig. 6.19). Finally, he made a pilgrimage to Canterbury, where he kissed St. Thomas' tomb, prayed, and drank the water given to supplicants for healing. Some of his subcutaneous abscesses burst, discharged their matter, and resolved; other lesions merely disappeared, leaving his skin dry and wrinkled, but his skin became clear in a matter of hours. C. H. Talbot's comments bear repetition for readers in a skeptical age:

> Whatever one may think of this story, one cannot doubt the sincerity and conviction of those who recorded it both in words and glass. The impression made on the herdsman's contemporaries

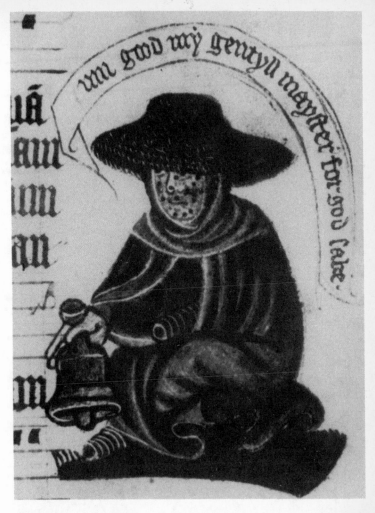

Figure 6.20. Leper begging alms. English, late fourteenth century. British Museum MS. Lansdowne 451, fol. 127. Courtesy of the Trustees of the British Museum.

must have been great for them to record the cure for all posterity to see, and though they may have been misled about the nature of the malady and the ability of the medical profession to cure it, they could not have been so utterly mistaken about the sudden change in the patient's condition.[16]

Before returning to the Continent from England, one ought not overlook the poignant illustration in the Exeter Pontifical, a late-fourteenth-century English illumination of a leper begging alms (fig. 6.20). He is swathed in protective garments; only his face is exposed. The familiar red spots are diagnostic, and he carries a bell-shaped clapper in his right hand while his left forearm is heavily bandaged, the left hand missing, presumably amputated. The isolated figure of the forlorn outcast has more emotional valence than any number of depictions that

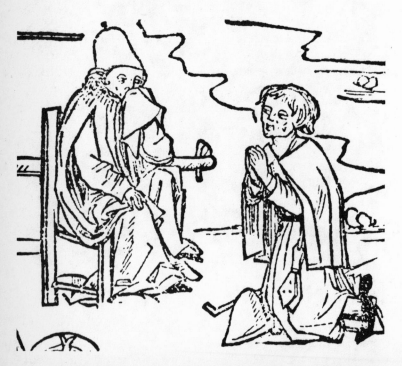

Figure 6.21. Leper confessing to a priest. Detail from the Nuremberg broadside. German, 1493. Woodcut.

show a leper among other sufferers or being cured among a crowd of onlookers. Previous depictions of leprosy were designed to show Christ's mercy. For the first time we see an icon that says, "Here is a leper. Take pity!" It is matched only by a late-fifteenth-century German woodcut showing a leper in rags, identifiable only by his clapper and a single spot on his face, confessing to a priest who has covered his mouth with a handkerchief lest he contract the disease by inhalation (fig. 6.21).

In medieval illuminations anonymous artists depicted anonymous lepers, but with the Renaissance maxim that man was the measure of all things, artists whose names are familiar began to portray lepers as individual human sufferers. With the change of style came a change of heart. But as usual, one must approach specific works of art with caution. A sequence of frescos in the Spanish chapel of S. Maria Novella at Florence shows an assortment of the lame, the halt, and the blind appealing to St. Dominic for relief. (He died in 1221 and was canonized in 1234; construction of the church began in 1278. The frescos date from 1355 and are generally ascribed to Andrea di Firenze.) One badly crippled figure in the foreground has traditionally been categorized as a leper, but the stigmata of the disease are not clearly painted, and the artist's intentions remain unknown. Likewise, Masaccio's frescos in the Church of S. Maria del Carmine on the south side of the Arno, executed over half a century later, show as one of St. Peter's miracles his healing of a cripple who exhibits none of the obvious lesions of leprosy, though reproductions of that painting often assert that diagnosis. Also in a doubtful category is a painting by Niklaus Manuel Deutsch in Basel.

That Italian Renaissance artists painted lepers as human sufferers does not imply that the subject was a popular one. Illuminations in medieval manuscripts far outnumber Renaissance frescos, and easel paintings of leprosy are almost nonexistent. With few exceptions, patrons who commissioned paintings for churches and monasteries had little desire to see leprosy displayed *coram publico,* nor would a king, prince, cardinal, duke, or wealthy merchant choose to hang such a subject in a public room of his castello. Bol's painting of Elisha refusing Naaman's gift was an exception, but it was commissioned for a leper house where the subject was appropriate. Even there the leper has no spots; in fact, he is not in the picture. (We have no record to indicate the purpose for which Englebrechtsz' painting was executed.) Leprosy was a loathsome disease, only slightly less terrifying than bubonic plague. Few Renaissance artists took a close look at a leper, and fewer still may have sketched one as a note for potential commission. Not even Leonardo da Vinci's voluminous notebooks contain drawings of cutaneous lesions or disfigured limbs, yet he was not repelled by organs dissected at autopsy. Conversely, Renaissance artists had no qualms about portraying martyrdom by any number of gruesome means—St. Sebastian well flèched, St. Lawrence grilled, St. Bartholomew flayed, St. Lucy's eyes plucked out, St. Agatha's breast cut off with a hot iron, and any number beheaded. Sadism, particularly when related to religion or the remote past, was acceptable, but the current ills of the flesh, by and large, were not. Except under special circumstances, leprosy and lepers had little audience appeal.

One exception to the general rule of taste followed in the wake of the Black Death that ravaged Tuscany as well as most of Western Europe in 1348–49. Millard Meiss has described in detail the profound effect of that epidemic on Tuscan artists as well as on religious outlook and the general attitude toward life.[17] It is difficult to imagine the effect of the sudden death of 30 percent of the population of a prosperous, productive society; anxiety, guilt, and consciousness of the fragility of human life were the inevitable sequelae. It was fitting that large frescos treating the Triumph of Death were painted for the churches and burying grounds that had to be expanded to accommodate the plague's victims. Only fragments remain at S. Croce at Florence of Orcagna's treatment of the theme, but Francesco Traini's coeval fresco (ca. 1350) was preserved at the Camposanto at Pisa until it was almost destroyed by an Allied artillery barrage in 1944. The surviving portions were taken to the Museo Nazionale for safekeeping, and studies there after World War II succeeded in establishing its proper attribution. (For almost four centuries it had been attributed to Orcagna on Vasari's authority, but Vasari lived two centuries later and was probably misled by the similarity in morphographic detail between Orcagna's work at Florence, which was then intact, and the one at Pisa, with which he was less familiar.) The frescos are now housed in a separate building near the Camposanto and are being restored.

Much of Traini's elaborate working of the narrative is devoted to scenes showing the tragedies wrought by bubonic plague. Frequently reproduced is the group of three young noblemen out hunting with falcons and dogs who come upon three coffins, each with a corpse in

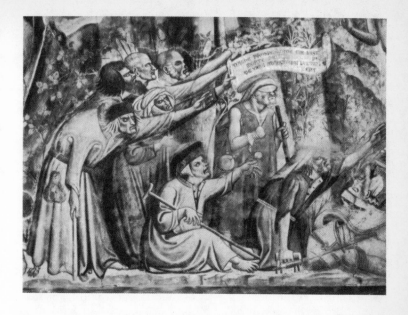

Figure 6.22. Detail from *Il trionfo della morte*. Francesco Traini, ca. 1355. Fresco from Camposanto, Pisa. Photo Anderson.

various stages of decomposition. An anchorite hermit stands opposite them at the head of the coffins, holding a scroll reminding them of the vanity of life and the ubiquity of death. In addition to dealing with the plague, Traini shows a group of eight figures in the lower central foreground (fig. 6.22) composed of cripples and lepers, the latter identifiable by amputations, blindness, saddle noses, and other deformities. The medieval red spots are absent. Traini shows their anger and despair as well as their physical damage. The scroll flaunted by one leper reads:

> Dache prosperitade cia las [ati] Morte medicina [d'ogni] pena
> De vieni a darci omai l'ultima cena
>
> (Since prosperity has abandoned us, Death, medicine for every pain, Come and gives us now the Last Supper.)

The text was inspired by the "Triumphs" by Petrarch, and its literary antecedents have been examined in detail by Morpurgo.[18]

Little purpose would be served by an encyclopedic census of lepers in representations of the Triumph of Death and other Italian Renaissance paintings. The pepper-pot sprinkle of red spots all but disappeared from the painter's vocabulary during the fourteenth century, surviving only in manuscripts and works deliberately based on medieval models. From mid-fourteenth-century Tuscany to late-fifteenth-century Rome is four generations, a giant leap in art history, but the next significant step in the iconography of leprosy is found in the Sistine Chapel, so named for the della Rovere pope who ordered it built. Late in 1481 and early in 1482, Giovanni dei Dolci, *superstans operibus* (master of works), signed contracts with such famous artists as Perugino, Botticelli, and Ghirlandaio to paint frescos on the side walls. They were assisted by others whose names are only slightly less familiar: Pinturrichio, Piero di Cosimo, Luca Signorelli, and Cosimo Rosselli. The project was executed speedily, and Sixtus IV consecrated the chapel in 1483. (Michelangelo's ceiling was not added until 1508–12, when Sixtus' nephew Julius II was pope, and his apsidal Last Judgment, commissioned by Clement VII [Giulio de Medici], was not completed until 1541 during the papacy of Paul III [Alessandro Farnese].)

The plan for the frescos called for an equal number of scenes from the life of Moses and the life of Christ in more or less parallel passages. Among them are Cosimo Rosselli's (1439–1507) conflation of the Sermon on the Mount with Christ Healing the Leper, the sequence as set forth in Matthew 5–8, and Botticelli's conflation of the Purification of the Leper with scenes showing the Temptations of Christ, two unrelated subjects, though a vague parallel might be drawn between Moses' trials and Christ's temptations before each received his divine ministry. Scenes from the life of Moses were not frequent in the canon of Renaissance painting, and Sixtus IV's choice of the contrapuntal juxtaposition of Moses and Jesus in the fresco cycle reflects his conception of the trinitarian role of the pope as priest, ruler, and lawgiver.

Rosselli's fresco presents a conventional treatment (fig. 6.23). Christ delivers the sermon from a small hillock and stands set apart from carefully arranged groupings of the members of his audience. Behind him on the left is a formulaic landscape including a small town rising from a river's edge. In the foreground a child plays with a lamb, the symbols of innocence and peace. The lower right quarter is given over to Christ healing the leper. Surrounded by a semicircle of his followers, Christ stands close to, but not touching, the kneeling leper, his right hand raised in blessing, his left extended in fellowship. The leper's disease is shown by fairly large, brownish macules and papules distributed dif-

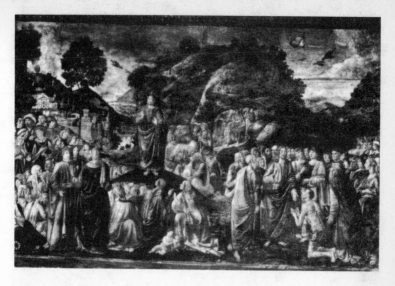

Figure 6.23. The Sermon on the Mount and Christ Healing the Leper. Cosimo Rosselli, 1482. Fresco from the Sistine Chapel, Vatican City. Photo Alinari.

fusely and symmetrically over his trunk, arms, and legs (fig. 6.24). The lesions are darker in the center than at their periphery and suggest more than would a superficial spot of paint. One senses that Rosselli was trying to indicate deeper involvement of subcutaneous tissue, that is, nodules of leprosy. The scene with its many characters is relatively static, but it is easily comprehended from the floor level of the nave, its essential elements plainly visible to the upward gaze of the viewer who is separated from close inspection by about fifteen feet of intervening, graduated pews.

Botticelli's (1445–1510) fresco is complex and subtle, not readily appreciated from ground level. It is based on the rite of purifying the leper according to the directions set forth in Leviticus 14 (fig. 6.25). The scene, bustling with activity, takes place in front of a splendid Renaissance-style temple with Northern Renaissance touches in the upper-story windows. Its facade is modeled after that of the Ospedale de Santo Spirito, founded a few years previously by Sixtus IV to provide care for the sick poor of Rome. (That facade is no longer extant, having been sacrificed for newer additions, but old engravings establish

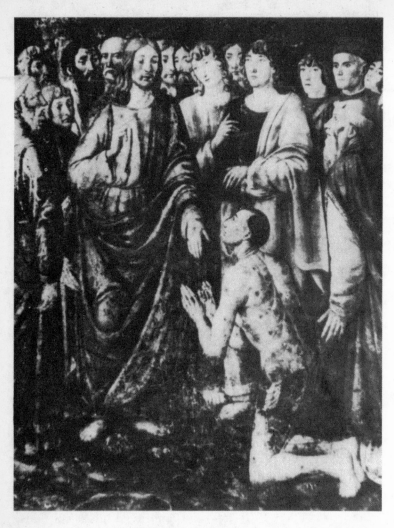

Figure 6.24. Detail of fig. 6.23 showing the leper receiving Christ's blessing. Cosimo Rosselli. Photo Alinari.

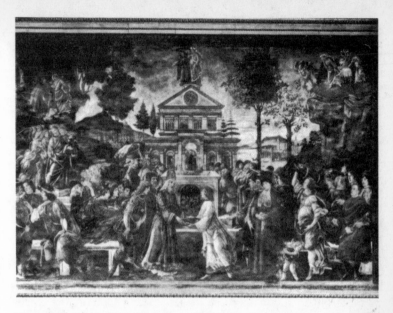

Figure 6.25. Purification of the Leper. Allessandro Botticelli, 1482. Fresco from Sistine Chapel, Vatican City. Photo Alinari.

the resemblance.) One of Botticelli's intentions was to relate the ancient ritual to recent events. In front of the "temple" stands a large altar in which the required cedarwood is being burned in a cauldron suspended over a blazing fire. The fragrant smoke was supposed to purify the air tainted by the leper's breath. A grateful throng surrounds the altar, some of the individuals kneeling (not a Hebrew posture), while a woman, presumably the wife of the healed leper, carries two fowl in a covered basket and is making her way to the running water in the right central background. Mosaic law prescribed that one of these birds be sacrificed and its blood collected, the other see free. In the foreground stands the high priest, who is being handed a golden bowl by a young priest or acolyte; perhaps the high priest suggests the patriarchal Moses and the young priest Christ, who is to follow as lawgiver. The interaction between them represents the directions in Leviticus 14:5–7:

> And the priest shall command that one of the birds be killed in an earthen vessel over running water. As for the living bird, he shall take it and the cedar wood, and the scarlet, and the hyssop,

and shall dip them and the living bird in the blood of the bird
that was killed over the running water. And he shall sprinkle
upon him that is to be cleansed from the leprosy seven times, and
shall pronounce him clean, and shall let loose the living bird into
the open field.

We do not actually see the bird being killed, but we may infer that its
blood is in the bowl. The high priest is actually dipping a bunch of
myrtle (*Vinca*) tied with scarlet thread into the bowl so he may later
sprinkle the cured leper with blood a magical seven times (cf. the number of times Elisha told Naaman to dunk himself in the river Jordan).
Myrtle had replaced hyssop in the customs of the Church for reasons
that are not entirely elucidated. Belief in the therapeutic powers of
freshly shed blood did not originate with the Hebrews but was common to many ancient religions.

The Israelites were less concerned with *tzara'ath* as a disease than as
an emblem of ritual uncleanliness; consider, for example, an illumination in a thirteenth-century French *Bible moralisée* in which Moses and
Aaron forbid a leper to approach the tabernacle (Bodleian MS. 270b.
fol. 63v D1). The ritual Botticelli painted carried only minor therapeutic implications; the emphasis is on purification after the disease had
been cured. It goes without saying that true leprosy was not curable or
cured in biblical times, but psoriasis, eczema, and other dermatoses
overdiagnosed as leprosy did remit, and it was for victims of such diseases that the ritual was carried out.

Botticelli's blending of an Old Testament rite with the contemporary
state of the Church takes account of Sixtus IV's origins in the Francis-
can order, hence his interest in leprosy as the archetypal disease cured by
faith. Giuliano della Rovere, the pope's nephew, later Julius II, appears
in the painting, just to the right of the central scene, standing with
crossed hands and carrying a white cloth. Girolamo Riario, then the
gonfaloniere, stands in the lower right corner with his gold-mounted
wand of office, and it has been claimed that the other figures, no longer
identifiable, are members of the Confraternity of the Santo Spirito
which Sixtus IV had founded to maintain his hospital after it was built.
It was a gracious way in which to commemorate the charitable works
of the pontiff who had commissioned the erection of the chapel and its
decoration.

But we seem to have lost sight of the leper who occasioned all this
ritual and the iconography peripheral to it. He is there in the crowd,

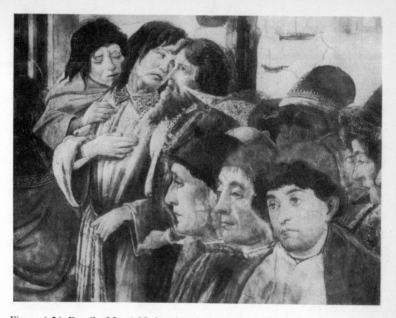

Figure 6.26. Detail of fig. 6.25 showing the leper being escorted to the altar. Alessandro Botticelli. Photo Alinari.

approaching the altar hesitantly from the right. Supported by two friends, he has just mounted the first step leading to the altar where he is soon to be sprinkled with the blood of a fowl and purified (fig. 6.26). His drawn mouth and wan countenance suggest his having passed through a recent illness. The friend on his right side seems a bit incredulous and is moving the leper's shirtwaist aside to convince himself that the lesions have actually disappeared. There are no skin lesions; Botticelli suggests the nature of the disease by showing that the terminal phalanges of the digits on his left hand have been amputated. (Such an even distribution of amputated phalanges on one hand only is not clinically plausible.)

Ettlinger has called attention to parallels between the Sistine Chapel frescos and a sermon preached on All Saints' Day, 1482, by the Spanish Cardinal Bernardino Carvajal, who was *cameriere d'onore* to Sixtus IV.[19] He compared Moses' lawgiving on Mount Sinai with Christ's lawgiving in the Sermon on the Mount, and his theological outlook has much in common with the imagery of the paintings: "[P]assages in his sermon suggest that he knew the two frescos in question, which by November 1482 would have been completed. It is impossible to say, however, whether the preacher alluded to pictures commissioned by the Pope, or whether he himself had been involved in planning them." It is difficult to judge to what extent theological subtleties influenced Botticelli, but one suspects that at that stage of his development he was more concerned with the niceties of painting than with postscholastic exegesis.

Two later Renaissance works require mention. A brush drawing by Parmigianino (1503–40) in the Devonshire Collection at Chatsworth of Christ healing ten lepers (ca. 1530) is a bold Mannerist treatment dramatically contrasting opposed masses of figures, using much swirling drapery to create the illusion of movement in the postures of Christ, his apostles, and the lepers. The only evidence of leprosy is seen on the gray-haired man in the foreground whose back is half turned from the viewer; he has a single leprous spot over his right scapula and another on his upper arm. A rather formal painting in the Galleria Sabauda at Turin by Bernart van Orley (1492?–1541), a Flemish painter strongly influenced by the Italian style, shows a French king being consecrated and healing the sick, one of whom is traditionally supposed to be a leper. He shows no cutaneous lesions or amputations, but he is on crutches, carries a beggar's bowl, wears ragged clothing, and has a badly damaged left leg. It is not a convincing image of a leper, and one hesitates to admit it to the canon.

The development of woodblock printing during the latter half of the fifteenth century provided artists with a new medium. An edition of the *Regimen sanitatis* published at Ulm in 1482 contains a woodcut of two physicians examining a leper (fig. 6.27). It is a completely secular picture with no hint of religious atmosphere. For the first time in a published book we see another human being actually touching a leper; by chronological irony it appeared in precisely the same year Rosselli and Botticelli were celebrating Christ and Moses, neither of whom is shown laying on hands. The patient is flanked by two physicians in long gowns, the one on the right with his hand upon the patient's chest, the other with the uroscopy flask. The patient's body is free of stigmata of leprosy; the diagnosis is established by the location of the woodblock print in the text. A little-known early-thirteenth-century manuscript catalogued as *Medica* (Trinity College MS. 0.1.20) gives an even better portrayal of a physician examining and actually touching a

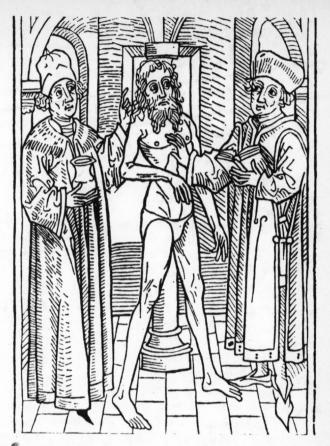

Figure 6.27. Two physicians examining a leper. German, 1482. Woodcut from *Regimen sanitatis*. Ulm: Conard Dinckmut, 1482.

leper (fig. 6.28). The disease is denoted by the punctate spots on the patient's face; the physician is holding the head still with his left hand and examining the skin lesions with an instrument held in his right hand. It is too much to ask that the physician is scraping the skin lesions to demonstrate bacilli, but perhaps he is trying to see whether the lesions are actually scaling. A more realistic portrayal is found a generation later in von Gersdorff's *Feldtbuch der Wundtarztney* (1517) showing leprosy diagnosed by a committee (fig. 6.29). Making due allowance for the limitations of the woodcut medium, one perceives the skin

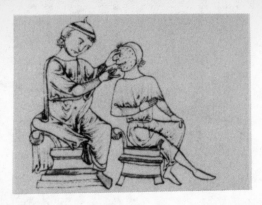

Figure 6.28. A physician examining a leper. Marginal sketch in an early-thirteenth-century manuscript. Cambridge: Trinity College, Cambridge MS. 0.1.20, fol. 262a. Reproduced by permission of The Master and Fellows of Trinity College.

lesions as nodules, some of them perhaps ulcerated. The patient is being examined by a physician whose left hand masks a possible judgment with respect to a leonine facies. Again, another physician with the uroscopy flask is present, also an older man merely looking on, perhaps one of the town's elders. On the left a servant rinses a concave object, perhaps the patient's wig, in a basin.

Another woodblock print of the period is the popular Nuremberg broadside of 1493, which combines religious with secular motifs. In several vignettes it commemorates Maundy Thursday, the day set aside annually for opening the walled city to lepers. They are shown hearing Mass, receiving Holy Communion, confessing to a priest (fig. 6.21), and feasting at the expense of the city treasury. The medieval convention of depicting leprosy by randomly scattered spots persists as part of the woodcutters' idiom. A colored woodcut in the Lübeck Bible of 1494 shows victims of the sixth plague of Egypt covered with boils (*schechin*) (fig. 6.30). The apogee of this convention was reached by Hans Burgkmair (1473–1531), who executed a series of paintings of diverse saints on commission from Maximillian I. They are best known from the late-eighteenth-century engravings of the series. Grön comments that

> [o]f 199 paintings, no fewer than 12 provide some representation of leprosy [with] little artistic value . . . characterized by a boring

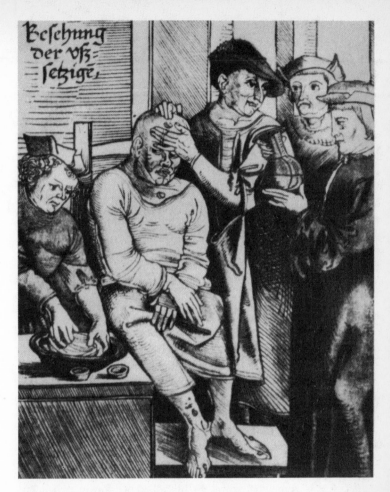

Figure 6.29. Leprosy being diagnosed by a committee. German, 1517. Woodcut from H. von Gersdorff, *Feldtbuch der Wundtarztney*. Strassburg: J. Schott, 1517.

schematism. . . . In them one sees small deformed cripples who are covered with spots and whose limbs are oddly twisted. His portraits of Edward the Confessor and Edmund, King of England, show both subjects distributing money. [St.] Thomas Becket . . . is shown in front of a sufferer from leprosy; St. Louis IX (King of France) nearing a table where many afflicted are eating; St.

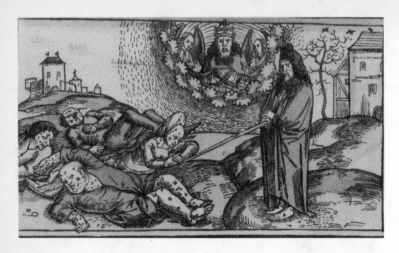

Figure 6.30. Egyptians smitten with boils, the sixth plague. German, 1491. Colored woodcut from the Lübeck Bible. Courtesy of Leonard J. Hansen, Englewood, N.J.

Adelaide (Queen of Italy) begging for such diseased; St. Adelard (Abbot of Corbia [where there was a leprosarium]) helping those with leprosy [fig. 6.31.]; St. Veronica as she refreshes a leprous woman by pouring water over her hands; St. Wandrille teaching a leprosy sufferer; St. Iduberge passing out alms; and St. Itte distributing money. The holy Abbess Sigualeine is shown bathing a person with leprosy while Saints Oda and Elizabeth are each shown as distributing food and drink to the sufferers.[20]

It is a tiresome catalogue of virtue unrelieved by Burgkmair's earnestness, made somewhat risible by his adherence to the archaic custom of making the saint (or hero) of his canvas conspicuously larger than the other figures, a device designed to emphasize his importance ("larger than life") but actually one that destroys any sense of verisimilitude by its disproportion (fig. 6.32).

Inclusion of St. Elizabeth of Hungary in Burgkmair's gallery was to be expected inasmuch as her manifold acts of charity were a frequent subject for sixteenth-century artists. Born the daughter of King Andreas of Hungary, she married Duke Louis of Thuringia, and in her short life (ca. 1207–31) managed to feed 900 paupers daily as well as minister personally to the sick, especially lepers. According to Grön, she even placed lepers in her husband's bed without his permission. After his death she joined the Third Order of St. Francis and built a hospice at Marburg. The Alte Pinakothek at Munich has two wings from a triptych of St. Sebastian painted by Hans Holbein the Elder in

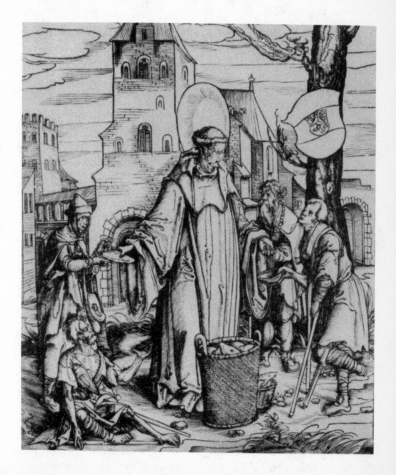

Figure 6.31. St. Adelard of Corbia ministering to cripples and lepers. Hans Burgk-mair, 1517. Woodcut.

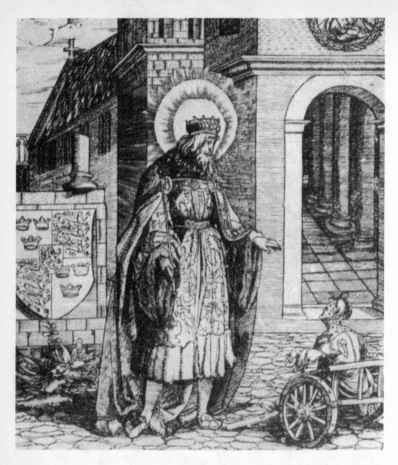

Figure 6.32. King Edward the Confessor giving alms to a leper. Hans Burgkmair, 1517. Woodcut. The royal coat of arms is one used by later kings of England.

1516 for the Church of St. Salvator in Augsburg. One panel shows St. Elizabeth holding a loaf of bread in her right hand, pouring wine from a ewer in her left hand into a bowl held by a beggar. Kneeling on her right is a leper with conspicuous spots on his forehead and a deformed facies. Even before that she had been depicted by Cologne artists, and her reputation extended as far south as Spain, where a large Murillo painting at El Hospital de Caridad at Seville shows her delousing a young person while another one scratches himself; a cripple and a leper are seated in the foreground. Murillo's usual sentimentality is modified by the natural poses of the afflicted, though he reserves the sickly sweet face of piety for St. Elizabeth herself. Most of these sixteenth-century paintings indicate leprosy by facial and skeletal deformities. Coarsened features simulate the leonine facies, though none actually achieves an accurate image. Cutaneous lesions are infrequent; unlike the woodcutters, the painters tended to avoid the obvious and "graphic." One caveat must be applied to the usual canon of the sixteenth-century leprosy paintings. The votive painting of St. Anne with Virgin and Child by Niklaus Manuel Deutsch (ca. 1484–1530) in the Kunstmuseum at Basel shows two sets of donors in the lower corners. Traditionally, the man in the lower left with crossed arms supported by a sling is supposed to be a leper because his left foot is deformed and some ill-defined lesions are present in the skin of his right arm. But the foot deformity is certainly nonspecific, and on close inspection what we are told is a skin lesion seems to be damage to the paint. St. Anne is flanked by St. Roche, who was called on in time of plague, and by St. James, who had general tutelary powers but was not especially associated with leprosy. In fact, at that time and even later, St. George was the patron saint of lepers. Precisely what Deutsch had in mind is not clear, but that he attempted to indicate leprosy as the disease St. Anne had or was supposed to have cured is dubious. The painting was executed circa 1517, coeval with Burgkmair's saints, Holbein's St. Elizabeth, and the illustrations for von Gersdorff's *Feldtbuch der Wundtarztney*.

Also painted in the same decade was Mathias Grünewald's famous Isenheimer altarpiece, now in the Unterlinden Museum at Colmar, probably begun in 1512, completed 1515–16. We have less biographical information about Grünewald (ca. 1460–1528) than any painter of comparable stature. Apart from the fact that the altarpiece was painted for the church of the Antonine Order at Isenheim and includes scenes from the life of St. Anthony, we can only surmise at the details that were meaningful at the time, either locally in Alsace or personally to Grünewald himself. The Antonine order was founded in 1093 by a French nobleman whose son had been cured of St. Anthony's fire (ergotism) by the intercession of that saint. The order became influential because of its good works, notably the establishment of hospitals. Treatment of patients with skin diseases was supposedly one of the specialties of the monks though inevitably they provided care for all manner of sufferers. Grünewald's altarpiece is a complex work with many

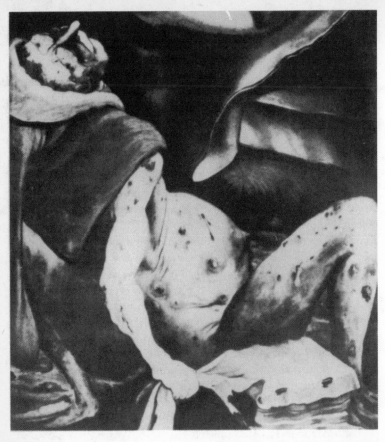

Figure 6.33. Detail from the Temptation of St. Anthony panel in the Isenheimer altarpiece showing a figure with ulcerated nodular skin lesions, etc. Mathias Grünewald, 1512–15. Colmar: Unterlinden Museum.

panels, the most famous of which is the Crucifixion. When the inner movable panels are opened, a panel usually called the Temptation of St. Anthony is revealed. It shows him beset by devils, demons, and beastly winged creatures. At the lower left corner of this panel is the sprawled figure of a man with nodular, ulcerated lesions distributed over his trunk and extremities and even involving the face, which is distorted by supraorbital thickening and a misshapen nose, consistent with the leonine facies of leprosy but also with foreshortening because of the perspective required by the figure's position (fig. 6.33).

Citing Charcot's opinion that the lesions represent tertiary syphilis and Richet's opinion that they represent nodular leprosy, J-K. Huysmans concludes that the lesions are supposed to represent ergotism, not so much because of clinical resemblance but because of the history and aims of the Antonine Order:

> And is this creature a larva or a man? Whatever it may be, one thing is certain: no painter has ever gone so far in the representation of putrefaction, nor does any medical textbook contain a more frightening illustration of skin disease. This bloated body, moulded in greasy white soap mottled with blue, and mamillated with boils and carbuncles, is the hosanna of gangrene, the song of triumph of decay!
>
> Was Grünewald's intention to depict a demon in its most despicable form? I think not. On careful examination the figure in question is seen to be a decomposing, suffering human being. And if it is recalled that this picture . . . comes from the Antonine Abbey at Isenheim, everything becomes clear. A brief account of the aims of this Order will, I think, suffice to explain the riddle.[21]

Even allowing for the hyperbole common to Huysmans' period in art history and analysis, not everything becomes clear. The lesions simply do not look like those of ergotism, which are usually confined to the extremities, especially fingers and toes, and result from ischemic gangrene. Secondary abscesses (imposthumes) could and did occur, but multiple ulcerated nodules did not. But none of the three diagnoses offered—ergotism, syphilis, or leprosy—can explain the distended abdomen and periumbilical cellulitis (phlegmon). Perhaps the solution to the enigma is "none of the above," a term borrowed from the jargon of psychometrics. Grünewald may not have had a specific skin disease in mind nor have been trying to depict a clinical entity; he was a painter, not a doctor. His aim may well have been to paint a figure with a disease so loathsome and disfiguring that even the least initiated observer would recognize it as emblem of the putrefaction Huysmans so rightly assigns it, an image designed to evoke terror and pity in the beholder. The figure is clearly that of a dying man whose gaze is heavenward, hence the inscription of a scrap of paper in the lower left corner directly opposite him: "Ubi eras, Jesu bone, ubi eras, quare non affuisti ut sanares vulnera mea?" (Where were you, good Jesus, where were you? Why did you not come to dress my sores?) It is an icon of *terribilitá* communicating the vulnerability of human flesh, the agony of dying, and the search for spiritual consolation. Perhaps we can also read it as an image of the incurable wound.

Can it be mere chronological coincidence that all these representations of lepers—the works of Grünewald, Holbein, Burgkmair, von Gersdorff's illustrator, and others—were produced in a five-year period from 1512 to 1517? Did a sudden outbreak of leprosy call the disease forcibly to artists' minds? Was some prominent public figure stricken with leprosy? There seems to be no record of a sudden increase of the disease in the Rhineland at the time, and one searches in vain for a social or biographicohistorical reason. McNeill comments that the incidence of leprosy in Europe declined steadily after the Black Death of 1348–49, perhaps because the reservoir of disease, lepers in their leprosaria, was all but wiped out by bubonic plague.[22] If this idea applies, the impact should have been felt and its repercussions seen in art a century earlier. Can one assign this high-water mark in the iconography of leprosy to a general climate of religious ferment, the background also for Luther's act of defiance in 1517? The notion is safely vague, but it is a feeble one. The relation of art and artists to society in the Rhineland in the early sixteenth century was quite different from that in Tuscany in the middle of the fourteenth century, and one must eschew the facile explanations that come to mind. The medieval notion of leprosy as a punishment for specific forms of sin had vanished.

As leprosy slowly waned in incidence and virulence, its interest for artists also declined, and with rare exceptions their emphasis was secular. The vogue for paintings and woodcuts of St. Elizabeth of Hungary can be explained as filling the need of a special cult. Rossigliani's engraving of Parmigianino's brush drawing was widely distributed, probably admired more for its dramatic artistry than anything to do with leprosy. Bruegel's painting of cripples (ca. 1568), now in the Louvre, shows four badly crippled men, one possibly achondroplastic, the others with amputations and deformities. Despite their facial peculiarities they have never been labeled lepers, and there is no ambiguity about them. A frequently reproduced engraving by Jan Visscher dated 1608 shows a group of lepers begging for alms. Skin lesions are not shown, but some have skeletal deformities from contractures; the leprous nature of their disease is denoted by a clapper in the hand of the first in line. Like the illustration in von Gersdoff's Feldtbuch, it shows leprosy as a disease in a social context, completely secular, far removed from any religious connotation.

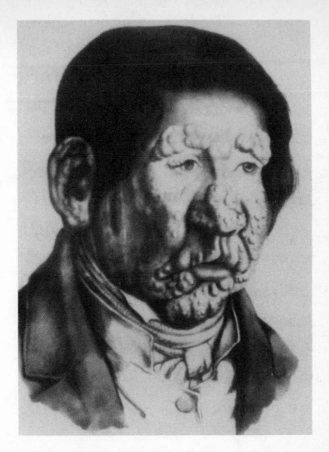

Figure 6.34. Chromolithograph of a man with the leonine facies of lepromatous leprosy. From D. C. Danielssen and C. W. Boeck, *Om spedalskhed,* vol. 2. Bergen: Gröndahl, 1847.

Gradually, the iconography of leprosy entered the "modern era." Richard's recent monograph reproduces drawings and paintings of lepers by a number of amateur artists in Scotland and Scandinavia dating from the end of the eighteenth century to the 1830s. They are individual portraits, varying in skill of execution, but all showing the clinical features of the disease with some fidelity, and certainly reflecting the "human interest" the lepers had for the unsophisticated artist. With the advent of lithography in the 1820s it was inevitable that the disease would soon be depicted as a disease, in icons of clinical accuracy. This

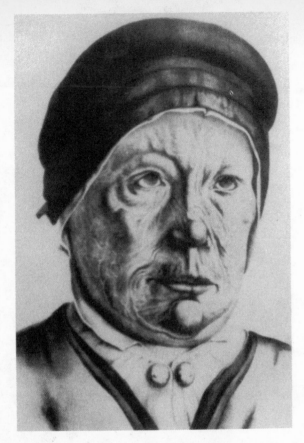

Figure 6.35. Chromolithograph of a woman with the saddle nose deformity of leprosy. The nasal septum has been destroyed. From Danielssen and Boeck, *Om spedalskhed*.

event took place in 1847 when Danielssen and Boeck published *Om spedalskhed,* the second volume of which was a set of chromolithographs drawn from life (figs. 6.34, 6.35).[24] The icons of leprosy became part of medicine, not part of art.

This essay began with an interrogative note in its title: "*Can the Leper Change His Spots?*" To this we can supply an affirmative: Yes, even to the vanishing point. To support the claim, there are two paintings of St. Francis of Assisi, the saint who more than anyone was concerned

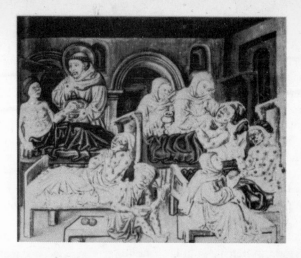

Figure 6.36. St. Francis in a lazarette. Italian, mid-fifteenth century. Gouache. Perugia: Biblioteca Municipale MS. 1238, ca. 233[4].

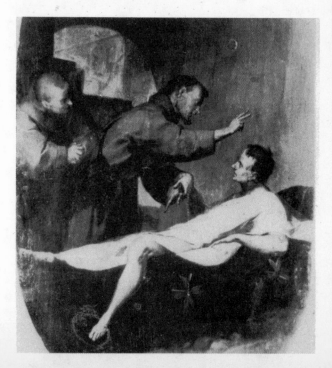

Figure 6.37. *St. Francis Healing the Leper.* Giovani Battista Crespi, detto Il Cerano, ca. 1610. Milan: Museo Civico, Castello Sforzesco.

with the care of lepers and who has been deliberately avoided up to this point. A mid-fifteenth-century gouache from a manuscript in the Biblioteca Municipale at Perugia (fig. 6.36) shows the saint and three of his monks ministering to the ills of half a dozen lepers whose bodies are covered with large ulcerating sores. The leper in the upper left has a saddle nose and a distorted facies. The leper in the lower right has small spots on his face and large spots on his chest and arms. The leper in the enter foreground holds his beggar's bowl and his clapper. The painting has been called the most terrifying late medieval image of leprosy. Certainly the skin lesions are the largest and most florid until Grünewald. The diagnosis is obvious. Contrast it with the seventeenth-century panel by Giovanni Battista Crespi (1572–1632) sometimes titled *St. Francis Healing the Leper,* now in the Museo Civico at Milan (fig. 6.37). It shows St. Francis in his monastic habit, accompanied by another monk, stretching out his hand to bless an emaciated man lying on a pallet, partly covered by a sheet. The patient has no deformity, no skin lesions; he is spotless, *immaculato*. If the cure is to be taken on faith, so is the diagnosis.

7
The Iconography
of Fanny Hill:
How to Illustrate
a Dirty Book

*I*n 1966 the United States Supreme Court reversed deci-
sions by lower courts and found that the G.P. Putnam's
Sons 1963 publication of John Cleland's *Memoirs of a Woman of Pleasure*
had sufficient redeeming social importance to qualify for protection
under the First Amendment. In short, it was no longer obscene, although in the etymological sense it remains pornography; it is a writing about whores. Because years of clandestine publication and the
vicissitudes of surreptitious typesetting had produced any number of
editions with corrupt texts, in 1985 both Oxford University Press and
Penguin Books, independently of each other, published critical *Urtext*
editions, each supervised by a qualified scholar in eighteenth-century
literature.[1] Each edition is equipped with a potted biography of Cleland, an introduction placing the novel among other fiction of the period, comments on the mores of the time, and a critical glossary to explain words now obsolete or whose meaning has changed. Like the
original edition of 1749 neither of these new editions contains any illustrations, but over the years many illustrated editions have appeared.
They vary in style, quality, selection of incident, and other features.
Like any depictions of a set piece, say the Last Supper, their variety is
contingent upon time and place, prevailing values and fashions in book
illustration, and, of course, the artist's skill. It is treatment, not subject
matter, that distinguishes a work of art, and some insights into the
creative process may be gained from examining the illustrations.

Little is to be gained by retelling the life history of John Cleland
(1709–89) except to note that he was educated at Westminster School,
served briefly as the British consul at Smyrna, worked in Bombay for
the East India Company, returned to England, where he could not earn

a living, and wound up in debtor's prison. He wrote *Memoirs of a Woman of Pleasure* while in prison and sold the manuscript for twenty pounds to Ralph Griffiths, better known as the publisher of the *Monthly Review*. Griffiths probably assumed the balance of Cleland's debts in addition. The book was advertised in November 1748 as "printed for G. Fenton in the Strand." Documents of the time refer to Fenton Griffiths, presumably Ralph's brother, but he remains a shadowy figure and may have been an invention. The novel was published in March 1749.

It is possible that the plot is based in part on a manuscript read at a meeting in 1737 of the Beggar's Benison Society, a Scottish sex club, of which Robert Cleland, a relative of the author, was a member.[2] Cleland claimed that the first part of the story was based on a plan "originally given me by a young gentleman . . . above eighteen years ago," and Peter Sabor identifies him as Charles Carmichael, a colleague of Cleland at Bombay.[3] But there is no doubt that the text of the 1749 edition was the product of Cleland's pen, and the second part is clearly his own invention. Cleland's purpose in writing was simply to get enough money to settle his debts and get out of prison. He pretended to no high literary aims, as did D. H. Lawrence for *Lady Chatterley's Lover* or James Joyce for *Ulysses*, nor can he be considered as anything more than a minor literary figure. His only other novel, *Memoirs of a Coxcomb*, is tedious, and his other publications disastrous. No special pleading can rebut the judgment that Cleland's intent was to whet his readers' prurience.

Yet the appeal to prurience does not vitiate *Fanny Hill*'s virtues as a novel. Its plot is well constructed, and incident follows incident logically and purposefully. It can be considered as the parable of the prodigal daughter who is finally redeemed by love. As the story unfolds, the characters of the central figures develop, and Cleland succeeds as few male novelists do in exploring female psychology. Though the action in most of the scenes is indelicate, Cleland clothes it in language that is euphemistic, even periphrastic; he never uses a coarse word or expression. As Sir Allen Lane, founder of Penguin Books, commented about the trial of his publication of *Lady Chatterley's Lover:* "Either I'll go to prison or I won't. I don't expect to. The only features of the book that anybody could possibly object to are the four-letter words, and there is not one of them that has not appeared in print in this country before."[4] There is more latitude in publishable vocabulary today than in Cleland's time, but his scrupulous avoidance of words that would give offense must be counted as one reason why it is not obscene. The only questionable item is the heroine's name. "Fanny" is a slang word denoting the female pudenda, and "Hill" alludes to the mons veneris. Charles Rembar points out that in one sense well-written pornography can be considered more dangerous to public morality than crudely written pornography.[5] He equates this with the notion that "the greater the truth, the greater the libel," adding that up to the eighteenth century truth was no defense against the charge of libel. Time has reversed that position, and by the same token a well-written account of explicit sexual behavior is no longer obscene. What commends *Fanny Hill* to the twentieth-century reader is that it is reasonably well written.

It is noteworthy that throughout the book's checkered career only two people have actually been convicted for publishing or selling it. Both Cleland and Griffiths, as well as Thomas Parker, who printed it, were haled before Lovel Stanhope, Law Clerk to the Secretary of State, and Cleland's letter to him is a model of special pleading.[6] It is much in the vein of the epigraph Griffiths lifted from Cleland's final paragraph and used on the title page of the 1750 edition, in which explicit descriptions of the sexual act were deleted: "If I have painted Vice in its gayest Colours, if I have deck'd it with Flowers, it has been solely in order to make the more worthier, the solemner Sacrifice of it to Virtue." To which a twentieth-century reader might inquire, whose tongue is in whose cheek? Lord Newcastle, the Secretary of State, referred the matter to the Attorney-General for prosecution, but there is no record that charges were brought. Soon after, Newcastle arranged an annual pension of £100 for Cleland as an inducement for him to write in the government's interest. However, in 1757 a London bookseller named Drybutter was sentenced to the pillory for selling the book.[7] Precisely which edition was involved is not known, but he was stated to have altered the language considerably for the worse. Whether the edition was illustrated or not also remains unknown. In 1821 at Boston, Peter Holmes was convicted and sent to prison for "publishing a lewd and obscene print contained in a book entitled *Memoirs of a Woman of Pleasure*"—and, almost as an afterthought, "for publishing the same book."[8] Whether Holmes had the book printed in Boston or imported copies from England is not certain, but the wording of the indictment leaves no doubt that it was illustrated.

For many years bibliographers disputed which was the first edition of the *Memoirs,* that is, which of several versions bearing the date 1749 was closet to Cleland's original intent. In 1885 Spencer Ashbee described an edition without place or date of publication that contained an account of an act of sodomy between two young men that Fanny witnesses at an inn when her coach breaks down en route to Hampton Court.[9] This edition bears the subtitle "from the Original Corrected Edition, etc." and cannot be the *editio princeps*. Several writers have claimed that the passage was inserted by Drybutter, but this hardly matches the charge of altering language. Moreover, Cleland carefully constructed the narrative to lead up to the incident, and the two paragraphs describing the act are thoroughly consistent with his style. David Foxon has identified a 1749 edition "printed for G. Fenton in the Strand" in the British Library (P.C. 27.a.44) as a copy of the first edition. It contains the detailed account of sodomy, and further identification is established by the woodcut ornaments.[10] Other copies are to be found at Yale, the Bibliothèque Nationale, and the Bayerische Staatsbibliothek at Munich. Perhaps the two paragraphs describing sodomy were deleted from later editions because at the time sodomy was a capital offense.

Cleland's novel is picaresque in form as incident is piled upon incident, and its heroine's development is a primitive form of *Bildungsroman*. It can be taken as the counterfoil to Richardson's *Pamela, or Virtue Rewarded* (1740–41). Cleland states the opposite case: promiscuity is also rewarded. From Richardson, as well as from Fielding's parody *Shamela* (1741), Cleland learned how to prepare a scene and develop it to its climax; it is a deliberate imitation, not an ironic parody. Unlike Richardson, Fielding, and Sterne, he does not "draw the curtain" on his amorous scenes; a novel of erotic realism perforce must follow Donne's maxim:

> Who does not the right true end of love propose
> Is one who goes to sea for nothing but to make him sick.

Fanny is not the first woman in literature to be portrayed as a willing, sexually accessible female after her libido has been quickened. Her illustrious predecessors include Tamar, Helen of Troy, Petronius' Quartilla and Tryphaena, even Moll Flanders (1722), and her successors include Emma Bovary, Constance Chatterley, and Molly Bloom, as well as any number of innocent maidens betrayed and suburban adulteresses of less distinguished fiction. But from Tamar and Helen we do not hear their *ipsissima verba,* and Quartilla tells us only that "he who carries the calf may well carry the bull." It is not until the eighteenth century that we hear from Polly Peachum in the *Beggars' Opera* (1728) why and how women respond to men, as she confesses to her mother that she has yielded to Macheath:

> But he so teased me
> And he so pleased me
> What I did you must have done.

The mood and motive for Cleland's novel is hedonism, and its moral is that sexual gratification is a worthy end in itself, though gratification plus love is even more satisfactory—scarcely a profound theme but one that has sufficed for more novels than one could bear to read. Not the least of Fanny's merits as a literary heroine is that Cleland presents her as a woman who is as willing to give pleasure as to receive it, a reciprocity of hedonism not commonly found in fiction before World War II. A simple change of sex is all that would be required for her to fit Auden's quatrain:

> Let us honor if we can
> The vertical man,
> Though we value none
> But the horizontal one.

With respect to the substance of any novel of erotic realism, the number of organs and orifices is finite, and the sexual menu is limited. Cleland was well aware of this, and at the beginning of the second part Fanny, using the epistolary-autobiographical mode, expresses the desire to avoid monotony and addresses the recipient of her letter:

> I imagined indeed, that you would have been cloy'd and tired
> with the uniformity of adventures and expressions, inseparable
> from a subject of this sort, whose bottom or ground-work being,
> in the nature of things, eternally one and the same, whatever vari-
> ety of forms and modes, the situations are susceptible of, there is
> no escaping a repetition of near the same images, the same fig-
> ures, the same expressions, with this further inconvenience added
> to the disgust it creates, that the words *joys, ardours, transports,
> extasies,* and the rest of those pathetic terms so congenial to, so
> received in the *practice of pleasure,* flatten, and lose much of their
> due spirit and energy, by the frequency they indispensibly recur

with, in a narrative of which that *practice* professedly composes the whole basis.[11]

Cleland's principal tropes are hyperbole and a specialized type of euphemistic-periphrastic metaphor applied to sexual organs and the sexual act. He carefully avoids the demotic words. Hyperbole is pornography's most characteristic idiom. The male sexual organs are always larger than average, sometimes larger than life; orgasms are more frequent and more intense than in one's wildest adolescent fantasies, and copulatory positions often require a degree of athleticism not to be found even in champion gymnasts. Considering that the readership of such literature is almost exclusively male, one speculates why such prodigies of nature do not produce feelings of inadequacy or inferiority in the common reader, but perhaps identification with the male protagonist and wish fulfillment overcome such responses. Cleland takes pains to provide an abundant variety of metaphors for the penis—e.g., "master member of the revels"—and for the vagina—e.g., "the soft laboratory of love." Sabor points out that "one of Cleland's favourite rhetorical strategies is matching metaphors for the sexual act with the occupations of Fanny's partners, . . . [e.g.] the sailor who 'seiz'd me as a prize,' 'fell directly on board me,' and 'drown'd in a deluge all my raging conflagrations of desire.'"[12]

Hyperbole and metaphor are of little value to the artist who engages to illustrate a text of this sort. If anatomic structures, particularly genital organs, are disproportionately exaggerated, the effect becomes caricature of the coarser variety. What the artist must aim for is anatomy that, to apply the vocabulary of the clinical laboratory, is at "the upper limit of normal." The purpose of illustrations to a work of fiction is to render visible, to reify, the action. The artist's imagination is controlled in large measure by the text; an illustrated version of *Le Morte d'Arthur* requires a knight in armor on horseback, not a London bobby, rescuing a damsel in distress. The artist has some latitude in selecting which incidents to depict, but his finished representation must bear a recognizable relationship to the writer's narrative. In the case of illustrations for a novel like *Fanny Hill*, the illustrations are designed to enhance the reader's response to the eroticism of the text, a visual embroidery upon its sexual ostinato. It is interesting to speculate whether the Putnam 1963 edition would have been declared not obscene had it been illustrated.

Patrick Kearney's *The Private Case* lists fifty editions of Fanny's *Memoirs* in the British Library, sixteen of which are illustrated.[13] No illustrated editions are catalogued in the Bodleian Library, the Cambridge University Library, the Widener Library at Harvard, or the Dartmouth College Library. Two illustrated editions purportedly in the New York Public Library cannot be located. Additional illustrated editions are located at the Library of Congress, Beinecke Library at Yale, Firestone Library at Princeton, and Olin Library at Cornell.[14] Editions indexed in the catalogues of several university libraries have disappeared. Through the courtesy of Dr. James Basker of Harvard University I have been allowed to examine a unique, otherwise uncatalogued edition published in England circa 1820. Inevitably, when one examines books labeled *curiosa,* it becomes evident that bibliographical information is unreliable because the publisher wishes to mislead the authorities. The classical example is *Poems on Several Occasions* by the Right Honourable E[arl] of R[ochester], which the title page assures us was published in Antwerp in 1680; no copy has ever been found in Flanders. Publishers of the eighteenth and nineteenth centuries were just as anxious to conceal the place and date of publication, and when it comes to the names of artists who supplied illustrations, anonymity is the rule. One cannot credit that an edition in French was printed "chez G. Fenton dans le Strand" in 1770 nor that a much truncated text in Italian, titled *La meretrice inglese,* was set in type at Parigi. Only in recent years, especially when the illustrations are less than explicit, does the publisher provide the artist's name. The ascription of specific sets of illustrations to Gravelot, to Elluin after designs by Borel, and to Paul Avril follow information given by Kearney which is generally accepted by connoisseurs and collectors of such books.[15]

The foregoing provides us with a census of twenty-two editions for analysis, but duplication of the illustrations reduces this number to eighteen. With one exception they can be divided into two groups: those that conscientiously depict the incidents in the text versus those in which the artist merely furnishes decorative vignettes of a quasi-erotic nature. The one exception is the Paris edition of 1933 with an introduction and bibliographical essay ascribed to Guillaume Apollinaire, then fifteen years dead. The publisher chose to illustrate the book with reproductions of Hogarth's *The Harlot's Progress* (1732), which have the safe advantage of being "of the period," topically related, and clearly not subject to a charge of obscenity. The decorative vignettes in the six editions in which the artist does not follow the text consist of a variety of affectionate or amorous poses in which the figures are more or less clothed, the sexual organs not exposed, only an occasional bared female bosom being visible or a wanton thigh displayed.

The first problem facing the illustrator is to select incidents or scenes from the narrative. Cleland's novel is shaped in the form of two long letters by Fanny Hill addressed to a "Madam" who does not appear in the tale. The first letter recounts how Fanny, from a small village near Liverpool, is orphaned at the age of fifteen. She leaves for London, where she presents herself at an "intelligence office" and is hired by Mrs. Brown, the madam of a house of ill fame. Mrs. Brown introduces Fanny to Phoebe Ayres, an experienced young woman of twenty-five, whose duty is to "bear such young fillies to the mounting block." Fanny shares Phoebe's bed and is there introduced to oral caresses and mutual masturbation. After several incidents, including an unsuccessful attempt on Fanny's maidenhead, Fanny meets Charles, a young man who had come to patronize the establishment but who had passed out from too much liquor and was unable to perform. She falls in love with Charles, who takes her to an inn at Chelsea, where he also takes her virginity. Their affair flourishes in a flat near St. James's for eleven months. Then, with Fanny three months pregnant, Charles is maneuvered out of the country by his father, and Fanny soon miscarries.

At this point their landlady Mrs. Jones arranges for Fanny to have an affair with Mr. H. With some reluctance Fanny agrees, and Mr. H. sets her up in an attractive flat. This relationship comes to an end when Fanny returns home one afternoon to find Mr. H. carrying on with her maidservant. She does not make her presence known, and takes her sauce for the goose by initiating an affair with Mr. H.'s liveried messenger, a sturdy nineteen-year-old youth. They enjoy each other several times but are finally caught *in flagrante delicto* by Mr. H., who dismisses Fanny with fifty guineas. Fanny takes lodgings in Covent Garden next to Mrs. Cole, who operates a "house of conveniency" disguised as a millinery establishment. Most of this half of the novel is probably based on the story line given to Cleland by Charles Carmichael at Bombay. It contains about a dozen episodes or scenes that lend themselves for depiction.

The second letter, containing a sequence of episodes of Cleland's own invention, is even richer in the number of characters and their sexual exploits. The other young women in Mrs. Cole's establishment,

Emily, Harriet, and Louisa, are introduced, and each relates at length her account of innocence, arousal, and betrayal followed by promiscuity. A decorous party is held for the four young women and their four young "sparks," a voyeuristic incident in which each couple takes turns copulating while the other three look on. Then Mrs. Cole arranges an affair between Fanny and Mr. Norbert, whose preferred activities include much voyeurism and occasional acts of fetishism, but not much coition. An interlude is provided when Fanny picks up a sailor in the street; he attempts to have her *a tergo,* claiming "any port in a storm," but Fanny directs his efforts to a more natural orifice. The next sequence finds Fanny in a flagellation episode with Mr. Barville, during which she enthusiastically participates in an act requiring considerable athleticism. Her next lover is an elderly man whose pleasures revolve around hair fetishism and white kid gloves. At this point Cleland inserts the sodomy episode, which takes place when Fanny goes to Hampton Court to visit Harriet, who has married respectably. Delayed en route, Fanny waits at a pub where she watches a youth of nineteen years bugger a lad about two years his junior; Fanny notes her disapproval of homosexual encounters. An interlude is provided by an account of Louisa's torrid fling with Good-Hearted Dick, a somewhat retarded youth who sells flowers; Fanny enjoys the voyeur's role, but out of prudence refrains from participating. We next see Fanny in the company of Emily and two young men who escort them up the Thames for bathing and an al fresco frolic in Surrey. Finally, Mr. Cole decides to retire. Fanny, whose fortune now amounts to £800, moves to Marylebone, where she befriends an elderly man and becomes his mistress; eight months later he dies and leaves her his estate. The finale comes when Fanny, now a well-to-do young woman, by chance meets Charles, her first lover, returned from exile. Their reunion causes their love to blossom afresh; they marry and raise a family, the conventional happy ending to so many romances, be they novels, short stories, plays, films, even ballets and operas.

Some of the artists to whom illustrations for *Fanny Hill* have been attributed are well known. Hubert-François Gravelot (1699–1773) was a French designer and engraver of book illustrations. He helped introduce the rococo style to England, where he was active from 1732 to 1755. In London he was acquainted with Hogarth and Gainsborough, and he illustrated an edition of Gay's *Fables* as well as an edition of Shakespeare and one of Dryden. He was one of the first artists to illustrate novels, designing illustrations for *Pamela* (1742) and *Tom Jones* (1750). His forte was depicting scenes from contemporary life rather than tragic subjects of classical and allegorical themes that were then fashionable. He returned to Paris circa 1755 and could easily have been available to illustrate the 1766 edition. Gravelot's illustrations were also published and sold separately, and Isaiah Thomas and Benjamin Gomex of New York offered plates in America.[16] Half a century later was François Elluin (1745–1810), a French artist much influenced by Boucher and Greuze; a well-known book illustrator, Elluin's career spanned the end of the Capetian monarchy and extended into the Napoleonic era. Antoine Borel was a French engraver who flourished in the 1770s and 1780s. Although Kearney states that a number of Parisian editions were engraved by Elluin after designs by Borel, the opposite may be true. Franz von Bayros (1866–1924) was a Viennese printmaker and book illustrator, best known for his illustrations for an edition of Aretino's poems and for Dante's *Divine Comedy*. His illustrations for the 1906 Vienna edition of *Fanny Hill* are in a style reminiscent of a music hall or cabaret setting, each in an elaborate cartouche. Female nudity is partly concealed by wisps of drapery and he avoids the actual depiction of sexual union. Edouard Chimot, who is reputed to have illustrated the 1954 Paris edition, was born at Lille and flourished between 1913 and 1943. The date of his death is not certain, but if he actually executed the illustrations, it was a work of his *vieillesse*. Paul (actually Edouard-Henri) Avril (1849–1928), who illustrated the exemplary 1923 Paris edition, was a versatile book illustrator in Paris during the heyday of the Third Republic. Liselotte (Lilo) Rasch-Nägele, who supplied the innocuous vignettes for the 1964 Vienna-Munich-Basel edition, was born at Stuttgart in 1914 and became a well-known artist and illustrator during the Third Reich and thereafter. It is not so much surprising that a majority of the artists are French but that none of the identifiable ones is English.

Certain unwritten conventions govern the artist's imagination. Great emphasis is placed upon the setting. All but one of the scenes take place indoors; the only exception is the al fresco frolic up the Thames. The rooms and their furnishings are depicted as elegant and fashionable. Gravelot's rendition of the gymnastic encounter between Fanny and Mr. Barville is set in a chamber with finely worked wood-paneled walls; the action takes place on a patterned Turkish carpet in front of an elaborate marble fireplace where a brisk, warming fire is lit (fig. 7.1).

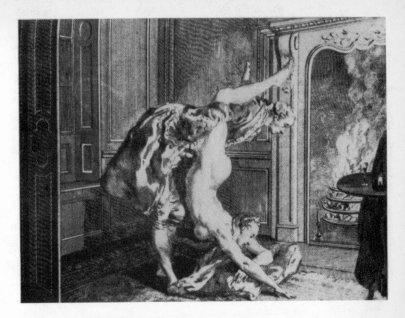

Figure 7.1. Mr. Barville in action with Fanny Hill after he has flogged her. Attributed to Gravelot. London, 1766.

Gravelot is the only illustrator who has attempted to recreate this scene, one in which the position of the figures seems to defy the laws of gravity and kinetic energy. A similar treatment of furnishings marks the earlier scene in which Fanny flogs Mr. Barville (fig. 7.2), and the anonymous copper-plate engraver of the 1770 Paris edition portrays Fanny and Charles embracing on a Madame Recamier couch in front of a decorative oriental screen (fig. 7.3).

Occasionally the artist will enhance the scene with ornaments compatible with the action; the anonymous artist of Dr. Basker's copy introduces a phallic candlestick on the mantle of a well-proportioned fireplace, and the handle of the poker as well as the hands of a nearby clock are also phallic. In general the chambers are far more luxurious than one might have found in a London bordello of the period. The Elluin-Borel treatment of the outdoor frolic shows the two couples in amorous embraces in a grotto veiled by a canopy; a picnic hamper with two wine bottles sits on the ground between the lovers (fig. 7.4). Gravelot's treatment of the same scene is comparable, set in a garden with well-

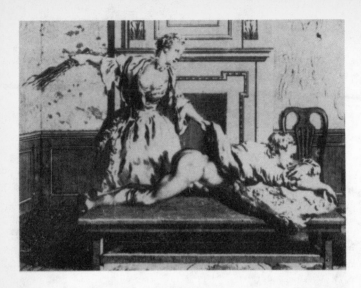

Figure 7.2. Fanny Hill birching Mr. Barville. Attributed to Gravelot. London, 1766.

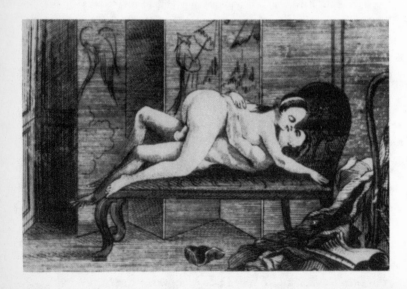

Figure 7.3. Fanny Hill astride Charles on a Madame Recamier couch. Anonymous copper-plate engraving. Paris, 1770.

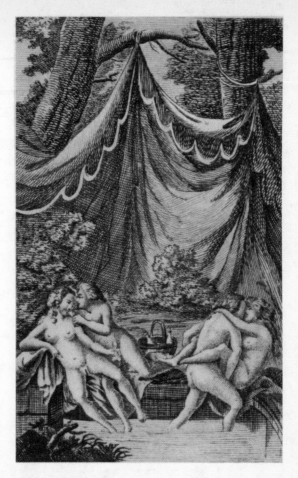

Figure 7.4. Fanny and Emily frolic with two young men in a grotto at Surrey. Attributed to Elluin after designs by Borel. Paris, 1786.

arranged shrubs and flowers. The frontispiece of the 1770 Paris edition shows a nude female figure, her arms outstretched, in front of a classical herm, the setting being a spacious colonnade and rotunda with Doric columns (fig. 7.5). Whenever possible the artists make use of expensive-looking fabrics, usually as draperies for canopied beds. The footstools in Paul Avril's frontispiece for the 1923 Paris edition are upholstered in striped silk satin complete with piping (fig. 7.6).

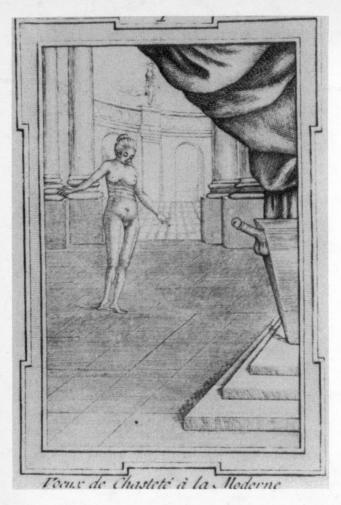

l'oeux de Chasteté à la Moderne

Figure 7.5. Frontispiece showing a nude female figure in front of a classical herm. Attributed to Elluin after designs by Borel. Paris, 1770.

The eighteenth-century French editions display the participants in costume of the period. A frequent detail is to show the man's three-cornered hat lying on the floor (fig. 7.7), but in Avril's 1923 representation of the scene between Fanny and the sailor, the hat is on his head (fig. 7.8). However, the anonymous artist of the 1861 Italian edition

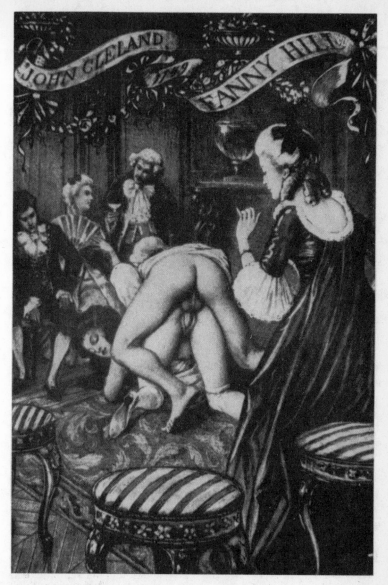

Figure 7.6. Frontispiece showing Mrs. Cole supervising a voyeuristic session in which four couples take turns while the others look on. Attributed to Paul Avril. Paris, 1923.

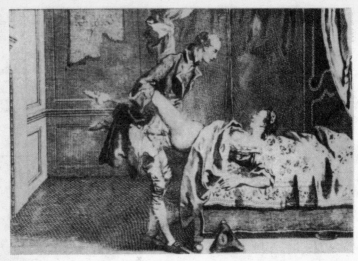

Figure 7.7. Charles and Fanny in action. Attributed to Gravelot. London, 1766.

from "Parigi" shows Mr. H. surprising Fanny in the arms of his liveried servant in a room fitted with mid-nineteenth-century furnishings. Mr. H. appears at the doorway wearing a stovepipe hat and a cutaway frock coat, while Fanny and the young man also are dressed in contemporary fashions (fig. 7.8). Complete nudity is not commonly shown. In general, the man's breeches are open and the woman's dress and petticoats rucked up, exposing her pubis, pudenda, and thighs (figs. 7.7–7.9). Often the woman reclines at the foot of the bed; in scenes depicting penetration *a tergo*, the woman is often shown bending over a table. The Elluin-Borel illustration of Fanny's first encounter with Charles is one of the few to show both participants completely nude in a setting marked by meticulous rendition of the drapery (fig. 7.10).

The figure drawing of the eighteenth-century French editions derives from the classical style of the period, the most familiar example being Boucher's provocative portrait of Kitty O'Shea. Both male and female bodies are portrayed as well proportioned, youthful, graceful, and vigorous. Even in the scenes showing Fanny with older men and the occasional one of Mrs. Brown with her young lover, the older figures appear to be somewhat less than their stated age. There is no attempt to

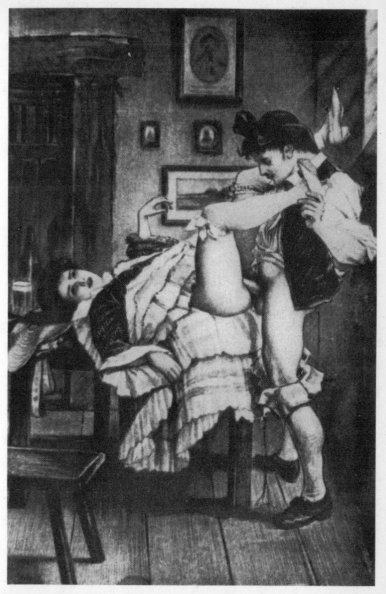

Figure 7.8. Fanny in action with a sailor. Attributed to Paul Avril. Paris, 1923.

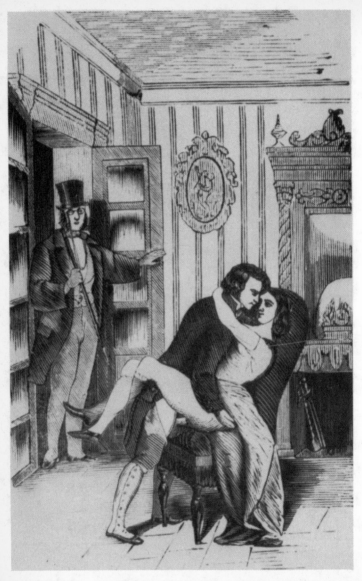

Figure 7.9. Mr. H. surprises Fanny in the embrace of his servant. Anonymous. Parigi, 1861.

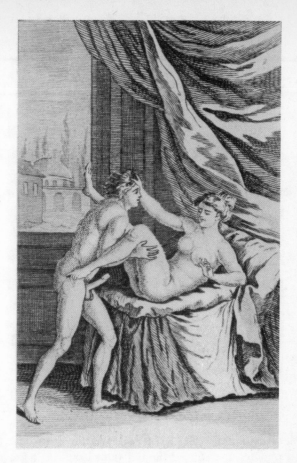

Figure 7.10. Charles about to penetrate Fanny. Attributed to Elluin after designs by Borel. Paris, 1786.

exaggerate the size of the breasts or buttocks, and needless to say, the breasts are always firm and not pendulous. With male figures, the penis is always erect, whether it is about to penetrate or has already done so. A small or flaccid organ would be incongruous. The erect penis is usually shown at the upper limit of normal size; exaggeration again would be incongruous. The only exception is the example of Good-Hearted Dick, the size of whose equipment so agitated Louisa (fig. 7.11). The

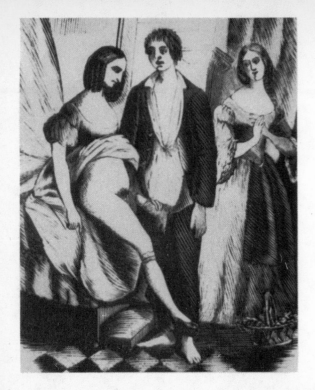

Figure 7.11. Louisa, Good-Hearted Dick, and Fanny. Anonymous. Parigi, 1861.

anonymous artist of the 1907 Kamashastra edition has no reluctance to portray the nude female figure, but his young ladies are in the tradition of Charles Dana Gibson and Howard Chandler Christy, and he never shows actual copulation.

Another convention governs the portrayal of pubic and axillary hair. The general rule is that it is not highlighted, being either absent or only lightly suggested. This tradition continued into the nineteenth century in both French and English art—for example, the nudes of Ingres and Etty. Delineation of pubic hair was the prerogative of artists who specialized in pornography or studies directly from the model and not for further promulgation.[16] The same taboo was followed by Lewis Carroll, who limited his voyeuristic photographs to nude, prepubescent

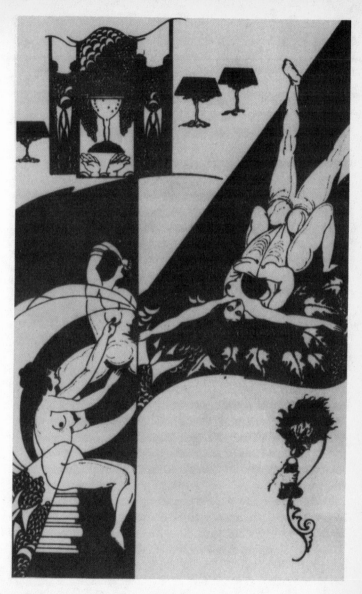

Figure 7.12. *Left,* Phoebe Ayres masturbates Fanny; *right,* Charles in action with Fanny. Anonymous. Hoboken, N.J., 1929.

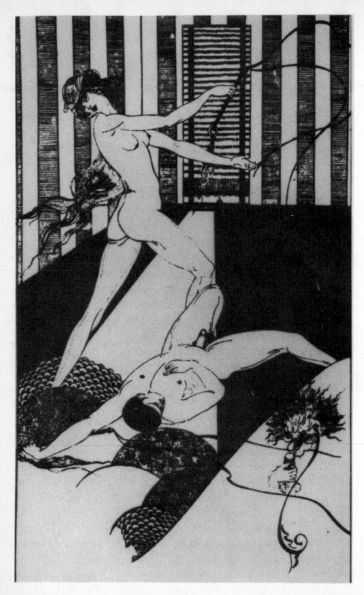

Figure 7.13. Flagellation scene, modeled on Fanny's flagellation of Mr. Barville. Anonymous. Hoboken, N.J., 1929.

girls. It has been speculated that Ruskin was unable to consummate his marriage to Effie Gray when he discovered on their wedding night that she had a normal female complement of pubic hair. Exceptions to the rule can be found in the crude illustrations for the so-called seventeenth edition of 1813 and in the 1861 Italian edition, where the pubic hair is heavily drawn. Attitudes toward pubic and axillary hair are culturally determined; a glance at the advertisements in any woman's magazine of this century will show that the taboo persists in England, France, and the United States. Even as recently as the 1920s there was a moderate public outcry when Henri Matisse exhibited his *Odalisques* with strokes of black paint to indicate the presence of axillary hair.

In a different tradition are the illustrations for the 1929 Hoboken edition by an anonymous artist who seems to have been influenced by Aubrey Beardsley. The nude male and female figures are highly stylized, and the incidental decorations owe their curling shapes to the *art nouveau* movement that was then in its ascendancy (figs. 7.12, 7.13). It should be noted that in the flagellation scene, the male is supine and the female figure is merely brandishing the whip. The pose is unsuitable for the actual act; it promises more than it can give.

Apart from the functional purpose of illustrating the novel and enhancing the reader's enjoyment, this gallery of erotic scenes shares in common with the erotic images of Greece and Rome what is common to erotic art of all times and places. As Catherine Johns puts it, they are "representations of lovemaking which seems to have no hidden meaning or purpose, but simply to depict an enjoyable activity in a straightforward manner." [17]

Part
Three
The

Sublimation

of

Psychopathology

8
Johnson and Boswell: "Vile Melancholy" and "The Hypochondriack"

Depression has replaced *melancholia* as a psychiatric term because we no longer credit the humoral notion of "black bile" as its cause. Yet Timothy Bright's *A Treatise of Melancholie* (1586) is the first monograph in English on a psychiatric topic. He recognized melancholia as an emotional disturbance not accompanied by dementia; in keeping with Tudor humoral theory, he wrote that "melancholic humor . . . settled in the spleane and with his vapour annoyeth the harte and passing up to the brayne, countersetteth terrible objects to the fantasie . . . causeth it without externall occasion to forge monstrous fictions . . . the brayne hath plentifully drunke of that spleneticke fogge . . . and the pure and bright spirites so defiled and eclipsed."[1] Bright's humoral ideas were adopted by Elizabethan and Jacobean writers, notably in Robert Burton's *Anatomy of Melancholy* (1621). The Puritan movement in Britain, allied to Calvinist doctrines of total human depravity and the lack of remission of sin by contrition or confession, contributed to the widely held sense of despair and impending doom that permeates much literature of the first six decades of the seventeenth century.

Only with Thomas Willis' post-Restoration insights in *Pathologiae cerebri et nervosae* (1667) and *De anima brutorum* (1672) did the first steps toward "modern" neuropsychiatry appear. He laid the groundwork for an organic and mechanical concept of mental disease. That his "explosive particles" and "animal spirits" have given way to more refined biochemical ideas about the neural impulse does not diminish their importance in the history of ideas. When Willis wrote, "Melancholy is commonly defined to be a raving without a Feavor or fury, joined with fear and sadness . . . it is a complicated Distemper of the Brain and Heart," he was assigning reason to the brain and emotion to the heart much as we do today.[2]

In the eighteenth century depression had such synonyms as low spirits, the spleen, and the vapours, as well as such classical terms as hysteria and hypochondriasis. In 1682 Thomas Sydenham denied the traditional idea that hysteria was due to a disturbance of the womb and peculiar to women. Its symptoms, he noted, were identical with hypochondriasis, then thought to be peculiar to men, and he insisted they were the same disease. The descriptions of symptoms range from mild anxiety states through organic conversion complaints to true depressive psychosis. Humoral vocabulary persisted; *The Spleen, a Pindarique Ode* (1701) by Anne, Countess of Winchilsea, who suffered from it:

> Falsely the Mortal Part we blame
> Of our deprest and pondrous frame. . . .
> The Cause indeed is a defect in Sense,
> But still the Spleen's alleg'd and still the dull pretence.[3]

Physicians such as John Purcell, Sir Richard Blackmore, Bernard Mandeville, William Stukeley, and Nicholas Robinson published monographs that attempted to describe and explain depression, reconciling humoral and mechanical theories with variable success. But the most influential treatise that dominated eighteenth-century ideas about the disease was George Cheyne's *The English Malady* (1733). The malady, he argued, was peculiarly English because of "the Moisture of our Air, the Variableness of our Weather . . . the Richness and Heaviness of our Food . . . the Inactivity and sedentary Occupations of the better Sort . . . and the Humour of living in great, populous and consequently unhealthy Towns."[4] Particularly dangerous was the cold, damp, penetrating east wind sweeping in over England from the North Sea.

Thomas Gray, who "trembled at an east wind," described his prevailing mood as "a white melancholy, or rather *Leucocholy,* and confessed to episodes of deeper depression.[5] His "Elegy, Written in a Country Churchyard" tells us that "Melancholy had marked him for her own," referring to the youth who lies buried there. William Cowper, who suffered from religious melancholia and weathered three suicide attempts, agreed with Cheyne, Gray, and others about the role of climate, "the unhealthful East that breathes the spleen," and depression's predilection for England: "It pleased God that I should be born in a country where melancholy is the national characteristic; and of a house more than commonly subject to it. To say the truth, I have often wished myself a Frenchman."[6] An astonishing statement from a writer so quintessentially English!

Samuel Johnson

But the writers who examined themselves and their depressions most closely were Samuel Johnson and James Boswell. Most people who read Johnson are immediately struck by how firm his ideas are and the force with which he expresses them. Few writers so consistently achieve such good sense and sound judgment. Yet one of the ironies of biography is that a mind so resolute when applied to life and letters suffered such anguish when it came to mastering its owner's emotions. The outline of his early struggles is familiar—not enough money to continue for an Oxford degree, "mental breakdown" on returning to Lichfield, failure as a schoolmaster, years of penury writing in London, his wife's death, loneliness, despair. His medical history is also familiar—scrofula as a child, poor eyesight, compulsive neurotic tics, asthma, and a variety of sicknesses. But recognition and reputation came with his *Dictionary* (1755), when he was in his mid-forties, then *Rasselas* (1759), and a royal pension (1762). Despite accumulated honors, despite a circle of loyal, devoted friends, many of them distinguished, during most of his adult life Johnson was subject to episodes of depression, usually characterized by self-reproach for indolence, feelings of guilt, and almost constant fear of insanity. As an intellect, Johnson towered above his melancholic predecessors, yet he too was a victim.

Boswell first met Johnson in 1763 after the successes cited above, and we are much better informed about the last two decades of his life than the first five. Unlike Boswell's journals, Johnson's diaries are not given to extensive self-revelation; they are reticent. Recent research has revealed more data about the external circumstances of Johnson's younger years than we knew a generation ago, but we have only fragmentary information about his psychic turmoil as a young adult. What we know about his formed adult psyche comes from his own writings and the posthumous biographies by Boswell, Hester Thrale Piozzi (who knew him only after he had turned fifty), and Sir John Hawkins (who had met him somewhat earlier).

Johnson returned to Lichfield from Oxford at the end of 1729. It was an unhappy household, and Johnson's bitter disappointment at leaving Oxford was compounded by the failure of his father's bookselling business and his father's declining health. Johnson rapidly sank into a state of depression. At the outset it seemed like a reactive depression with adequate external cause in the circumstances of a young man with few prospects. But it lasted two years in its profound form and persisted, though slowly improving, three years more. During the phase of profound depression Johnson was apathetic. Writing many years later, he said he could look at the town clock for an hour and not know what time it was, as good an image as any to convey the immobilizing effect of depression on perception, intellect, and initiative. There is a vague hint that he might have entertained thoughts of suicide, but the phrase "fearful that there was something wrong in his constitution, which might impair his Intellects, or shorten his Life" can equally well be inerpreted as fear that he was suffering from an organic disease.[7]

Boswell's comments are descriptive rather than analytical, and, given Johnson's reticence about that period of his life, wisely so:

> [H]e felt himself overwhelmed with an horrible hypochrondria, with perpetual irritation, fretfulness, and impatience; and with a dejection, gloom, and despair, which made existence misery. From this dreadful malady he never afterwards was perfectly relieved; and all his labours, and all his enjoyments, were but temporary interruptions of its baleful influence. . . . That it was, in some degree, occasioned by a defect in his nervous system, that inexplicable part of our frame, appears highly probable.[8]

Boswell and a few of Johnson's intimate friends knew that he lived in almost continual fear of insanity, and he exculpates his hero:

> But let not little men triumph knowing that Johnson was an HYPOCHONDRIACK. . . . Though he suffered severely from it, he was not therefore degraded. The powers of his great mind might be troubled, and their full exercise suspended at times, but the mind itself was ever entire. . . . I am aware that he himself was too ready to call such a complaint by the name of *madness*. But there is surely a clear distinction between a disorder which

affects only the imagination and spirits, while the judgment is sound, and a disorder by which the judgment is impaired.[9]

Boswell makes a major psychiatric distinction. Though Johnson was severely depressed in 1730–31 and on later occasions, he never lost his reason. He was never agitated in the technical sense; he experienced no hallucinations. Unhappy though he was, he could cope with daily living. Nonetheless, the apathetic depression of those years must be reckoned as a major psychiatric illness, and it set the pattern for subsequent episodes, mercifully shorter and less severe. During later episodes, Johnson's major symptom was what today we would call work inhibition, which he called sloth or idleness.

For Johnson, sloth had a specific theological significance, that is, despair of (hence inactivity toward) achieving a spiritual good: *tristitia de aliquo bono spirituale*. Bate has summarized more than a dozen entries from his diaries in which he either prays to God to deliver him from sloth or makes a resolution to develop a program to keep himself from idleness.[10]

Young Johnson was fully aware of his predicament and sought medical advice. He composed a long letter in Latin to his godfather, Dr. Swynfen, then practicing in Birmingham, presenting a detailed account of his symptoms and their evolution. Swynfen seems to have been baffled, and his reply (as paraphrased or summarized by Sir John Hawkins, who probably found the letter in Johnson's papers after his death) could only have depressed Johnson more deeply: "[F]rom the symptoms therein described, he [Swynfen] could think nothing better of his disorder, than it had a tendency to insanity; and without great care might possibly terminate in the deprivation of his rational faculties."[11] It was the most damaging comment he could have made. Small wonder that Johnson lived in fear of insanity for the rest of his life. What probably helped Johnson overcome his depression was religion. At Oxford he had read William Law's *A Serious Call to a Devout and Holy Life*. Up to then Johnson had been indifferent to religious principles and practices; Law's persuasive, well-written arguments made him a convinced Christian. Later he was to refer to the book as "the finest piece of hortatory theology in any language." We cannot reconstruct Johnson's dialogue with the text, but it provided the young man in his distress both with comfort and strength and a motive to face the problems of life and to make something of himself and his God-given talents.

Later, Johnson was reluctant to discuss details of this black period during his twenties. But he freely admits his melancholy temperament in two letters to Joseph Warton while he was still at work on the *Dictionary*. The first alludes to the death of Dodsley's wife:

> . . . I believe he is much affected. I hope he will not suffer so much as I yet suffer for the loss of mine.
> "Why should I lament? Man is born to sorrow."
> I have ever since seemed to myself broken off from mankind, a kind of solitary wanderer in the wild of life, without any certain direction, or fixed point of view. A gloomy gazer on a World to which I have little relation.[12]

Wharton's reply must have contained news of their mutual friend William Collins, by then in a state of irreversible depressive psychosis and confined. Johnson answered: "Poor dear Collins—Let me know whether you think it would give him pleasure if I should write to him. I have often been near his state and therefore have it in great commiseration."[13]

Johnson's most explicit statement of his greatest fear is found near the end of *Rasselas* (1759) in the conversation in which the astronomer tells Imlac, "Of the uncertainties of our present state, the most dreadful and alarming is the uncertain continuance of reason." Johnson's mother died in March 1759, and *Rasselas* was published in April. A few days before the book came from the press, Johnson's prayer for Easter Day included the following supplication: "Let me not sink into useless dejection; but so sanctify my affliction, O Lord, that I may be converted and healed."[14] Converted to faith he was and had been for thirty years, but healed, alas, for only a short time.

MELANCHOLIA IN JOHNSON'S *DICTIONARY*

But these letters and prayers were private. It is profitable to examine Johnson's public statements about the nature of depressive disease, and these are conveniently found in his *Dictionary*. He defines *hypochondriacal* and *hypochondriack* as "Melancholy; disordered in the imagination"—fair enough as a capsule definition, though scarcely illuminating. But to one's dismay he defines *hysterical* and *hysterick* as "1. Troubled with fits; disordered in the region of the womb," to which he subjoins a century-old quotation from Harvey that the symptoms of hysteria suggest possession by the devil. Perhaps this was intended as a tribute to the historical nature of lexicography, but the second definition reads, "2. Proceeding from disorders of the womb," which he supports by Pope's couplet,

> Parent of vapours, and of female wit,
> Who have th' hysterick or poetic fit.

Nowhere does the *Dictionary* take account of Willis' or Sydenham's views that hypochondria and hysteria are the same disorder.

When one looks at the relevant definition for *vapours,* it reads, "5. [In the plural]—Diseases caused by flatulence, or by diseased nerves; hypochondriacal maladies; spleen." This has the advantage of combining neural etiology with gastrointestinal symptoms and was consistent with contemporary medical opinion. But the supporting quotation for the usage is from Addison's *Spectator* essay of 1711, "To this we must ascribe the spleen, so frequent in studious men, as well as the vapours to which the other sex are so often subject," which contains both the obsolete Aristotelian idea relating melancholy to the life of the intellect and the distinction between the sexes so roundly dismissed by Sydenham three score and ten years before.

Johnson remains on traditional ground when he defines *spleen* as "1. The milt; one of the viscera, of which the use is scarcely known. 2. Anger; spite; ill-humour. 3. A fit of anger. 4. Melancholy; hypochondriacal vapours." By now the definitions seem circular, defining subjects in terms of themselves. But most revealing of all is his definition of *melancholy,* the central part of his own most human condition, "1. A disease, supposed to proceed from a redundance of black bile; but it is better known to arise from too heavy and too viscid blood: its cure is evacuation, nervous medicines, and powerful stimuli." Shades of Bright and Burton! Willis, Sydenham, Robinson, and Cheyne might never have written a line! Nor would any contemporary physician concur except tangentially with the second entry, "2. A kind of madness, in which the mind is always fixed on one object." Possibly Johnson had in mind his friends Richard Savage and Christopher Smart, but in his accounts of their lives, written two decades later, he does not refer to them as melancholics and seems to have a clear grasp of their monomania, though that term was not then in general use. We can forgive Johnson his terminological inexactitudes for the sake of his quoting

Jaques' speech from *As You Like It* to illustrate the many faces of melancholy:

> I have neither the scholar's melancholy, which is emulation; nor the musician's, which is fantastical; nor the courtier's, which is proud; nor the soldier's, which is ambitious; nor the lawyer's, which is politick; nor the lady's, which is nice; nor the lover's, which is all these, but it is a melancholy of mine own, compounded of many simples, extracted from many objects, and, indeed, the sundry contemplation of my travels, in which my rumination wraps me in a most humorous sadness. (4.1.10–29)

It is a Burtonian catalogue, but Johnson—like Shakespeare and Burton—recognized that melancholy, though not quite all things to all men, took a variety of shapes and guises depending on its victims' circumstances. Jaques' speech may have struck a responsive chord because Johnson saw himself obliquely included. But his definitions of the various terms then in use to describe depression were old-fashioned even in 1755, and Johnson did not take into account newer medical ideas that had been current for a generation.

JOHNSON'S PADLOCK

Johnson's melancholia gradually returned in 1764–65, and by 1766 he was considerably depressed. Literary production was reduced, though Johnson was well enough to attend meetings of The Club regularly. Boswell was in Scotland for most of this period, and the *Life* tells us little. Johnson preferred solitude when he was depressed. His friend Dr. William Adams came to London on a visit and called on Johnson; his housekeeper told him that no one had been admitted for several days except Bennet Langton. Johnson agreed to receive Dr. Adams, who found him with Langton, and he reported that Johnson "looked miserable[;] his lips moved, tho he was not speaking[;] he could not sit long at a time—was quite restless, sometimes walked up and down the room, sometimes into the next room, and returned immediately." [15] By this time Johnson had met the Thrales and was their frequent guest at Streatham and Southwark. His mental state was so precarious that Henry Thrale insisted he leave London and stay with them under Hester's care, which he did, staying at Streatham from the end of June to the beginning of October 1766, by which time he was somewhat improved.

There is no doubt about the affection between Johnson and the Thrales, the benefits each received from the other, and the solicitude each had for the other's welfare. With respect to Johnson's physical and emotional health, Hester Thrale was at her best, a warm-hearted, capable, cultivated woman who did her utmost to keep her valued friend and intellectual mentor as well and as happy as he could be. Which brings us to the curious question of the padlock (cf. Conan Doyle's curious incident of the dog—it did nothing during the night). To paraphrase Katharine Balderston's lucid account, at the sale of Hester Thrale's library and personal effects in 1823, one of the items catalogued was a padlock, with an attached note in her handwriting, "Johnson's padlock, committed to my care in the year 1768."[16] Literary scholarship associates this with a note in her diaries for 1779, "the Fetters & Padlocks will tell Posterity the Truth," as well as with a letter written in French to her by Johnson while he was staying at her house which closes with, "Je souhaite, ma patronne, que vôtre autorité me soit toujours sensible, et que vous me tiennez dans l'esclavage que vou[s] sçavez si bien rendre heureuse."[17] Her reply to this letter concludes, "do not quarrel with your Governess for not using the Rod enough."[17]

To twentieth-century readers inured to the innuendos of psychopathology, allusions to slavery and the rod suggest that Johnson was a masochist who fancied bondage and flagellation and that he had prevailed upon Mrs. Thrale to assume the role of "Governess" and satisfy these erotic needs. It seems improbable that such carryings-on could have taken place at Streatham or Southwark, in a house filled with children and servants, and there is nothing to suggest surreptitious meetings elsewhere for clandestine purposes. Nor does Johnson's frequent use of the image of chains and shackles (e.g., *De pedicis et manicis insana cogitatio,* or chained by sin) suggest anything more erotic than the language of *The Book of Common Prayer.* Bate has adumbrated the implausibility of Johnson's being chained and beaten, and perhaps it is significant that no chains or fetters were included in the auction catalogue, just the padlock.[18] However, during the half-century inverval between 1768 and 1823 the chains might have been used for some other purpose.

What does the padlock signify? Hester Thrale associated it with "a Secret far dearer to him than his Life," which more plausibly than any masochistic impulses or their acting out could have been his almost constant fear of insanity and confinement. At that time it was still common practice to chain lunatics to the walls of their padlocked cells. Between Johnson and Mrs. Thrale, the padlock was most likely a symbol of what might befall him were he not to keep his melancholia in check. At most, when he felt the melancholy fit might fall, she may have padlocked him in his room for an hour while he composed his thoughts and feelings. But the greatest likelihood is that it was merely a symbol, a reminder, and was never used at all. This is not to be taken to indicate that Johnson was free of erotic impulses; Johnson was a man of strong but disciplined passions. In his prayers he frequently asks to be delivered from licentious thoughts, because such impulses conflicted with his moral principles as well as his status as a widower. Nor was Johnson unacquainted with pain. His much quoted comment about his boyhood schoolmaster, "He whip't me well," does not, however, indicate an adult predilection for being flogged. In a conversation with Boswell on madness in 1777 he remarked: "Madmen are all sensual in the lower stages of their distemper. They are eager for gratifications to sooth their minds and divert their attention from the misery which they suffer; but when they grow very ill, pleasure is too weak for them, and they seek pain. . . ."[19] Johnson directed his energies to escape madness; to have requested the painful infliction of the rod would have confirmed his worst fears about his sanity.

The above remark closes with one of Johnson's insights into managing depression: "Employment, Sir, and hardships, prevent melancholy." He was speaking from personal experience; many of his milder depressions had dissipated when he lost himself in his work. The point is valid; many people with a tendency to mild depression stay on a more or less even keel by keeping busy. But when depression becomes more severe, work inhibition is common, and the sufferer is as helpless as Johnson in the two dark episodes of 1730–31 and 1766. Another of Johnson's insights was, "I inherited a vile melancholy from my father, which has made me mad all my life, at least not sober."[20] Of all major mental disorders, manic-depressive disease, cyclical alternation of mood, is the most likely to be familial. Johnson must have been familiar with the symptoms from early childhood.

Johnson was not self-analytical about his melancholia in the sense that Boswell was about his. Many components played a part in its pathogenesis, among them heredity and sexual guilt. More important were the frustration of Johnson's youthful hopes at Oxford and his struggles to establish himself and realize his talents. This led him to believe in the essential unhappiness of human life. Even more central was the conflict between the independence of his ego and the tenets of his orthodox Christianity with its emphasis on submission to God's will. He set high standards for himself and was his own severest critic; any feeling that he had not given of his best could precipitate a sense of failure and despondency. To be sure, his moderate Anglicanism did not commit him to belief in eternal damnation or that sin was unforgivable, as did the Calvinism that was inflicted on Boswell as a boy, but it did demand unfaltering obligations to "Duty, stern daughter of the voice of God."

James Boswell

Born three decades later than Johnson, Boswell, a man of many moods, can be proposed as the epitome of the late-eighteenth-century attitude toward melancholia, a role earned by his regular habit of self-scrutiny as well as by the name he gave his monthly column in *The London Magazine* (1777–83), *The Hypochondriack*. His comments reveal the prevailing temper of his time; he was more than a barometer of the period; he was its polygraph. Thanks to the publication of his private papers, we have a more detailed medical record of him than of any man of the era. Perhaps it is illuminating to consider first Boswell's own appraisal of his personality.

In 1764, when on the Grand Tour, he sought an interview with Rousseau, then living near Geneva. Rousseau's reputation as a savant was international, and Boswell wanted advice about how to order his life and plan his career. Before the interviews he wrote out a sketch of his life, a revealing document with more emphasis on character traits than specific autobiographical data, to some extent a self-serving declaration. After two paragraphs of special pleading, Boswell begins his self-analysis:

> I was born with a melancholy temperament. It is the temperament of our family. Several of my relations have suffered from it. Yet I do not regret that I am melancholy. It is the temperament of tender hearts, of noble souls. But such temperaments require a

very careful education. There is danger either that they will fall into a debility which will completely destroy them, or that they will form a habit of viewing everything in such colours as to make their lives miserable.[21]

Boswell's statement about his family was certainly true. Of his father's twin younger brothers, the older was John Boswell, M.D., who was subject to episodic depression and indulged in eccentric behavior. According to Pottle, "he forsook the Kirk for the more 'primitive' society of the Glassites, preached the extreme doctrine of salvation by faith, demonstrated his antinomianism practically by frequenting bawdy houses, and was excommunicated by his sect." Boswell had many conversations with his physician uncle about melancholia. The younger twin, James, is described as "idle, given to keeping to his bed, and finally had to be put in a strait-waistcoat."[22] By 1764, when Boswell wrote his sketch for Rousseau, his younger brother, Johnny, had shown signs of mental instability, and soon thereafter confinement proved necessary; he suffered from "violent or morose insanity" for the rest of his life. Given that family history, small wonder that Boswell entertained fears about his mental equilibrium. It is of passing interest that his first cousin, James Boswell, son of Dr. John, took his M.D. degree at Edinburgh, and the subject of his thesis was *De malo hysterico* (1776). Sadly, the budding young physician died the following year at the age of twenty-three, and we have no details about his personality. However, it is not unreasonable to state that Boswell came from what we would call a psychogenic family.

Boswell's comment that "such temperaments require a very careful education" suggests he was unhappy about the way he was reared. His father, Lord Auchinleck, eighth Laird of the family's Ayrshire estates, had risen through intellectual merit and force of character to become one of the leading judges in Scotland. When Boswell was fourteen, his father was appointed one of the fifteen Lords of the Court of Session, hence the nonhereditary title Lord Auchinleck, and a year later was elevated as one of the six members of the High Court of Justiciary. He was a staunch Whig, a convinced Presbyterian, stern, upright, inflexible, and he had neither the time nor the interest to be a warm, affectionate father. One gets the impression that he liked his children provided they did exactly as they were told and fulfilled his level of expectation. Boswell respected him but he also feared him.

Boswell's mother is less clearly defined. Her father was sixty years old when she was born, the only child of a third marriage. Her mother died when she was two, and her father became a helpless paralytic a few years later. She was raised in seclusion, and Boswell himself describes her as "an extremely delicate girl, very hypochondriac . . . her notions were pious, visionary, and scrupulous."

Growing up in such a household incurs its penalties, and in his memoir to Rousseau Boswell recites some of them: "I was brought up very tenderly. Consequently I began at an early age to be indisposed, and people pitied me as a delicate child. . . . When my health was restored, my slavery would begin again. I knew it, and I preferred being weak and ill to being strong and healthy." Religious observance was important to the Auchinlecks, as it was for many other conservative upper-middle-class Scots: "My mother was extremely pious. She inspired me with devotion. But unfortunately she taught me Calvinism. My catechism contained the gloomiest doctrines of the system. The eternity of punishment was the first great idea I ever formed. How it made me shudder. . . . I became the most timid and contemptible of human beings." On Sundays the family attended divine service regularly: "I was obliged to hear three sermons in the same day, with a great many impromptu prayers and a great many sung psalms, all rendered in a stern and doleful manner. In the evening I was made to say my catechism and to repeat psalms translated into the vilest doggerel." [23]

Boswell's first tutor awakened the boy's interest in literature by introducing him to *The Spectator* as well as to the Roman poets. He provided some comfort about religion: "He told me that if I behaved well during my life, I should be happy in the other world." The next tutor was a dogmatic disciplinarian with little sympathy for the boy's developing interest in literature. His tenure was short because an undefined illness supervened:

> In my twelfth year I caught a very severe cold. I was given a great many medicines, and my naturally weak stomach became so upset that I could scarcely digest anything. I confess that the fear of having to go back to what were called my studies made me hope I could stay ill. The greatest doctors in Scotland were called in.
> . . . I could somehow control the operations of my stomach, and I immediately threw up everything they made me take. The Faculty decided I was suffering from an extraordinary illness. . . . I

laughed heartily to myself after their consultations. I was weakened in body and mind, and my natural melancholy increased.[24]

Clearly, the prepubescent boy was deliberately aggravating his symptoms as a defense against tutorial and domestic discipline. Escape came when his father sent him to Moffat, the Spa of Scotland, where he regained his health and good spirits in the company of "many lively people." He had used illness to manipulate those in charge of him.

Boswell matriculated at the University of Edinburgh at the age of thirteen, continuing to live in his father's house in Parliament Close. About this time he entered puberty. Spontaneous ejaculations gave him pleasure at first, but he soon learned masturbation from a friend and developed the usual guilt feelings, even to the point of contemplating self-castration: "I was always in fear of damnation. I thought what I was doing was but a small sin, whereas fornication was horrible. . . . But the madness passed." As a young bachelor he fornicated many times, and after his marriage he was a chronic, recurrent adulterer. The sense of guilt persisted, accompanied by self-reproach. Further problems arose from his studies: "Unluckily a terrible hypochondria seized me at the age of sixteen. I studied logic and metaphysics. . . . I looked upon the whole human race with horror. That I passed, I know not how; I think by yielding to received opinion For even now it does not seem clear to me." The importance of this episode of depression in 1756–57 ought not be underestimated. His illness at the age of twelve may have begun as an organic disease, though his reaction to it was emotional. His guilt about the dawn of adolescent sexuality was normal for a boy of that age and in that environment. But when "he branched from language and literature [and] his limitations became apparent"—that was a serious blow to his self-confidence.[25] Until then he had been able to compensate for the restrictions of his early years, even for the enforced religiosity, by good academic performance, but now his performance did not equal his level of aspiration.

The prescribed courses at Edinburgh in logic and natural philosophy compelled students to pursue systematic dialectic and abstract reasoning. Boswell was not gifted in rigorous intellectual discipline; his forte lay in language and literature and in analyzing "the variety of human nature." Even beyond successfully passing his examinations, the actual questions raised in logic and metaphysics disturbed his ego and the image he had formed of himself: "The study of metaphysics forced him to think of the problem of determinism, or to state the problem in terms in which it usually presented itself to him, of God's foreknowledge and man's free will. He found that he could not reconcile the two logically, and with the realization lost forever the foundations of his peace."[26] In some respects, this conflict resembles what is currently called an "identity crisis," but in Boswell's case, given the religious orientation to which he had been subjected, it disturbed not only his self-image but his relation to the cosmos. He felt rudderless in a sea of intellectual and moral doubt, alienated from those beliefs and values that had been integral elements in his daily life. Such crises of self-doubt, loss of self-confidence, and alienation are common among adolescents in all societies. One recognizable pattern for resolving them is for the perplexed young man to attach himself, or to identify with, a father-image, a prophet, even a vocation. At this time John Williamson, a self-educated farmer interested in the transmigration of souls, vegetarianism, mysticism, and alchemy, was Boswell's "guru." In later life more distinguished men served him as a father-substitute—General Paoli, Dr. Johnson, Sir John Pringle. Even his interviews with Rousseau and Voltaire are part of this pattern.

One reason Boswell sought such relationships was the inadequacy of his relations with his own father. Lord Auchinleck had entertained high hopes for his oldest son, and when Boswell's intellect proved unequal to such aspirations, he surely felt that he had failed his father's expectations and that his learned father would neither sympathize with his doubts and uncertainties nor excuse an indifferent academic performance. This was his second *crise de nerfs,* which affected Lord Auchinleck's attitude: "[H]e had to balance two possibilities: either his son was behaving in a culpably flighty manner, or he was not wholly responsible. Lord Auchinleck acted on the first of these suppositions and feared secretly that the second was true."[27] There is every justification for this view; he had before him the sad examples of his two younger brothers and the incipient breakdown of his youngest son. In any case, the failure of rapport between father and son was decisive for much of Boswell's conduct as an adult: recurrent episodes of depression, sexual promiscuity, excessive drinking, and compulsive gambling. Nor could his father-substitutes save him from those.

That Boswell is not explicit about how he resolved his crisis in 1756–57 reinforces the notion that this episode was so profoundly traumatic that he repressed many of the circumstances connected with it. His yielding to "received authority" is confirmed by his return to Edinburgh, where he took his degree in 1758.

His next escapade led not to another episode of melancholy but to additional strain upon his relations with his father. He became attached to an actress who happened to be a Roman Catholic, and he considered conversion to that faith. Lord Auchinleck was dismayed; civil and political disabilities for professed Roman Catholics at that time included debarment from any public career or entrance into any learned professions and even devolution of certain types of property. Had Boswell pursued such a course, he could not have inherited Auchinleck nor could he become a member of the Scottish bar, which was precisely what Lord Auchinleck had decided his son should and would do. Accordingly, he packed him off to Glasgow to break up the potential mésalliance and to begin studying law. Boswell had no choice but to comply.

Glasgow had little social life and no theater. Though Boswell applied himself earnestly to his studies and proved an adequate law student, he was unhappy and low-spirited. He continued to study the Roman Catholic position and announced that he intended to convert and become a priest or a monk. Disregarding a peremptory summons to return home, he fled to London, where he heard Mass for the first time and was admitted to the Church. How firm his convictions were can be gauged by his "rescue" by Lord Eglinton, his father's Ayrshire neighbor, who took the young rebel to his Mayfair home and introduced him to the delights of London society and speedily convinced him that a life of ascetic Christianity was less attractive than the pleasures a metropolis could provide. Boswell also consummated his first sexual experience, needless to say, with a prostitute. Also, needless to say, he suffered no attacks of hypochondriasis. He fell in love with London, and his regular revisits and final move there are too familiar to require retelling.

Lord Eglinton's intercession established a truce between father and son. Lord Auchinleck allowed Boswell his fling in London, and Boswell agreed to return to Edinburgh to take his degree in law. Boswell did pass the examination in civil law in 1762, but his conduct during the two years of Edinburgh scarcely permitted his father to revise his opinion of his son's unstable character. Boswell continued to associate with theatrical folk and other "undesirables"; he indulged in a few literary efforts, none likely to advance a young lawyer's reputation; he was publicly promiscuous and sired an illegitimate child. Having fulfilled his part of the bargain, Boswell persuaded his father to give him a year in London to try for a commission in a regiment of guards (cf. his *London Journal,* 1762–63). It was on this visit that he met Johnson, but they had scarcely time for more than a brief acquaintanceship, the budding of friendship, before Boswell set off for Utrecht in August 1763 to complete his legal studies.

Utrecht was as dull as Glasgow, and Boswell's journal for the period (*Boswell in Holland,* 1763–64) is filled with entries recording episodes of hypochondriasis and symptoms we now recognize as psychosomatic. He "kept his good resolutions by writing them down, and redressed his backslidings by copying them out."[28] An unfulfilled romance with Belle de Zuylen provided interest to an otherwise tiresome interval. On completing his legal studies in Holland, Boswell persuaded his father to underwrite a Grand Tour through Germany and Switzerland, where he had interviews with Rousseau and Voltaire, then Italy and France before returning home. Travel to new and exciting places took Boswell's mind from the fluctuations of his moods, and his journals (*Boswell on the Grand Tour,* 1764) record the observations of a well-educated young man preparing to meet the world on its own terms. By one device or another he extended his stay on the Continent, postponing the inevitable return to Edinburgh, where he would assume his predetermined position. He returned in 1766, passed the examination in Scottish law, and was admitted to the bar. He passed the next few years establishing himself in his profession and in search of a wife.

Returning to Edinburgh and beginning to practice law in a court where his father was so prominent again put Boswell's ego in jeopardy. He was not unsuccessful as a neophyte trial lawyer, but he probably sensed at the outset that the large prizes were beyond him and that he could not hope to attain anything like his father's eminence. So, probably, did his father, and Boswell's journals record recurrent episodes of low spirits. He relieved these by a series of sexual and alcoholic adventures and misadventures, none of which gained him a reputation for prudence. In his quest for a wife he fared somewhat better. He courted and married in 1769 Margaret Montgomerie, a first cousin on his father's side. Quite naturally, Lord Auchinleck had hoped his son and heir would marry a young woman of good family and good fortune. He could not complain of the family connection, for it was his own— none better. But the bride was a poor relation without a farthing to her name. Lord Auchinleck did not attend the wedding. A widower for several years, he chose that day to marry for a second time, his choice falling on his own first cousin, Elizabeth Boswell, a spinster.

Margaret Montgomerie made Boswell an excellent wife, and for the first few years they were happy. His journals record only brief, isolated episodes of melancholy. But he was never fully at ease in Edinburgh; as often as he could, when court sessions rose, he quickly departed for London, leaving his wife and children behind. As the responsibilities of a husband and father increased, attacks of melancholy and psychosomatic symptoms reappeared, and with them promiscuity, drinking, and gambling became more frequent. His wife was forgiving and supportive up to a point, but the need for such forgiveness and support only underscored his sense of inadequacy. His psychological status deteriorated slowly.

Boswell was fully aware of his problems and frequently sought advice on how better to order his life and conduct. The best advice came from Johnson: "You are always complaining of melancholy, and I conclude . . . you are fond of it. . . . [M]ake it an invariable and obligatory law to yourself, never to mention your own mental disease; if you are never to speak of them, you will think on them but little, and if you think little of them, they will molest you rarely."[29] This is in one sense equivalent to saying, "Disregard them, and they will go away," which is not always the case, but Johnson was also telling Boswell to discontinue his habit of morbid introspection, which did aggravate his symptoms. He was also counseling from examination of his own case. Consider Burton's apologia for writing: "I write of melancholy, by being busy, to avoid melancholy." In addition, Johnson told Boswell to stop drinking to excess; he had done so himself, substituting vast quantities of tea for wine and spirits. Perhaps he had in mind the example of William Collins, of whom he later wrote, "with the usual weakness of men so diseased, he eagerly snatched that relief with which the table and the bottle flatter and seduce."[30] He advised Boswell to keep occupied: "The safe and general antidote against sorrow, is employment."[31] In an age when psychotherapy and mood-altering drugs were unknown, the advice of "forget it and keep busy" was as sensible as any remedy. Again, recall Burton's precept: "Be not solitary, be not idle." But Boswell's sense of inadequacy and continuous feelings of guilt for his innumerable lapses were too strong for such counsel to be of more than temporary value. His wife died in 1782, leaving him a handful of children whose rearing and education he tried to supervise. Johnson died in 1784, and, as Boswell's fortunes declined, the only redeeming feature of his life was his steadfast devotion to writing the *Life of Johnson*. This self-imposed assignment kept him busy, but even so he required moral and intellectual support from Edward Malone before his melancholy days came to an end in 1795.

BOSWELL'S MELANCHOLIA DOCUMENTED

Boswell's journals are a diary-catalogue of the vicissitudes of the melancholic man, often moderately depressed but always well this side of psychosis despite his erratic behavior. However, to illuminate the question of eighteenth-century spleen one must examine his one venture into regular systematic journalism. In 1771 Boswell acquired part interest in the *London Magazine* and, starting in October 1777, began a series of monthly essays in a column titled *The Hypochondriack*.[32] Each short piece was written on a single theme in the form of the familiar literary essay modeled on *The Spectator, The Rambler,* and other specimens of the genre. One cannot charge Boswell with sloth; he always met his deadline and wrote to full measure. He continued these essays for almost six years, the seventieth and last appearing in August 1783. As self-therapy they were an application of Johnson's advice to keep busy. The epigraph to the first essay is from Horace:

> Sunt verba voces quibus hunc lenire dolorem
> Possis, magnam morbi deponere partem.

Boswell translates this as:

> Words will avail the wretched mind to ease,
> And much abate the dismal black disease.

The essay is an apologia explaining and justifying both the column's title and its purpose.

> From my title of *Hypochondriack* I would not have it thought that I am at present actually labouring under that malady, but as it is a saying in feudal treatises, *semel Baro semper Baro,* "Once a baron always a baron;" or as one who has had a commission in the army is ever after called captain; so I call myself the Hypo-

chondriack from former sufferings. I am so well acquainted with the distemper of Hypochondria, that I think myself qualified to assist some of my unhappy companions who are now groaning under it.

Among other points, Boswell refutes the idea that hypochondria is peculiar to Britain. Without mentioning Cheyne by name, he takes a position contrary to *The English Malady,* noting that the disease is found in France as well and is widely distributed among the nations: "We may trace it in all countries in one shape or another." The essay concludes with the not ignoble sentiment that Boswell intends to offer his readers: "[W]ithout ever offending them by an excess of gayety, insensibly communicate to them that good-humour, which if it does not make life rise to felicity, at least preserves it from wretchedness."

Four of the essays deal specifically with hypochondria as a disease, though scattered allusions to it are found in other essays. In essay No. 5 (February 1778) Boswell specifically refutes Aristotle's notion that melancholy is "the concomitant of distinguished genius":

> Melancholy, or Hypochondria, like the fever or gout, or any other disease, is incident to all sorts of men, from the wisest to the most foolish. . . . I do not dispute that men are miserable in a greater or lesser degree in proportion to their understanding and sensibility. It is not every man who can be exquisitely miserable, any more than exquisitely happy. But the distemper indubitably operates, though in different degrees, upon every species or constitution, as fire produces its effects, though in different degrees, upon every species of matter, however much or however little of a combustible nature.

Boswell also has a sound grasp of both the psychosomatic presentation of depression and its protean symptoms: "Hypochondria affects us in an infinite variety of ways; for, disordered imagination teems with a boundless multiplicity of evils; and the disorders of the body which I believe always attend the direful disease, make such diversities of combination, that it is scarcely possible to specify all the sufferings of a Hypochondriack." He concludes the essay with comments on Matthew Green's "The Spleen" (1737), "an elegant and most useful didactick poem, as it not only points out in a very lively manner the ordinary effects of the disease, but also suggests excellent methods of cure, so smartly, and at the same time so pleasingly, that the patients cannot fail to take them." To this he adds favorable comments on John Armstrong's "Art of Preserving Health" (1744) and James Thomason's "Castle of Indolence" (1748) and notes that Fielding's description of an attack of the vapours in *Amelia* (1751) struck him with the "justness of the representation."

Essay No. 6 (March 1778) is a continuation of the preceding essay. One of Boswell's finest insights opens the argument: "Nothing characterizes a Hypochondriack more peculiarly than irresolution, or the want of power over his mind." Had he been a metaphysician, he would have launched into a discussion of the will, whether it was free or determined, and the relation between reason and emotion, but he chose instead to develop the metaphor of a watch to explore the question, "What that power is by which the conscious spirit governs and directs the various mental faculties, is, it must be confessed, utterly inexplicable as long as our souls are enclosed in material frames." He identified ego psychology and placed it in the framework of the mind-body relationship, trying to resolve it on a mechanical basis, somewhat Newtonian in origin, but his approach is literary rather than scientific. He does note the inadequacy of language to convey what the hypochondriac suffers, particularly when he tries to describe his symptoms after they have abated: "He will find his language quite inadequate; so that he must use those strong indefinite phrases which do not particularly specify any thing, convey any distinct meaning, or excite any lively perception." He concludes the essay with a social rather than a clinical description of "languor" and its effects rather than pursue an analytic approach.

Boswell did not return to the subject of hypochondria for two and a half years, but essay No. 39 (December 1780) finds him writing "at this moment in a state of very dismal depression," and he decides to share his symptoms with his readers. As expected, they include such characteristics as: "His opinion of himself is low and desponding. His temporary dejection makes his faculties seem quite feeble. . . . He regrets his having ever attempted distinction and excellence in any way. . . . Nor has he any prospect of more agreeable days when he looks forward. . . . He is distracted between indolence and shame." He repeats from Hamlet (somewhat garbling the quotation),

How weary, stale, flat, and unprofitable
To me seem as the uses of this world!

Surprisingly, Boswell closes this essay by suggesting that a firm religious faith can dispel melancholy: "How blessed is the relief . . . from the divine comforts of religion! from the comforts of GOD . . . who graciously hears the prayers of the afflicted." Despite this capitulation to faith, Boswell remains somewhat cautious: "Dreadful beyond description is the state of the Hypochondriack who is bewildered in universal skepticism. But when the mind is sick and distressed, and has need of religion, that is not the time to acquire it." One cannot plead *de profundis* merely because one finds one's self in the bottomless pit. One must have paid one's dues in advance for the prayer to be effective. We ought not consider this a harsh judgment on the unbelieving. Boswell was genuinely shocked when he visited David Hume on his deathbed and found him an unregenerate nonbeliever, and we must remember that Boswell had been listening to Johnson for almost two decades. However we may judge Boswell's plea for faith, we cannot disregard the value to be placed on the essay's concluding lines: "While writing this paper, I have by some gracious influence been insensibly relieved from the distress under which I labored when I began it. May the same happy change be experienced by any of my readers, in the like affliction, is my sincere prayer." It appears that Johnson's work ethic was effective. Having occupied his mind with the task of writing his essay, Boswell's low spirits dissipated. What he did not comprehend is that alternation of mood and relief from depression are of uncertain cause and that apparent remission after a prescribed regimen may be misleading, if not due entirely to chance. We are not much wiser about the cause of melancholia today, but current psychiatric thought does not advocate treatment by faith and prayer.

The last of Boswell's essays on hypochondria (No. 63, December 1782) was written a few months after his father's death, and it begins auspiciously: "I have for so long a time been free of the fireful malady from which the title of this periodical paper is taken, that I almost begin to forget that I ever was afflicted with." He was either too tactful or lacked enough insight to relate his remission to Lord Auchinleck's death and inheriting his estate. Much of the essay is devoted to an encomium of Burton's *Anatomy of Melancholy,* which he doubtless read on

Johnson's recommendation. He recommends it to his readers not so much for its exposition of humoral theory but because of its admonition, *Sperate miseri, cavete felices,* "Let the wretched hope and the happy take care." The second half of the essay is a disquisition on the mind-body problem. Boswell disagreed with Revillon's recent *Recherches sur la cause des affections hypochondriques* (1779), which emphasized the influence of the body upon the mind: "That man is composed of two distinct principles, body or matter, and the mind, I firmly believe; and that these mutually act one upon another, is, I think, very certain. That the body influences the mind is commonly admitted; and it is equally certain that the mind influences the body." He supports that view with references to Frank Nicholl's *De anima medica* (1750) and William Battie's *Treatise on Madness* (1758). Apparently, Boswell was able to resolve his uncertainties about the mind-body problem, but whether he ever reconciled free will with determinism cannot be judged.

Even though Boswell's essays in *The Hypochondriack* are more literary exercises than psychological analyses, he was more modern and better conversant with medical ideas than was Johnson in the *Dictionary*. Boswell's ideas may not have been original, but he examined reputable sources and was sufficiently confident of his opinions to refute popularly held beliefs that were in error. Like most literary figures who wrote on melancholia, he drew upon his personal experience with the disease. Unlike Johnson, who, except for rare occasions, reserved his thoughts on melancholy to himself and his prayers, Boswell used both his journals and his essays in the persona of *The Hypochondriack* to gain some degree of self-knowledge and self-therapy. In his penetrating study of Boswell's imagery and melancholic stance, Allan Ingram comments:

> The imagination . . . maintains a permanent and inescapable relationship with the tendency to melancholy. . . . [I]t organizes the experience of melancholy using those elements of external reality which most correspond to the sensations of the condition. This is what constitutes the rhetoric of melancholy upon which Boswell is able to draw in *The Hypochondriack* in order to touch the common imagination of fellow sufferers and so inspire a sort of community of consciousness among his readers. But secondly, the imagination itself produces . . . the phantasms and fancies

that inhabit the melancholy vision, or else casts the melancholic's distempered ideas in so powerful a way that his weakened judgment is induced to take them for valid representations of reality.[33]

This contemporary statement is not so far removed from Timothy Bright's comment in 1586 that the "monstrous fiction[s] . . . which the judgment taking as they are presented by the disordered instrument, deliver over to the hart, which hath no judgment of discretion in it self, but giving mistaken credit to the report of the braine, breaketh out in the inordinate passion against reason. . . ."[34]

And the wheel has come full cycle.

Conclusion

Frank Brady says that *The Hypochondriack* is Boswell's only long work to be a failure because it brought out his weaknesses rather than his strengths.[35] This is true if, as Brady later admits, one reads them in batches rather than singly. True enough, as an essayist Boswell lacks Bacon's command of aphorism and Johnson's ability to abstract from experience (which accounts for the enduring value of the *Rambler* and *Idler* essays), but as a contributor to a monthly magazine he writes at no lower a level than Addison and Steele in the *Tatler* or the *Spectator*. With respect to his comments on hypochondria, twentieth-century readers must remember that he was not describing a state of imaginary invalidism or a neurosis, but what for his century was a specific disease with a rich variety of definable symptoms that culminated in disabling depression, an "impotence of Mind." Brady points out that Boswell could not understand why Johnson, a fellow sufferer, could think his depression an affectation. Though Johnson had heard Boswell complain of hypochondria often enough, he had never seen him in a fit of depression. The Boswell Johnson knew was in high spirits, enjoying London with loquacious exuberance, perhaps even hypomanic with respect to his gambling and compulsive whoring. The difference seems one of tone: Johnson presents his melancholia with a stoic facade; Boswell whimpers with self-indulgence.

9

Margery Kempe:
Hysteria and
Mysticism Reconciled

> But I, except in bed,
> Wore hair-cloth next the skin,
> And nursed more than my child
> That grudge against my side.
> Now, spirit and flesh assoil'd.
> Against the wild world
> I lace my pride in,
> Crying out odd and even.
> —Howard Nemerov, "A Poem of Margery Kempe"[1]

Margery Kempe (ca. 1373–ca. 1440) was a fifteenth-century Englishwoman whose *Book* is a narrative of her pilgrimages and spiritual experiences. With a poet's insight Howard Nemerov tells us clearly that her incurable wound was sustained in childbearing and delivery, that the damage to her ego (pride, first of the deadly sins) was as much spiritual as physical, that it set her against the world, and that she cried out against it, appearing odd to her neighbors but keeping even with her pilgrimage through life. The epigraph for this essay is the final strophe of Nemerov's poem, but the refrain that recurs after each stanza is

> Alas! that ever I did sin.
> It is full merry in heaven.

These words she uttered one night after hearing a melody "so sweet and delectable, that she thought she had been in Paradise."[2] Her past sins debarred her from heaven, and she repented of them. Coupling this insight with what is known of Margery's biography, what we can learn from her writing, what medical inferences can be drawn, perhaps we can approach a more detailed, if less poetic, definition of her particular problem and illuminate some of the medical aspects of mystical experience.

Until 1934 all that was known of Margery Kempe was seven pages in a quarto pamphlet printed by Wynkyn de Worde in 1501, titled *A shorte treatyse of contemplacyon taught by our lorde Ihesu cryste, or taken out of the boke of Margerie kempe of Lynn*. A single copy was preserved in the Cambridge University Library, and its contents were selected passages so chosen as not to offend the religious sensibilities of early Tudor readers. These extracts gave a flavorless impression of Margery's character and spiritual development. In 1934 Colonel William Butler-Bowdon, the representative of an old recusant Roman Catholic family in Yorkshire, sent for examination by experts at the Victoria and Albert Museum a manuscript book that had been "in the possession of [his] family from time immemorial."[3] Hope Emily Allen identified it as the lost *Book* of Margery Kempe. Marginal notes in the manuscript as well as analysis of the handwriting, paper, and watermarks indicated that it had been written at King's Lynn between 1440 and 1450 and had been in the possession of the Yorkshire Charterhouse of Mount Grace prior to the dissolution of the monasteries. Colonel Butler-Bowdon published a modern English version of the text in 1936, and a full critical edition supplemented by extensive annotation by Miss Allen was published by the Early English Text Society in 1940.

Appearing *de novo* from five centuries past but lacking an established niche in the English mystical tradition, Margery Kempe was not warmly received by the public; even the Anglican and Roman Catholic press was reserved. To be sure, the late 1930s was not the optimal time to introduce a new mystic. The economic depression that began in 1929 was slowly improving, but political events in Europe were ominous. Waiting for the gun-butt on the door often precludes mystical contemplation, though Sir Thomas More's *Dialogue of Comfort* and John Bunyan's *Pilgrim's Progress* are notable exceptions. The general level of spiritual aspiration in the 1930s was no higher than the moral rearmament advocated by the Oxford Group. Prophets, let alone mystics, were not wanted.

In her prefatory note Miss Allen quotes Father David Thurston, S.J., who wrote soon after the *Book* appeared, "That Margery was a victim of hysteria can hardly be open to doubt." In an earlier definition of hysteria Thurston had written that it was "chiefly . . . an exaggeration of suggestibility," a concept derived from the relation between hysteria and hypnotic states by the nineteenth-century studies of Charcot, Janet, and their predecessors.[4] But Miss Allen tempers that diagnosis with her own judgment:

> I do not believe that Margery's book can be explained, as I first thought, as merely the naïve outburst of an illiterate woman, who had persuaded two pliant men to write down her egotistical reminiscences. . . .
>
> . . . Obviously, many factors forbid her idea of herself as a great mystic from being accepted. . . . [I]t has seemed to me that . . . the best chance of understanding her life and work lay along the line of ascribing to her some degree, at least, of endowment with the spiritual graces (or psychological phenomena) which are called mysticism. I would call her a minor mystic.[5]

Two decades later Martin Thornton attempted to reconcile Margery's mysticism with the realities of everyday life:

> [S]he may not be much of a mystic but she was a first-class parishioner, with all the faults and failings that first-class parishioners usually have. . . . [L]et us call her an ordinary Christian matron, . . . who nevertheless did some very extra-ordinary things. . . . I do not wish to deny that [she] knew "mystical" experience, but that does not make her a "Mystic." True mystical experience is notoriously difficult to describe in words—some would say that it was impossible—and on the occasions when Margery claims to have reached it she wisely refrains from attempting any such description. What she does explain, so vividly and accurately, are the "ordinary" ascetical processes of recollection, meditation, and colloquy.[6]

To say that she "wisely refrains" is to impute to her a verbal sophistication to which she could not and did not pretend. If anything, the flow of words and sentences in the *Book* is unrestrained. As for the "ordinary" processes of asceticism, one can only mildly ask just how common they were in the first half of the fifteenth century, or indeed, our own.

Admittedly it is difficult to assess or even communicate the nature or quality of a mystical experience, but Dom David Knowles attempts both a rating scale and a comparison: "[T]he book is not in any real sense a treatise on contemplation, and Margery herself, however interesting a figure she may be to the student of religious sentiment or psychology, is clearly not the equal of the earlier English mystics in depth or perception or wisdom of spiritual doctrine, nor as a personality can she challenge comparison with Juliana of Norwich."[7] To complain that the *Book* is not a treatise on contemplation is to subscribe to the title Wynkyn de Worde fixed to his inadequate extract seventy years later. Margery Kempe made no such claim. The "Proem" describes the *Book* as "a short treatise and a comfortable [i.e., reassuring one], for sinful wretches, wherein they may have a great solace and comfort to themselves and understand the high and unspeakable mercy of our Sovereign Saviour Christ Jesus" (p. 1). By dictating her spiritual biography Margery Kempe intended only to provide comfort to others who were troubled in heart and mind. Knowles is not precise about the scale on which he rates depth of perception, but even conceding that point, a personality challenge does not settle the merits of a pointless comparison. By what criterion can one judge which mystic had the more mystique?

It would be presumptuous for a physician to gauge spiritual depth, but there are other dimensions to Margery Kempe. A synopsis of the major events in her life may serve to orient her in time and place. Born circa 1373 at King's Lynn, then an important commercial center in Norfolk, she was the daughter of John Brunham, who had been the town's mayor in 1370–71 and would be mayor three times later. We are told nothing about her mother or any siblings. About 1393 she married John Kempe, whose antecedents are unknown, but who served as one of the town's chamberlains in 1394–95. The family was prosperous, and all auguries pointed to a conventional life in the mercantile class. Disaster struck when Margery developed a prolonged psychotic episode after the birth of her first child, but she was cured when Christ appeared to her in a vision, saying, "Daughter, why hast thou forsaken Me, and I forsook never thee?" (p. 11). Following this experience she resumed life with her husband and had sufficient stability to go into business, first as a brewer, then as a miller. Both ventures proved unsuccessful. She became preoccupied with religious ideas and desired to live in celibacy with her husband. At one point in the text she writes of having borne fourteen children to him, but whether this total includes miscarriages or how many children survived infancy is not stated; late in the text she does write about one son who grew to adulthood, married a German woman, and had a daughter, but died young. In 1413

John Kempe finally acceded to Margery's wish to live chaste. One condition he made was that she pay his debts; apparently he was equally unsuccessful in trade. Perhaps twenty years of marriage to an unresponsive woman who complied only passively with his physical demands made him lose interest in pursuing their physical relationship.

At this point Margery was free to follow her spiritual vocation. She did penance, wore a haircloth, and had interviews with Philip Repington, Bishop of Lincoln, and Thomas Arundel, Archbishop of Canterbury, trying to secure their permission to wear a white mantle and a ring to symbolize her chastity and to represent it to the world. In his perceptive introduction, R. W. Chambers writes: "And note how Margery got them both on their weak spot. She charged Philip Repington . . . with want of moral courage: the very thing that his enemies were saying at the time, and historians have said ever since. She charged the high-born Arundel with not rising to the responsibilities of the supreme position to which he had been called. If Margery had tried to 'dally' in this way with two English prelates of the nineteenth or even of the twentieth century, I am not sure that the interview would have gone off so pleasantly" (p. xxv). In the event, both fifteenth-century prelates gave her money, and she set off on a pilgrimage to Italy and the Holy Land. The *Book* recounts her experiences there, including her mystical marriage to the Godhead in the Apostles' Church at Rome in November 1414. In 1417 she made a pilgrimage to the shrine of St. James of Compostella. The following year she returned to Lynn, which became the base for numerous visits to religious establishments in England for the next decade. Some of these excursions landed her in trouble. At both Leicester and York she was charged with Lollardy, but she defended herself bravely and with wise words against the hostile Mayor of Leicester, the Archbishop of York, and the Duke of Bedford's underlings. John Kempe died in 1431, as did their son shortly after his return from Germany with his wife and daughter. In 1433 Margery embarked on further travels, visiting Norway and Germany. She began dictating her *Book* to a priest in 1436; when her amanuensis died in 1438, she found another priest to take down the short section titled "Book II." The following year she was admitted to the Guild of the Trinity, a semi-conventual house at Lynn, and she probably died there around 1440.

Margery supplies no details of her childhood or adolescence. Her *Book* begins with the statement that she was married at twenty years of age "or some deal more" and was with child within a short time. Labor and delivery might have been difficult, and they precipitated an episode that today would be classified as a postpartum depressive psychosis with features of agitation:

> [S]he despaired of her life, weening she might not live. And then she sent for her ghostly father, for she had a thing on her conscience which she had never shewn before that time in all her life. For she was ever hindered by her enemy, the devil, evermore saying to her that whilst she was in good health she needed no confession, but to do penance by herself alone and all should be forgiven, for God is merciful enough. . . .
>
> And when she was at any time sick or dis-eased, the devil said in her mind that she should be damned because she was not shriven of that default. Wherefore . . . she, not trusting to live, sent for her ghostly father, . . . in full will to be shriven.
>
> . . . And when she came to the point for to say that thing which she had so long concealed, her confessor was a little too hasty and began sharply to reprove her before she had fully said her intent, and so she would no more say for aught he might do. Anon, for the dread she had of damnation on the one side, and his sharp reproving of her on the other side, [she] went out of her mind . . . and laboured with spirits for half a year, eight weeks and odd days. (Pp. 9–10)

If Margery's recollection is accurate, her postpartum psychosis lasted somewhat more than eight months. The most plausible pathogenesis is that she had deep-seated feelings of guilt for an unconfessed sin she had committed prior to her marriage and that the sin was that of premarital sexual activity. It is tempting to conjecture that her partner was not the man she later married, for in the fourteenth century premarital sex between a betrothed couple was not considered a grave sin. Her confessor seems to have had limited psychological insight; he failed to allow her the catharsis of a full and complete confession and, when she became mute, would not grant her absolution. In Judaeo-Christian societies, feelings of sexual guilt are a common cause of emotional disturbance, and the Christian sacrament of penance which follows verbal confession is designed to lift the burden of guilt from the repentant and contrite. One would think a wiser or more experienced confessor might have been more sensitive to what, after all, must have been a frequent occurrence in his parish. Margery's attempt to secure absolution failed, and psychotic symptoms such as delusions and self-destructive behavior followed rapidly:

> [S]he saw, as she thought, devils opening their mouths all inflamed with burning waves of fire, as if they would have swallowed her in, sometimes ramping at her, sometimes threatening her, pulling her and hauling her. . . . [T]he devils cried upon her . . . that she should forsake Christendom, her faith, and deny her God. . . . She said many a wicked word, and many a cruel word; she knew no virtue nor goodness; she desired all wickedness; like as the spirits tempted her to say and do, so she said and did. . . . [S]he bit her own hand so violently, that the mark was seen all her life after.
>
> And also she rived the skin on her body against her heart with her nails spitefully, for she had no other instruments, and worse she would have done, but that she was bound and kept with strength day and night. . . . (P. 10)

At this point she had her vision of Christ, "clad in a mantle of purple silk, sitting upon her bedside, looking upon her with so blessed a face that she was strengthened in all her spirit" (p. 11). There is no objective criterion for distinguishing a vision from an hallucination, but the effect of the epiphany was almost instantaneous: "[A]non this creature became calmed in her wits and reason, as well as ever she was before, and prayed her husband as soon as he came to her, that she might have the keys of the buttery to take her meat and drink as she had done before" (p. 11). Acting against the advice of her attendants and servants, he did so.

Margery's recovery from the psychotic episode was complete. In a short while she was able to start the business enterprises that later failed. She interpreted her lack of success in worldly affairs as a sign from God that she should devote herself to matters of the spirit and spent much time in prayer and contemplation. She began to long for a celibate life, but her entreaties to her husband that they might live chastely together met with the reply that "it was good to do so, but he might not yet" (p. 16). With this reply he was in the goodly company of St. Augustine.

Margery relates an episode in which she was tempted to commit adultery, but when she finally consented, the man rejected her, saying "he never would for all the gold in this world" (p. 20). She was ashamed and felt that God had forsaken her; for the next year she was "afflicted with horrible temptations to lechery" (p. 20). It is difficult to interpret this episode in the history of a woman whose sexual impulses were so confused. Perhaps she misconstrued some friendly gestures by the man, projecting her unconscious desires upon him. Her conflicts were resolved when she was at prayer in a chapel "weeping wondrous sore" (p. 21); Christ appeared to her, reassured her of his love, told her to abstain from eating flesh, and recommended contemplation and meditation. This was the first of many conversations she reports having had with Christ. She also had conversations with the Virgin Mary and St. Anne, the Virgin's mother. It was after this that she and her husband struck their bargain: She would pay his outstanding debts in return for his abstention from sexual relations and his permission to make a pilgrimage to Jerusalem.

Much of the *Book* describes her tribulations as a pilgrim. She traveled the dusty and muddy roads dressed in white, the emblem of her purity but hardly the most suitable costume. Other pilgrims avoided her, chiefly because they found her frequent fits of "great weeping, boisterous sobbing, and loud crying" (p. 102) objectionable and distracting. These fits would occur whenever she took Communion, occasionally when she was at prayer, but also spontaneously: "Sometimes she wept full plenteously . . . for desire of the bliss of Heaven, and because she was so long deferred therefrom" (p. 25). Her fellow travelers in Venice misinformed her about their plans for arranging passage because they had no desire for her company in the close quarters of a sailing vessel. "[P]eople were oftentimes afraid and greatly astonished deeming she had been vexed with some evil spirit or a sudden sickness, not believing it was the work of God, but rather . . . simulation and hypocrisy . . ." (p. 106), a charge easily made by those whose religious fervor does not express itself with such doleful public exuberance. Her outbursts are not typical of English piety, which then as now was little inclined to extravagant self-expression. Margery records dozens of such incidents with what can only be called *la belle indifférence* to both her own symptoms and the reactions of other people. In the meantime her conversations with Christ continued, and in November 1414 the mystical marriage to Him was accomplished at Rome.

Margery's description of the postnuptial effects of the ceremony leaves no doubt that it was a sublimation of the physical aspects of marriage: "Our Lord gave her another token . . . and that was a flame of fire, wondrous hot and delectable, and right comfortable, not wasting but ever increasing, of love; for though the weather were never so cold, she felt the heat burning in her breast and at her heart, as verily as a man could feel the material fire if he put his hand or his finger therein" (p. 113). Concomitantly, she developed both olfactory and auditory symptoms as a penumbra to her state of grace:

> Sometimes she felt sweet smells with her nose . . . sweeter, she thought, than ever was any sweet earthly thing that she smelt before. . . .
>
> Sometimes she heard with her bodily ears . . . sounds and melodies . . . nearly every day . . . especially when she was in devout prayer. . . . (P. 112)

Likewise she had "divers tokens in her bodily hearing . . . a sort of sound as if it were a pair of bellows blowing in her ear. She, being abashed thereby, was warned in her soul no fear to have, for it was the sound of the Holy Ghost. And then Our Lord turned [it] into the voice of a dove, and later on, He turned it into the voice of a little bird which is called a red-breast, that sang full merrily oftentimes in her right ear" (p. 116).

Margery also developed visual symptoms. One day at Mass she saw that "the Sacrament shook and flickered to and fro, as a dove flickereth with her wings" (p. 61), but more distinctive was a recurrent vision: "She saw with her bodily eyes many white things flying all about her on every side, as thick . . . as specks in a sunbeam. They were right subtle and comfortable, and the brighter the sun shone, the better might she see them. She saw them many divers times and in many divers places, both in church and in her chamber, . . . in the fields, and in town . . ." (p. 113). The description suggests scotomata, common in migraine, but Margery did not complain of headaches. An epileptiform component accompanied some of her outbursts: "[W]hen they came up on to the Mount of Calvary, she fell down because she could not stand or kneel, and rolled and wrested with her body, spreading her arms abroad, and cried with a loud voice . . ." (p. 87). She records several such convulsive episodes, all of which took place in public, and apparently she sustained no injuries in any of her falls. She also retained consciousness and sufficient memory of them to record at least some of the details a quarter of a century later.

The fits of "boisterous sobbing" continued and were precipitated chiefly when she contemplated Christ's sufferings or when she was houseled, that is, received the Sacrament. In 1431 her husband died; in a touching chapter she describes his gradual deterioration over the period of a year following a fall downstairs, presumably the result of a cerebrovascular accident (pp. 235–38). Significantly, it was only after this bereavement that she prayed to be relieved of her crying fits.

> Lord, why wilt Thou give me such crying that people wonder at me therefor? . . . I had rather . . . be in a prison ten fathoms deep, there to cry and weep for my sin. . . .
> . . . I pray Thee, if it be Thy will, take these cryings from me at the time of sermons, . . . and let me have them by myself alone. . . .
> . . . give it me alone in my chamber. . . . (p. 238–39)

Thus the first breach in Margery's remarkable indifference, the first indication that she recognized that her outbursts of weeping were a nuisance to others, occurred after her husband's death had removed him as a potential sexual threat. Nonetheless, her symptoms must have served some need, for she reports Christ's denial of her petition: "[D]aughter, suffer the people to say what they will of thy crying, for thou art no cause of their sin. . . . [T]he people sinned over Me, yet was I no cause of their sin" (p. 241).

Even her repeated conversations with Christ and His reassurances of His love did not entirely quell her sexual impulses:

> [S]o now she had as many hours of foul thoughts and foul memories of lechery and all uncleanness, as though she had been common to all manner of people. . . .
> . . . horrible sights and abominable, for aught she could do, of beholding men's members. . . .
> She saw, as she thought verily, divers men of religion, priests and many others, both heathen and Christian, coming before her sight, . . . shewing their bare members unto her. (Pp. 189–90)

The comforts of her special relationship with the Godhead are recorded in the following speech she reports Christ as making: "[T]hou mayest boldly, when thou art in thy bed, take Me to thee as thy wedded husband, . . . and I will that thou lovest Me, daughter, as a good wife ought to love her husband. Therefore thou mayest boldly take Me in the arms of thy soul and kiss My mouth, My head, and My feet, as sweetly as thou wilt" (p. 116). Indeed, she claimed to have had the promised experience. In an ecstatic vision she saw "Our Lord standing right up over her, so near that she thought she took His toes in her hand and felt them, and to her feeling, it was as if they had been very flesh and bone" (p. 274).

However a psychologically more sophisticated readership may assess her emotional status some six and one half centuries later, there is no room for doubt that such conversations and visions were therapeutic. Her feelings of guilt may not have been repressed, but she had no recurrence of psychotic episodes. The *Book* also records her numerous acts of kindness and charity. She nursed the husband whom she had sexually rejected through the long year of his decline. She visited the sick and prayed at many sickbeds, sometimes successfully, but she made no claim of being able to perform miracles. Instead, she wrote, "[P]atience is more worthy than miracle-working" (p. 158). One remarkable incident is her encounter with a woman who had developed a postpartum psychosis, even as Margery herself had. The woman was violent and had to be restrained, so obstreperous that she had to be kept in a room on the outskirts of the town. Margery visited her daily, and when she spoke with her, the madwoman was "meek enough." Margery prayed for her recovery regularly, and after a while, "God gave her her wits and her mind again" (p. 234). Gradual recovery from postpartum psychosis is not unexpected, but that the woman could communicate rationally with Margery and no one else suggests a special gift and probably insight on Margery's part.

Not all of Margery's symptoms were emotional or psychosomatic. After her return to Lynn from refuting the charge of Lollardy, she was stricken by a severe "flux," or dysentery, so prostrated that she was given the last rites. Soon thereafter she developed recurrent attacks of what sounds like gallstones: pain "set in her right side, lasting the time of eight years. . . . Sometimes she had it once a week, . . . so hard and so sharp that she must void what was in her stomach, as bitter as if it were gall, neither eating nor drinking . . . till it was gone" (p. 180). It was during these attacks that she pleaded with Christ, "Lord, because of Thy great pain, have mercy on my little pain" (p. 180). A medical detective in the twentieth century could plausibly speculate that her dysentery had been typhoid fever and that, as often happens, it was followed by cholelithiasis.

At this point it would be easy enough to dismiss Margery Kempe with a diagnosis of religious hysteria. The elements for the diagnosis are explicit in her account of herself: the background of guilt for pre-marital, perhaps even juvenile, sexual experiences, for marital sexual relations and more especially for impulses to adultery, the fits of public weeping and sobbing, the migraine-like scotomata, the convulsions, the visions and other sensory disturbances, the conversations, and the bland acceptance of her symptoms and obliviousness of their effect on others. But there is more to Margery than to the usual religious hysteric.

Like diversely attributed medieval paintings, Margery Kempe has been "variously judged." Her *Book* has been read as anything from the work of a saintly mystic to that of an hysterical exhibitionist, and indeed both qualities are present. Knowles writes that

> In her favour . . . editors and most readers agree that her story gives an impression of basic sincerity. Margery may seem restless, talkative and self-centered, but she is at the same time a woman of faith and goodwill, charitable in word and deed; she never abuses her opponents and even suppresses their names, . . . when she can be checked, she is found accurate and truthful, and she displays courage, candour and good sense in many of her encounters with critics great and small.[8]

She made no attempt to proselytize, nor did she found a sect. When arrested and charged with being a Lollard, she proved her orthodoxy before a hostile ecclesiastical court.[9]

Unlike most hysterics, Margery did not repress her consciousness of sin. Early in the text, when she asked Christ how best she might love him, she records his reply: "Have mind of thy wickedness and think of My goodness" (p. 63). Her identification with the Godhead was complete in a mystical sense, and she repeats Christ's reassurances of it: "[F]or I am a hidden God in thee . . ." (p. 40) and "Daughter, how often have I told thee that thy sins are forgiven thee, and that we are united (in love) together without end" (p. 65). This sense of identity reached many daily experiences; when she would see a wounded man or animal, or when she would see a man beating a child or a horse, she would equate it with Christ being beaten or wounded (p. 88). From this mystical union she finally reaped her reward. On one occasion when she was in difficulty because of the hostility of her fellow towns-people, Christ comforted her: ". . . I must needs comfort thee, for now thou hast the right way to Heaven. By this way, came I to Heaven and all My disciples, for now thou shalt know the better what sorrow and shame I suffered for thy love, and thou shalt have the more compassion when thou thinkest on My Passion" (p. 204).

There is no reason to doubt Margery's intention that she was writing a book designed to bring comfort to other sinners. She used her own experiences, however we may judge them and their psychological roots, as the basis for a text of spiritual consolation for others similarly afflicted. It may be true that many passages do not rise above the level of "I love to tell the story / Of Jesus and his glory," but if her spiritual communications lack the depth of other English medieval mystics, that may reflect the weakness of her education and that of her spiritual advisers rather than the nature and quality of her subjective experiences.

Margery Kempe invites comparison with St. Juliana of Norwich, the anchoress whom she visited in 1413 shortly before departing for Rome. In 1373, then about thirty years old, Juliana had experienced sixteen "shewings" or visions during the crisis and defervescence of an acute febrile illness. We know nothing about Juliana's youth and early womanhood except that she was unmarried. Perhaps the effects of a high fever facilitated the appearance of visions of Christ and the Virgin Mary, but the images elicited by a toxic delirium could only have taken the forms they did in a mind already prepared to see them. She had no further visions but retired from the world and became an anchoress at Norwich. She lived in enclosed solitude but received the large number of people who sought her guidance. Under these circumstances she wrote her *Revelations of Divine Love,* meditations based on her visions. Unlike Margery's *Book,* it is not a narrative of her life's experiences in the world but a set of spiritual exercises. St. Juliana advised Margery that "the Holy Ghost asketh for us with mourning and weeping unspeakable, [and] He maketh us to ask and pray with mourning and weeping so plenteously that the tears may not be numbered," and she enjoined her to "fear not the language of the world, for the more despite, shame and reproof that ye have in the world, the more is your merit in the sight of God" (pp. 55–56). At least that is Margery's verbatim report of their conversation when she came to dictate it more than thirty years later. St. Juliana clearly believed, as do many Christians, that suffering, either by illness or alienation, was necessary to achieve God's grace, and Margery was quite ready to take literally her remarks about the Holy Ghost's mourning and weeping.

T. S. Eliot's *Murder in the Cathedral* reminds us that a Christian martyrdom is never the work of man; it is always the design of God. (A martyr has been described as someone who has to live with a saint.) Even so, God's instrument for producing martyrs seems to be human hands. It is a human being who lights the pyre, wields the axe, or initiates whatever means have been ordained to dispatch and thereby create the martyr. If we are to believe that mystical experiences are likewise the work of God, not willed by man, He has chosen the human mind as His instrument. The experience is *cognitive* and involves the entire consciousness. In addition to involving the psyche, it is commonly translated into sensory experiences and is frequently accompanied by expressive behavior. For such reasons, the mystical experience has exercised and frustrated the descriptive and analytic powers of psychologists and psychiatrists alike. A precondition of the mystical experience seems to be that it occurs only to those who are ready and willing to receive it. In that context, Margery's postpartum psychosis and her recovery from it set the stage for her continuing direct communication with the Godhead. I do not imply that she consciously sought this communication, but when the event occurred, she found that it gave her satisfaction, and she was ready and willing to experience it again.

A generation before Charcot's studies of hysteria, Robert Carter classified the disorder into three progressive changes. The initial paroxysm was "primary," and could be a nonrecurrent episode. If subsequent attacks appeared following induced or spontaneous recall of the emotions that had elicited the primary incident, these were "secondary." "Tertiary" attacks were those "designedly excited by the patient herself through the instrumentality of voluntary recollection, and with perfect knowledge of her own power to produce them."[10] Under such a rubric one would classify St. Juliana's sixteen "shewings" as a primary event and Margery's continuing dialogues and visions as tertiary hysteria. Carter's next point is that the patient most likely to develop the tertiary form is one who feels herself neglected and uncared for rather than a victim of sexual frustration; logically, her efforts are designed to bring her sympathy and solicitous attention. Margery may not have received much solicitude from most of her contemporaries, but she was in almost daily contact with her spiritual advisers, and they took her seriously.

From the earliest days of the Church, ecclesiastical authorities had reservations about communicants with mystical or ecstatic experiences.

Ronald Knox cites Athenagoras as writing that prophets were "lifted in ecstasy above the natural operation of their minds by the impulses of the Divine Spirit, . . . inspired to utterance, the Spirit making use of them as a flute-player breathes into a flute."[11] But the Church branded Athenagoras a heretic, and the patristic tradition held that a prophet must be conscious and in full command of his faculties. However, the tradition was not invariably followed, and Knox comments.

> The mystic tradition was that you were justified in thus abandoning yourself to the breath of the Holy Spirit. . . .
>
> . . . [Yet] no writers have insisted more strongly than the mystics themselves on the fact that ecstasy can be counterfeited by diabolic influence, or even by hysteria. One of the privileges of sanctity, it is not necessarily a mark of sanctity. . . . [T]he spokesmen of orthodoxy, not without excuse, were inclined to view with suspicion any kind of enthusiasm which was accompanied by alienation of the senses.

Margery's outbursts were a departure from conventional orthodox behavior, but she did not belong to any of the definable heretical sects of the Middle Ages. She was no Albigensian, Anabaptist, Catharist, Manichean, or Lollard. She traveled her own spiritual path, and the key to her unique pilgrimage is ecstasy, not doctrine.

Many writers have commented on the sexual aspects of mystical experience, and the erotic element is either explicit or implicit in many accounts. Margery's vision of priests "shewing their bare members to her" is easily understood as representing an unfulfilled wish. Materialists use the point to reduce mystical experience to a reflex or animalistic level, and Margery, like other mystics, leaves us no doubt about the sexual implications of her responses. But R. C. Zaehner cautions that "there is scarcely a form of *religious* mysticism . . . in which sexual imagery does not turn up. . . . Even—and indeed particularly—the Christian mystics who go into ecstasy over their spiritual espousals with God or Christ cannot accept the rapture . . . as anything but a diabolical caricature of the raptures of the spirit in which the soul is ravished by God. Yet 'ravishing' and 'rapture' are, after all, only a polite way of saying 'rape.'"[13] The sexual imagery in the *Book* does not invalidate Margery's experiences, subjective as they inevitably were.

Inevitably, an individual undergoing mystical experience interprets it in accordance with the religion or ideology in which he or she has been brought up. One can scarcely imagine that a Hindu mystic would have a vision of Christ crucified. Likewise, as Ilza Veith points out, hysteria "defies definition and any attempt to portray it concretely. . . . Whenever it appears it takes on the colors of the ambient culture and mores; and thus throughout the ages it presents itself as a shifting, changing, mist-enshrouded phenomenon that must, nevertheless, be dealt with as though it were definite and tangible."[14] It is in that sense that Charcot, Bernheim, Janet, Breuer, and Freud investigated the disorder, and we are indebted to them for a clear delineation of its varying clinical features and psychodynamics. Contemporaneous with them was William James, whose Gifford lectures at Edinburgh in 1901–2 form the basis for the twentieth-century view of mysticism.

"Mysticism," James wrote, ". . . is essentially private and individualistic. . . ." Feeling (the deeper source of religion than philosophical or theological formation)

> is private and dumb, and unable to give an account of itself. It allows that its results are mysteries and enigmas, declines to justify them rationally, and on occasion is willing that they should even pass for paradoxical and absurd. . . . To redeem religion from unwholesome privacy, and to give public status and universal right of way to its deliverances, has been reason's task.[15]

Rational discourse has long been highly valued on New England's stern and rockbound coast, and the Massachusetts Bay Colony was founded by religious dissenters who insisted on the public status of their faith. Yet there is a private aspect to one's devotion that scarcely merits the pejorative "unwholesome." In most faiths the individual prays directly to God and is personally accountable to Him, and many believers in such religions feel that God, or part of Him, is immanent within themselves.

James' application of reason to mysticism led to his justly famous characterization of mystical experience:

> 1. *Ineffability.*—. . . [The experience] defies expression, . . . its contents can[not] be given in words. . . . its quality must be directly experienced. . . .
> 2. *Noetic quality.*—. . . [S]tates of insight into depths of truth unplumbed by . . . intellect. . . . illuminations, revelations, full of significance . . . with . . . a curious sense of authority. . . .

3. *Transiency.*—. . . Except in rare instances, half an hour, or at most an hour or two, seems to be the limit. . . .

4. *Passivity.*—. . . [T]he mystic feels as if his own will were in abeyance, . . . as if he were grasped and held by a superior power.[16]

The formulation has stood the test of eight decades, but like so many descriptions, it does not explain, nor did James intend it to carry that burden. Margery Kempe's account fulfills most of its terms except that she was able to report, perhaps imperfectly, her experiences. However, her *Book* was not public knowledge until three decades later. James does not allude to hysteria specifically, nor did he attempt a clinical application of his ideas. A clue to his general approach can be found in his first lecture, titled "Religion and Neurology."

As regards the psychopathic origin of so many religious phenomena, that would not be in the least surprising or disconcerting, even were such phenomena certified from on high to be the most precious of human experiences. . . . Few of us are not in some way infirm, or even diseased; and our very infirmities help us unexpectedly. In the psychopathic temperament we have the emotionality which is the *sine qua non* of moral perception; . . . the intensity and tendency to emphasis which are the essence of practical moral vigor; and we have the love of metaphysics and mysticism which carry one's interests beyond the surface of the sensible world. . . .

If there were such a thing as inspiration from a higher realm, it might well be that the neurotic temperament would furnish the chief condition of the requisite receptivity.[17]

The key to susceptibility to mysticism appears then to be receptivity to whatever stimulus is sufficient to elicit the response. In Margery's case the stimulus was usually prayer, receiving the Sacrament, or meditation on the Passion, though her boisterous sobbing was occasionally precipitated by other sights and sounds. Her visions were those of Eros and of God, but unlike, for example, St. Teresa of Avila, who denied it, she heard and saw her visions "with her bodily eyes, . . . [and] her bodily ears."[18] If, under the light of Carter's concept of voluntary recollections and perfect knowledge of her power to produce them, we examine her receptivity, it becomes clear that the response of her sensorium was not so much a matter of heightened awareness or altered consciousness as one of increased autosuggestibility, and that is the denominator common to both hysteria and mysticism. That Margery did not repress recollection of her sin and that her fits recurred for over thirty years indicates that they were a necessary form of self-therapy to avoid recurrence of psychosis and that her passage through the three phases of the *via mystica* (*purgatio, illuminatio, unio*) was a valid solution to her emotional problems in the context of her time. The mystic sees the ineffable, but the psychobiographer sees the unspeakable.

10
All the Colours
of the Rimbaud

The short unhappy life and brief poetic career of Arthur Rimbaud (1854–91) invite comparison with the angel Lucifer, whom Spenser called "the brightest angel, even the child of Light." But most readers will recall Lucifer from *Paradise Lost* as Milton's demon of sinful pride (*hubris*). Milton derived his pejorative casting from St. Jerome, who misread a phrase in Isaiah and applied the name "Lucifer" to Satan, the adversary. But Isaiah 14:12 merely exclaims, "How art thou fallen from Heaven, O Lucifer, son of the morning!" an apostrophe to Nebuchadnezzar, who later ate grass. Indeed, Rimbaud's contrarieties include many variora. As son of the morning his poetic gifts blossomed early. Though he may not have fallen from Heaven, he fell from grace. He was the Child of Light, at least the bearer of *Les illuminations,* but he was also guilty of *hubris*. At times he was angelic, at times satanic. Readers may tire of melodramatic antitheses between good and evil, but the young French poet was a curious admixture of both, and in varying degrees, shades, and hues.

Until recent years Rimbaud has not been too well served by his biographers, and critics have read into his poems what they wanted to find. The few scattered medical comments on Rimbaud have been notable for a lack of information and inaccuracy. This essay examines Rimbaud from a medical point of view: a discussion of his psychosexual development, the influence of drugs and alcohol on his poetry, and the nature of his illnesses during his last years. The last are relatively unimportant *per se,* merely a rectification of the record. Except as noted by citation, I have relied on the 1972 Pléiade edition of his poems and correspondence, and Enid Starkie's useful biography.[1] Several sources have been used for translations; these are specifically cited in each instance.

Inevitably, when one focuses the retrospectoscope on such material, lacunae in the fabric become apparent. Specific evidence one would like to have is not only not available; much of it was never recorded. Unlike Boswell, Rimbaud did not keep a journal, and one is forced to infer not only the sequence of events but the events themselves from his poems and letters to friends. Circumstances limit choices, and circumstantial evidence must be relied on to considerable extent. One must also be on guard lest suppression or distortion of evidence by well-meaning relatives and friends alter significant detail. In the long run the exposition and analysis presented here must be judged on its plausibility, its internal consistency, its "goodness of fit."

Psychosexual Development

FAMILY CONSTELLATION, CHILDHOOD, EARLY POEMS

Rimbaud's father was an army captain who had spent most of his military career in Algeria and Morocco. He had a gift for languages and is said to have translated the Koran into French. In 1850 at the age of thirty-eight he was posted to Mézières, a town in the Ardennes region, just south of the Belgian border, lying across the Meuse from Charleville. He had the reputation of being a fine soldier, a trustworthy officer, and a conscientious and humane administrator. In Charleville he met Vitalie Cuif, the twenty-eight-year-old daughter of a well-to-do farmer, and married her, perhaps more attracted by her substantial dowry than her beauty. Captain Rimbaud is described as easygoing, good-tempered, and generous; presumably he wanted a comfortable, undemanding marriage, but such was not to be his lot.

Rimbaud's mother has earned a thesaurus of pejorative adjectives from her son's biographers: stingy, bigoted, rigid, humorless, authoritarian, austere, strict. She seems to have been a woman incapable of giving affection; she had a firm and certain knowledge of what was right and wrong, what was proper and improper, what was respectable and disreputable. She proved to be singularly incapable of keeping her menfolk at home, and in that home it was she, not the captain, who gave the orders. Quarrels and arguments between husband and wife were frequent. In November 1853, eleven months after they were married, the Rimbauds had their first child, a son named Frédéric, and eleven months after that, a second son, Jean-Nicolas-Arthur, whose unhappy career we shall follow. After an interval three daughters were born, one who died at three months in 1857, Vitalie in 1858, and Isabelle in 1860. Mme. Rimbaud's father, who had kept peace between husband and wife, died in 1858, and Captain Rimbaud, tired of domestic wrangling, took his departure in 1860, two months after the birth of their fifth child. The children were raised entirely by their mother, for Captain Rimbaud never saw his wife or children again.

One can summon a degree of sympathy for Mme. Rimbaud, left with financial anxieties and embittered by her huband's abandonment. She was determined to maintain her status in the community and be known as one of the respectable and respected bourgeoisie of Charleville. She saw to it that her children were well mannered, clean, neatly dressed, and regular in the performance of their religious duties. Perhaps the rigid, strict discipline with which she reared them was an attempt to avoid the unfortunate example of her two brothers, both of whom were ne'er-do-wells and from whom she had no difficulty in wresting control, then ownership, of their father's farm. Regardless of her intentions, Frédéric turned out to be a hefty lout whose disgraceful life matched those of his uncles. Vitalie died of tuberculosis at seventeen. Isabelle grew up in her mother's image, a woman of conventional piety and limited intelligence who married late. But Arthur was the exceptional child with all the latent potential for disaster the term implies. In defense of Mme. Rimbaud's motherliness, one ought to note that there were thousands of French households with similar standards and values, and many such women raised sons who led untroubled, uneventful lives—and have been forgotten.

Rimbaud's early life fulfills one term of the stock combination "absent father/binding mother," but Mme. Rimbaud was anything but a mother who bound by overt affection. True enough, she supervised her two sons so closely that she would wait for them at the schoolhouse gate and escort them home, lest they learn naughty ways from other boys. Close constriction breeds rebellion, and Rimbaud's indictment of his mother in *Les poètes de sept ans* describes his hidden hostility. It was written before he turned seventeen, and though it purports to recall his state of mind at the age of seven, one year after his father's desertion, it more likely describes his emotions at a somewhat later age:

Et la Mère, fermant le livre du devoir,
S'en allait satisfaite et très fière, sans voir,
Dans les yeux bleus et sous le front plein d'éminences,
L'âme de son enfant livrée aux répugnances.

(And the Mother, closing the exercise book,
Went off satisfied and proud, without seeing
In the blue eyes, beneath the pimply forehead,
The horror and loathing in her child's soul.)[2]

Early in life Rimbaud learned to dissemble his real feelings under a mask of compliance to escape the pressure imposed by his mother. One avenue of escape was to the outhouse. In the next stanza he describes himself as

. . . vaincu, stupide, il était entête
A se renfermer dans la fraîcheur des latrines:
Il pensait là, tranquille et livrant ses narines.

(. . . defeated, dull, he was bent
On shutting himself up in the cool outhouse:
There he meditated, peacefully, opening his nostrils.)

It is not difficult to trace the prominent scatological elements in his poetry to the fragrance of this juvenile ambience.

Rimbaud's formal education began in 1862 when he entered the Pension Rossat. He was a quick student with a good vocabulary, and in the spring of 1865, at the age of eleven, he was ready to enter the Collège de Charleville, where his academic progress was rapid. Within a year it was evident that he had outstanding gifts, and at the end of the academic year 1868–69, having finished the *classe de seconde,* he won no fewer than nine first prizes. Externally, he conformed to the expected mold; as he later put it, "I sweated obedience."[3] He was well liked by his schoolmates and made at least two close friends who were sufficiently well behaved and from sufficiently respectable families to meet with his mother's approval. His particular talents were in languages. He had his father's knack for grasping the structure and feeling of foreign tongues, and his schoolboy compositions were precociously fluent.

Perhaps the most revealing of his accomplishments was the poem with which he won first prize in Latin Composition in November 1868 at the age of fourteen. The assignment was to develop in Latin verse the theme outlined by Horace in Ode 4 from Book 13: "As a boy, once, beside the Vultur in Apulia, not far from my house, tired of games and of sleep, wonderful doves covered me with new leaves. . . . I was crowned with sacred laurel and with myrtle, not without divine intent." Using the text as his point of departure, Rimbaud describes himself as a youth in the midst of a pastoral reverie carried aloft by a flock of doves to a distant subcelestial height where they crown him with laurel. At this point Phoebus Apollo appears:

Divina vocale manu praetendere plectrum
Tum capiti inscripsit caelesti haec nomina flamma.
TU VATES ERIS . . .

(His divine hand offered me the sounding lyre,
And with fire from heaven he traced these words on my brow:
YOU WILL BE A POET . . .)[3]

Note that the Latin word Rimbaud uses for poet is *vates,* not *poeta.* Even at that early age he conceived of a poet as a prophet, *un voyant,* a seer, rather than a maker or artificer of words, phrases, and stanzas. It was a bold notion for a boy of fourteen to project, but he maintained it and developed it further during the next five years. One speculates whether in some fashion exposure to his father's translation of the Koran, a prophetic book in an alien tongue, had initiated the idea. If so, perhaps his youthful wish to be a poet-prophet reflected a desire to supply himself with the attributes of an absent father.

There can be no doubt that Rimbaud lacked a male figure with which he could identify, and the consequences of that deficiency will shortly become apparent. In January 1870 a new teacher arrived at the Collège de Charleville, Georges Izambard, then twenty-two years old, fresh from the university, just given his first teaching assignment as master of rhetoric. He was young enough to be of Rimbaud's generation and to share its ideals. He had an intense interest in contemporary French literature and a well-stocked library with many books that the promising, intellectually curious Rimbaud was eager to read. Izambard gave his prize pupil the run of his library, and for the seven months he was at Charleville he combined the roles of teacher, adviser, guide, older brother, and father substitute. In the light of Rimbaud's later experiences it is important to state that there is no evidence of a homosexual component to this relationship, latent or overt. But Mme. Rimbaud did not surrender her son's mind or a share in his affections without a struggle. She thought Izambard was a bad influence and accused him of giving her son a book to read that was likely to corrupt his morals, the volume in question being Hugo's *Les misérables*. Twentieth-century readers may smile, but in 1870 Hugo's name was in bad odor. He had been exiled for his political views, and the scene in *Les misérables* in which a bishop asks forgiveness from a convicted felon was a shock to conventional pieties. Nor is it fair to label Mme. Rimbaud provincial; the view was held by many conservative Parisians. In the long run literature prevailed, and in Izambard's library young Rimbaud read not only Hugo but Baudelaire, only three years dead, and the poems of the then prominent Parnassian school—Banville, Coppée, Leconte de Lisle, Verlaine. In these few months of his sixteenth year Rimbaud decided his true vocation: Poet. In a letter to Banville accompanying some poems he hoped to have published in *Le Parnasse contemporain* he referred to himself as "a child touched by the finger of the Muse."

Yet behind the facade of the diligent student lay smoldering emotions, an impasto of impulses and aspirations that were, as is common in adolescents, especially those with a creative gift, ambivalent and self-contradictory. One can readily contrast the attitude of the young poet in *Première soirée,* so eager to embrace the young girl's body ("Elle était fort déshabillée"—She was quite undressed), with the stance assumed in *Vénus Anadyomène* written a few weeks later, expressing disgust with the female body ("Belle hideusement d'un ulcère à l'anus"—Hideously beautiful with an ulcer on her anus). Precisely how a fifteen-year-old boy found the image of an anal ulcer is difficult to imagine. It is not a common lesion, one not seen outside of a medical setting, not usually an item discussed *sub rosa* by adolescent boys. Perhaps Rimbaud saw one illustrated in a medical book in the public library. The poem is a sonnet perfect in form and scansion, but its content seems designed for little more than *épater les bourgeois*. It marks the beginning of a distinctive element in Rimbaud's vocabulary—the anatomically explicit, scatological, and bluntly sexual, a language quite different from the reticent velleities used by other poets of the period. In England, Swinburne's *Poems and Ballads* (1866) had caused scandal, yet his vocabulary was far more restrained.

Again, at the end of the academic year 1869–70 Rimbaud led his class, winning all but two prizes in his form and the Concours Académique. Izambard was not present on Prizegiving Day; he had returned two weeks earlier to his aunts' home at Douai. Rimbaud had been left the key to Izambard's rooms and library, but he rapidly exhausted that resource, had no one to talk to, and was bored. External events soon began to impinge on his life as a student. The Franco-Prussian War had been declared in July, and it was apparent that the French army was giving ground. At some time in August, Rimbaud's brother Frédéric enlisted in the army. German troops were beginning to occupy nearby districts in northern France. In fact Napoleon III surrendered at Sédan about twenty miles southeast of Charleville on September 2, 1870. It was announced that the Collège de Charleville would not reopen for the fall term because of the military situation and civil confusion. Rimbaud chafed at the restricted life he led with his mother and two sisters and he complained of the stifling dullness of Charleville. Actually, the population of Charleville was 12,059 (census of 1872) and with its twin city of Mézières formed a sizable regional center. What Rimbaud disliked was not so much the size or geography of his birthplace but its stagnant state of mind and the absence of articulate people with intellectual curiosity. And, like so many adolescents, he found the conventional hypocrisies intolerable. He rebelled against them inwardly and was soon to do so openly. On August 25 he wrote to Izambard complaining of his *tedium vitae* and remarked in the postscript, "Very soon I shall give you some startling news of the kind of life I'm going to lead after the summer holidays."

Mme. Rimbaud had no idea of what was going on in the mind of her son, who seemed so promising, so docile, such a good performer. On August 28, three days after writing to Izambard, Rimbaud was escorting his mother and sisters for a walk along the river when he remarked that he wanted to return home to fetch a book. Instead, he went to the railway station and took the train for Paris without a franc in his pockets. Some biographers have described this episode as a fugue, but there is no sign that Rimbaud's consciousness was impaired, no sign of mental confusion. It was an escape, partly premeditated (*vide* the postscript to Izambard) but partly spontaneous. Even a boy brought up so closely under his mother's thumb as Rimbaud must have known that one cannot travel very far without money. It was a sudden flight conceived in a moment of panic, and it was the first of several. On arriving at Paris he was arrested for not being able to pay his fare and was committed to Mazas prison. After a week of trying to brazen it out he wrote to Izambard—"I hope in you as a mother! You have always been a brother to me! . . . I love you as a brother, I will love you as a father"—to come and bail him out. Izambard did not have to travel to Paris to fetch the errant youth. He wrote to the Procureur Imperial, enclosed the money, and arranged with the governor of the prison to have Rimbaud put on the train to Douai. While Rimbaud sat in jail, the Deuxième Empire had fallen. Travel conditions were now difficult and uncertain; Rimbaud stayed with Izambard's aunts at Douai. His poem *Les chercheuses de poux* (The Lice-Seekers) was written on the occasion. Finally, on September 26 Izambard was able to return Rimbaud to Charleville. Mme. Rimbaud received her son with a box on the ear and thanked Izambard brusquely.

Rimbaud did not stay at home for long. After about a week of his mother's ire he set forth on foot for Charleroi and on to Brussels, writing poems as he went. He had no money but managed to beg food and lodging, even presenting himself at the home of a friend of Izambard at Brussels whose name he had heard mentioned. About October 11 he managed to reach Douai, where he was glad to see Izambard and his aunts. Mme. Rimbaud was duly informed, but she rejected Izambard's offer to escort the boy home and insisted he be returned by the police. The poems from this period strike a happy note. In *Ma bohème* he is Tom Thumb in a daze, sowing rhymes as he wanders along. In *La maline* he shows a healthy appreciation of the sly serving maid who offered him her cheek, and in *Au cabaret vert* where he stopped in Charleroi (now part of the Hôtel de l'Esperance) he ogled the waitress, "La fille aux tétons énormes, aux yeux vifs" (The girl with huge tits and lively eyes), who brought him ham, bread and butter, and a mug of ale. He also wrote a handful of political poems inspired by the events of the day. Like any self-respecting young rebel Rimbaud thought the government was a pack of fools and rogues and that no good would come of them (he was right). Brief as his walking tour was, it was a happy escape.

The autumn and winter of 1870–71 were a fallow period. Rimbaud managed to make some form of viable truce with his mother. Prussian troops moved close, shelling Mézières and occupying it on December 31. Bismarck had Wilhelm I declared Emperor of Germany on January

18 at Versailles. In mid-February, a month later, the Collège de Charleville reopened, but Rimbaud refused to return to his studies. At the age of sixteen he became what we would call "a high-school dropout." Many Frenchmen were disgruntled and ready for some sort of revolt, few more ready than Rimbaud who expanded his hatred of his mother's discipline into a hatred of all government, all forms of authority. In today's terms he became "radicalized," albeit superficially, for like most literary adolescents he was a naif about politics and the art of government.

INITIATION AND ITS CONSEQUENCES

Rimbaud's next escape was somewhat better planned than his two previous adventures. He sold his watch and actually had some money in his pocket. Some confusion exists concerning the precise dates of this event. The chronology provided in the Pléiade edition gives the dates as April 19 to May 3, 1871, during the Commune. Starkie assigns an earlier time, February 25 to March 10, the period when the Thiers government was trying to arrange national election, but she notes that this does not preclude a later visit during April and May. From a medical point of view the precise dates are less important than what is supposed to have happened, namely Rimbaud's first sexual experience, a disastrous one at that.

There is no documentary evidence of what took place. We can only infer the events from a single poem and a few scraps of circumstantial evidence. Precisely how this event became incorporated in the oral tradition of Rimbaud's biography is not clear. There is no record of anyone's claim that he heard it from Rimbaud himself. Perhaps, somewhat later, during his affair with Verlaine, he recounted it to his lover, who, after the affair was ended, later disclosed it to some of his associates. It is a commonplace of biography that oral transmission leads to distortion and inaccuracy. However, given these caveats, it seems possible to reconstruct the supposed scenario. Inevitably, much of the reasoning is *post hoc ergo propter hoc,* but in historiographic reconstruction sometimes it is only possible to infer causes from their effects.

Rimbaud was a good-looking lad of sixteen with bright blue eyes, tousled hair, and a fresh country complexion. His physiognomy had not matured in pace with the rest of his body; one might even call him baby-faced. Verlaine's sketch of him a year later (fig. 10.1) suggests a

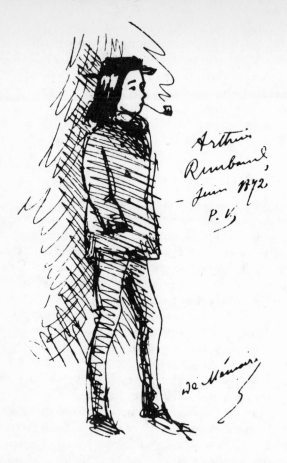

Figure 10.1. Pen and ink sketch of Rimbaud. Verlaine, 1872. Courtesy of Enid Rhodes Peschel.

boy about two years younger in appearance, and Fantin-Latour's famous portrait in *Le coin de table* (fig. 10.2) accentuates his ephebic appearance. So far as many biographers agree, Rimbaud fell in with some soldiers stationed at the barracks in the Rue Babylon. He was articulate and responded with obvious pleasure at being free and on his own in Paris with all the sights and novelties the metropolis had to offer. The soldiers treated him with bluff, easy camaraderie, making him feel more grown up and sophisticated than he was. Then a glass or two of wine to

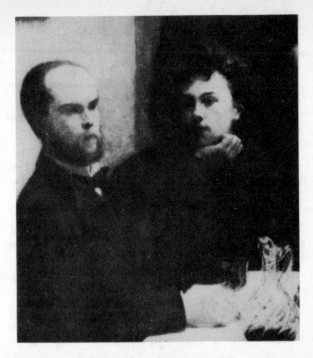

Figure 10.2. Detail from *Le coin de table,* showing Rimbaud (*right*) and Verlaine. Fantin-Latour, 1872. Galerie Jeu de Paume, Paris.

release inhibitions, a bit of lewd conversation to whet his prurience and make him randy, *e voi sapete quel che fa.* To the soldiers he was a young country chicken ready for plucking. At least one biographer has called it a homosexual rape, but the term is a bit strong; whatever may have happened was not entirely without Rimbaud's consent, at least in the preliminary stages. It may not have been an informed consent, to use the legal jargon of today, for, though Rimbaud had the usual farm boy's knowledge of barnyard copulation, he was inexperienced and uninstructed about human sexual behavior. Probably the only instruction he had at home was "Ne touchez pas." When it came to the inevitable conjunction of organs with orifices, he may not have known what was going to happen until it did.

Badly shattered, he returned to Charleville on foot, a difficult journey through territory still occupied by Prussian troops. He undoubtedly felt a profound sense of guilt and shame. Unlike many individuals who can rationalize away their own role in misconduct or displace the guilt on to others, Rimbaud knew that he had willingly encouraged the soldiers and bore some responsibility for the denouement. He may even have admitted to himself that in spite of the pain he had experienced a certain degree of pleasure. During that taxing journey Rimbaud may have conceded to himself that he had been an accomplice to his own seduction. If so, that may have only increased his sense of guilt. He felt defiled and on returning to Charleville he acted as if he were. He refused to wash, wore dirty clothes, let his hair grow long and unkempt, saying in effect: If I am unclean, I shall look unclean. He had no one to turn to for advice. He could scarcely have told his mother what had happened. Confession to the local curé would have been equally unthinkable and unhelpful. There were no psychiatrists or youth guidance centers in those days. He indulged in behavior that shocked the good people of Charleville. In addition to his disheveled appearance, he now smoked his pipe with its bowl turned upside down. He scribbled graffiti such as "Merde à Dieu" on park benches. His language became coarse and profane, and he put off attempts at conversation by brusque, bitter, sarcastic replies. Some writers have argued that this was an episode of schizophrenia, one that foreshadowed his later behavior with Verlaine. But there is no evidence of dementia, and his affect was not inappropriate to his real psychological circumstances. One might classify his behavior at this time as "character disorder, schizoid type," but beyond telling the reader that this was a young man torn by emotional problems whose behavior was unconventional, such a label means very little. There is little homogeneity among cases so pigeonholed. Taxonomy for its own sake offers little help in understanding his mental processes. One writer has gone so far as to suggest a neuroendocrine imbalance as a cause. The case seems to rest on the observation that Rimbaud grew about six inches between his fifteenth and sixteenth birthdays and that his hands were large. There is no endocrinological evidence to support the hypothesis, and the observations are consistent with a delayed adolescent growth spurt.

The poetic expression of the supposed incident in the barracks is found in a rondeau, first titled *Le coeur supplicé* and later *Le coeur volé*. It is written in slang and begins with "Mon triste coeur bave à la poupe" (My sad heart slobbers on the deck) and then describes the ithyphallic, barracks-lewd soldiers who laugh and jeer, covering his heart with tobacco spit. In the last three lines he asks:

> Moi, si mon coeur est ravalé:
> Quand ils auront tari leur chiques,
> Comment agir, ô coeur volé?
>
> (If my heart is degraded:
> When they have used up their quid,
> How shall I act, o plundered heart?)[4]

He sent a copy of the poem to Izambard in a letter dated May 13, 1871, but Izambard did not recognize the poem for what it was, a cry for help. He took the use of soldier's slang as a crude joke and returned a parody. That marked the end of the Rimbaud-Izambard correspondence, and the young man was left to resolve his sexual identity alone. Perhaps what disturbed him most in the spring and summer of 1871 was that despite the pain, then the feelings of guilt and shame, of having been violated, he recognized that he had, at least in part, wanted the experience and enjoyed it. Needless to say, this feeling was difficult to reconcile with what he had been taught about acts that were *contra legem et naturam*.

The one force that sustained Rimbaud during this period of emotional turmoil was his continuing dedication to the vocation of poet. In the letter of May 13 to Izambard he first enunciated his doctrine of "reaching the unknown by the derangement of *all the senses*." He expanded the theme two days later in a letter to Paul Demeny, the much-quoted manifesto known as the *Lettre du voyant:*

> Le Poète se fait *voyant* par un long, immense et raisonné *dérèglement* de *tous les sens*. Toutes les formes d'amour, de souffrance, de folie; il cherche lui-même, il épuise en lui tous les poisons, pour n'en garder que les quintessences. Ineffable torture où il a besoin de toute la foi, de toute la force surhumaine, où il devient tous le grand malade, le grand criminel, le grand maudit,—et le suprême Savant!—Car il arrive a *l'inconnu!* Puisqu'il a cultivé son âme, déjà riche, plus qu'aucun! Il arrive à l'inconnu, et quand, affolé, il finirait par perdre l'intelligence de ses visions, il les a vues! Qu'il crève dans son bondissement par les choses inouies et innommables: viendront d'autres horribles travailleurs; ils commenceront par les horizons où l'autre s'est affaissé!
>
> (The poet makes himself a *seer* by a long, gigantic, and rational *derangement* of *all the senses*. All forms of love, suffering, and

madness. He searches himself. He exhausts all poisons in himself and keeps only their quintessences. Unspeakable torture where he needs all his faith, all his superhuman strength, where he becomes among all men the great patient, the great criminal, the one accursed—and the supreme Scholar!—Because he reaches *the unknown,* and when, bewildered, he ends by losing the insights of his visions, he has seen them. Let him die as he leaps through unheard of and unnamable things: other horrible workers will come; they will begin from the horizons where the other collapsed!)[5]

The sixteen-year-old youth set himself a formidable role to play, and during the next two years acted out his program with such intensity and dedication that it drove him to the edge of disaster. A key word is that the *dérèglement des sens* is rational. Rimbaud's descent into the maelstrom was deliberate and planned. One sees in the manifesto the influence of his readings in cabalistic and mystical literature, a sense of following in Baudelaire's footsteps, a Promethean impulse, that notion being expressed in another passage in which Rimbaud calls the poet "the thief of fire." In his impetuous desire to capture the unknown he failed to recognize the old adage: He who plays with fire is often scorched. Rimbaud's formula for achieving "the unknown" carried with it a self-fulfilling implication of self-destruction: After gaining the prize, the poet would lose the value of the insights and visions he had gained. And this is precisely what happened: triumph followed by defeat. "His poetic adventure, which generally begins with rebellion, proceeds through extraordinary hope until it reaches a momentary, sometimes apocalyptic, vision and then terminates in defeat. But the defeat appears at times as a new beginning, a new affirmation."[6] Examined chronologically, Rimbaud's poems exhibit an almost unlimited capacity for self-regeneration.

He passed the summer of 1871 planning a safe entry into the literary life of Paris. When not engaged in writing, he passed his time in cafés, cadging drinks from anyone who would stand him a round. He repaid his hosts by telling risqué stories and lurid, probably fictitious, accounts of his adventures in Paris. From this period date the anticlerical poems *Les premières communions* and *L'homme juste,* which continue the theme first enunciated in *Le châtiment de Tartuffe* written the previous year. His two major poems were *Le bateau ivre* and the less familiar but revealing *Ce qu'on dit au poète à propos des fleurs*. The latter was dedicated to Banville and is a parody of the Parnassian style. Its quatrains are as polished as any of Gautier's *Emaux et Camées,* but Rimbaud broke from the conventional vocabulary of French poetry and wrote in a manner then peculiar to himself, using scientific terms, slang expressions, and many words not used in the salon. These verbal eccentricities served Laforgue and later poets as a model, but to the staid Parnassians they were a novelty. Probably no poet since Swift has had so close an interest in the excremental (cf. young Rimbaud's escape to the outhouse), and in *Ce qu'on dit* he gives ample play to the scatological. Lilies become "clystères d'extase" (enemas of ecstasy), and he asks whether any flower, rosemary or lily, alive or dead, is worth a seabird's droppings.

Le bateau ivre expands the boyhood fantasy in *Poètes de sept ans,* ". . . seul, et couché sur des pièces de toile/Ecru, et pressentant la voile!" (alone, and lying on pieces of unbleached/Canvas, and violently announcing a sail!). Now a year older, he follows the lead of Baudelaire's *Le voyage* and describes the loneliness and dangers of the poet's quest. In the sense that the drunken boat is on a voyage it is also a poem of escape. The imagery is striking and colorful, and one can understand why the surrealists of the 1920s claimed Rimbaud as an intellectual precursor. Particularly interesting in view of his later experiences with drugs is the synaesthesia explicit in his dream of "l'éveil jaune et bleu des phosphores chanteurs" (the yellow and blue awakening of singing phosphorus). But when the poet, not yet seventeen years old, informs us that "Tout lune est atroce et tout soleil amer" (Every moon is atrocious and every sun bitter), we can recognize his profound unhappiness and pessimism as well as what his future might hold. It is painful and frightening to see that an adolescent boy can summon such an idea from his personal stock of emotional experience.

In one of the cafés Rimbaud met Charles Bretagne, who had some acquaintance with Verlaine. Supplied with a note of introduction from Bretagne, Rimbaud wrote to Verlaine in Paris, enclosed some of his poems (*Le coeur volé* included), and soon received the generous reply, "Venez, chère grande âme, on vous appelle, on vous attend." The older poet sent Rimbaud some money for train fare and invited him to stay with him and his wife. It is doubtful that Bretagne knew Verlaine's character well enough to think he might be introducing Ganymede to Zeus, nor is it plausible that Verlaine intuitively grasped the meaning of

Le coeur volé and was planning a seduction when he extended his open-handed invitation. Rimbaud arrived chez Verlaine on September 10, 1871, and the stage was set.

THE AFFAIR WITH VERLAINE AND ITS CONSEQUENCES

At this juncture a few biographical words about Paul Verlaine are in order. Born in 1844, he was ten years older than Rimbaud, twenty-seven in contrast to seventeen, when they met in 1871. Like Rimbaud's, Verlaine's father had been an army captain who had met his wife when stationed in a provincial town, and like Rimbaud's parents the Verlaines were older than average; Captain Verlaine was forty-six and Mme. Verlaine thirty-five when their son was born. Unlike Rimbaud, Verlaine was an only child, born after three miscarriages; Mme. Verlaine kept the fetuses preserved in spirit on a shelf in her armoire. The Verlaines moved to Paris when Paul was seven years old. Unlike the Rimbaud household the Verlaines lived harmoniously, and Paul remained on good terms with his father until the latter's death in 1865, when the poet was twenty-one. Unlike Rimbaud's mother, Mme. Verlaine, according to Joanna Richardson, was a possessive mother who called him *le petit* years after he had outgrown the term and allowed him, perhaps wanted him, to remain weak and dependent.[7] He never outgrew his *garçonneries* which started about the time of puberty, and the majority of his sexual contacts were homosexual.

Again, according to Richardson, Verlaine in his early twenties was already bisexual and a potential alcoholic. Rimbaud's father was, to be sure, absent from the time the boy was six, but Verlaine's father was not absent, nor was he detached or hostile. Rimbaud's mother was anything but binding, but Verlaine's mother was. Such disparities in the parent-child relationship demonstrate the inadequacy of trying to construct such a simplistic formula as "absent father/binding mother" as the familial context in which homosexual preferences develop. Even when both terms of the equation are satisfied, the majority of children develop the customary heterosexual pattern. So far as one can judge, Verlaine's only heterosexual experiences up to 1871 were some adolescent experiments in bordellos and an ill-starred alliance with a naive, immature girl of seventeen whom he had married in the hope that successful matrimony would straighten out his life. After the marriage foundered on the rock of his relationship with Rimbaud, Verlaine had no sexual relations with women until *after his mother's death* in 1886, when the poet was forty-two years old.

When Rimbaud arrived in Paris in September 1871, Paul and Mathilde Verlaine (née Mauté) were living in the comfortable town house of her rentier parents in the Rue Nicolet. Verlaine had managed to achieve an unenviable reputation for cowardice in both the war and the Commune. He had quit his job at the Hôtel de Ville and was content to live on his wife's allowance from her father plus whatever money he could scrounge from his widowed mother. Rimbaud felt ill at ease, inadequate, and on the defensive in the atmosphere of such unaccustomed wealth, and he promptly managed to alienate Mme. Mauté and Mathilde by his boorish manners, uncouth vocabulary, and unkempt appearance. When M. Mauté, who had been absent on a shooting trip when Rimbaud arrived, returned home a few days later, he soon showed the sulky youth the door. To complicate matters, Mathilde, who had been married little more than a year, was in the eighth month of pregnancy. Perhaps Verlaine had not had sexual access to her for some time and his homosexual feelings, suppressed for almost two years, were aroused by the good-looking, intense country youth. Even before M. Mauté gave Rimbaud his *congé,* the two poets fell into the practice of leaving the house shortly after dinner, touring the cafés, and returning quite drunk to the Rue Nicolet.

Needless to say, Rimbaud looked up to Verlaine, not only because the older poet introduced him to his circle of literary and artistic friends, but because Verlaine was already the author of three important books of poetry, *Poèmes saturniens* (1866), *Fêtes galantes* (1869), and *La bonne chanson* (1870), written in honor of Mathilde. At first Verlaine arranged for Rimbaud to lodge with Charles Cros, but the youth's bad manners soon made him unwelcome. With assistance from his friends Verlaine rented and furnished attic quarters for the penniless Rimbaud in the Rue de Buci, off the Boulevard Saint-Germain. It was probably at that location that they became lovers. It is most likely that the first advances were by the older to the younger poet. The open question is why Rimbaud consented. From the outset it was apparent that this was not a casual affair like Rimbaud's supposed initiation but a commitment to a homosexual way of life. It is reasonable to believe that both parties conceived it as an enduring relationship. Certainly in the beginning Verlaine was the dominant figure for Rimbaud, competent in precisely those areas important to him—knowledgeable, widely read, an established figure in literary circles, a cicerone in the *coulisses* of Parisian night life, even a tutor in poetic technique. For the young man so unsure of himself that he almost bristled, Verlaine offered the security of an older friend with shared interests in an area of central importance to both of them. To this may be added that in the months since Rimbaud's supposed initiation he had come to recognize the homosexual component in his sexual identity and that he found the physical aspect of it satisfying. So far as we know, he had had no other form of sexual experience, nor were such outlets readily accessible; at this stage Rimbaud probably had no idea of how to approach a woman. Finally, he may have considered his participation as one of the first steps in experiencing "all forms of love."

There is little value in relating the vicissitudes of the affair, including Verlaine's recurrent vacillations about securing a reconciliation with his wife and Rimbaud's intermittent returns to Charleville and the family farm at Roche. A major event was Verlaine's violent quarrel with his wife in June 1872. He had a nasty habit of being physically abusive to women when he was angry or frustrated and drunk, and this attack caused the final break between them. By this time Rimbaud had made himself *persona non grata* to many of the figures in literary and artistic circles, and in July Rimbaud and Verlaine found it expedient to go to London. They lived together in Soho until November, when for unstated reasons Rimbaud returned to Charleville. He returned in January 1873 when Verlaine was taken ill, but they separated again in April—Verlaine to Paris, Rimbaud to his mother's farm in Roche. They were reunited in May and went back to London, but early in July they quarreled bitterly, and Verlaine left for Brussels.

Two such volatile personalities could not live together without squabbling. Verlaine left in anger, no longer able to endure Rimbaud's caustic tongue and mockery. He walked to the docks, announcing his intention to become reconciled with Mathilde. Rimbaud followed him and signaled to him to get off, but Verlaine stayed on board. Disconsolate, Rimbaud wrote to Verlaine:

> Come back, come back, dear friend, my only friend. I swear I will behave. If I was surly with you, it was a joke. . . . I am more repentant than I can say. . . . For two days I haven't stopped crying. . . . Nothing is lost. . . . We will live here again courageously.

. . . But why didn't you come when I signaled to you to get off the boat? We lived together for two years, to come to this moment. . . . If you don't want to come back here, do you want me to come to you? . . . Listen only to your good heart.[8]

Before receiving this Verlaine had written while at sea, reproaching Rimbaud and saying he could no longer put up with scenes and quarrels:

Only as I love you greatly (honi soit qui mal y pense!) I want to tell you that if at the end of three days I'm not reconciled with my wife, in perfect amity, I'm going to blow my brains out. . . . If, which is very likely, I'm obliged to perform this last pitiable act, I shall, at least, do it bravely. My last thought will be for you, for you who were beckoning to me, this afternoon, from the quayside, when I wouldn't go back, for it's necessary that I should die. Nevertheless, I embrace you before I die.[9]

He also wrote his mother that he would commit suicide if Mathilde did not return to him. Mme. Verlaine hastened to Brussels and was present at the denouement. Alone in London and without much money, Rimbaud received this characteristic example of Verlaine's capacity for self-dramatization and self-deception. He replied:

I have your letter dated "at sea." You are wrong this time. Your wife is not coming, or she will come in three months, or three years, or sometime. As for dying, I know you. So, while waiting for your wife and your Death, you are going to struggle, wander about, and bore people. . . . Do you think life with others will be happier than it was with me? . . . I am sorry for my part in the wrong. . . . I am fond of you. . . . Believe me, if your wife comes back, I will not compromise you by writing. I will never write. . . . The one true word is: come back, I want to be with you. I love you.[10]

He then packed his belongings and went to see Verlaine in Brussels. After a day of recriminations, protestations, and hysterical arguments Verlaine, quite drunk, shot Rimbaud in the left wrist and was arrested. Though Rimbaud's wounds were superficial (fig. 10.3) and he did not wish to press charges, the authorities prosecuted Verlaine, and he was sentenced to prison for two years.[11] Rimbaud returned to Roche and *Une saison en enfer,* which he had begun in April. The two lovers met

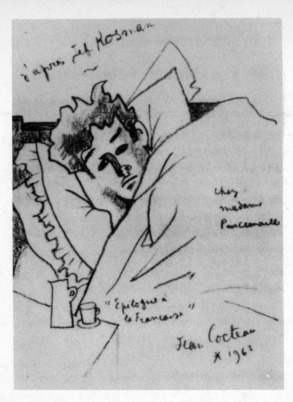

Figure 10.3. Rimbaud recovering from his wounds. Sketch by Jean Cocteau, 1962. Based on a contemporary painting by Jef Rosman.

only once again. When Verlaine was released in January 1875, he arranged to meet Rimbaud in Stuttgart, where the latter had gone to study German. Verlaine pleaded with him to renew their relationship, but Rimbaud refused. Our last view of Verlaine is a photograph taken in a Paris café in 1892, some twenty years later, looking like a dissipated, dirty old man.

Certain aspects of the Rimbaud-Verlaine affair require comment. Chronologically, it lasted twenty-two months during which Verlaine had no other male lovers, nor did Rimbaud. The emotional and physical bond between them was intense, and they were not promiscuous. When the affair began, Verlaine was probably the instigator and domi-

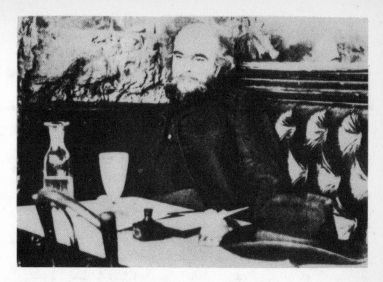

Figure 10.4. Photograph of Verlaine in a Montmartre café with a glass of absinthe, 1892. The café is identified variously as the Café de Lilas or the Café François 1ᵉʳ. Photo Harlingue.

nant partner, but as the affair continued Rimbaud's stronger personality came to the fore. Only a few of the bohemian literati of Paris were censorious; most were tolerant. However, Rimbaud's disruptive rudeness turned them against him. (At one evening of poetry reading Rimbaud offended everyone present by exclaiming "Merde!" after each line of one poet's offering.) When Verlaine returned to Paris alone in 1875, he was accepted by his fellow writers despite the known weaknesses in his character. There was no outcry against him for having led a youth astray; they blamed Rimbaud for the unpleasant ending. Verlaine continued his homosexual activities without censure. There is no evidence that Rimbaud had any further homosexual experiences in the two decades that followed. If he did, and surely opportunities were present, they were casual and without any emotional involvement. Ultimately he may have tried to establish heterosexual competence. Both poets were dedicated to their vocation and freely criticized each other's work. Received critical opinion is that in the long run Verlaine learned more from Rimbaud than conversely. The financial arrangements were simple:

Rimbaud had no money and almost no earning power; they lived chiefly on whatever money Verlaine could wheedle from his mother. In London they did give a few French lessons and had occasional odd jobs, but income from these sources was small and irregular. It was Verlaine who provided the means for Rimbaud to use hashish and drink absinthe in his role as would-be *voyant*. When Rimbaud left London to meet Verlaine in Brussels in July 1873, he was prepared to rejoin his lover. It was there he decided against it, chiefly because of Verlaine's weakness, vacillation, and ultimately his violence. In no sense was it based upon a moral rejection of homosexuality.

The major poetic consequence of Rimbaud's affair with Verlaine was, of course, *Une saison en enfer.* But first let us consider the autobiographical *Les remembrances du vieillard idiot* because it bears upon the psychosexual aspects of his childhood. (I have chosen, perhaps arbitrarily, to consider *Les illuminations* and other poems written while he was Verlaine's companion under the subheading of "Hashish and Absinthe.") *Les remembrances* was written in the *Album Zutique,* and Rimbaud's contributions to that manuscript volume were not fully published until 1962.[12] The poem is cast as a confessional piece, opening with "Pardon, mon père!" (Forgive me, father!), and continuing with Rimbaud's recollections of his long-repressed juvenile interest in a donkey's long penis, being stimulated by a crease in his mother's nightgown, his sister's urination, and finally a fascination by his father's penis followed by a comment on his delayed puberty.

> Car un père est troublant!—et les choses conçues! . . .
> Son genou, calineur parfois; son pantalon
> Dont mon doigt désirait ouvrir la fente . . . —oh! non!—
> Pour avoir le bout gros, noir et dur de mon père,
> Dont la pileuse main me bercait! . . .
>
> Puisque les sens infects m'ont mis de leurs victimes,
> Je confesse de l'aveu des jeunes crimes! . . .
>
> Pourquoi la puberté tardive et le malheur
> Du gland tenace et trop consulté? Pourquoi l'ombre
> Si lente au bas de ventre? et ces terreurs sans nombre
> Comblant toujours la joie ainsi qu'un gravier noir?
> Moi, j'ai toujours été stupéfait! Quoi savoir.

Pardonné? . . .
>   Reprenez la chancelière bleue,
Mon père
>   O cette enfance! . . .
>>>>   —et tirons-nous l³ queue!

(For a father is disturbing!—and the things imagined! . . .
His knee, at times coaxing: his trousers
Whose fly my finger wanted to open . . . —oh! no!—
To have the thick dark hard cock of my father,
Whose hairy hand rocked me! . . .

Since my infected senses have made me their victim,
I confess and avow my youthful crimes . . .

Why puberty so late and the disgrace
Of my tenacious and too often consulted glans? Why the dark
So slow at the base of my belly? and those countless terrors
Always burying my joy like black gravel.
I have always been astounded! What can I know?

Forgiven? . . .
>   Take back that blue hassock,
My father,
>   O that childhood! . . .
>>>   and let's jack each other off!) [13]

These recollections of juvenile sexual feelings were clearly released into Rimbaud's consciousness under the influence of his relationship with Verlaine. To be stimulated by one's mother's intimate garments or one's sister's micturition is commonplace, but Rimbaud is explicit about an interest in his father's *membrum virile* that must have occurred before he was six years old, an item not commonly reported in juvenile fantasies. There is a certain ambiguity in the phrase "avoir le bout gros." If we construe "avoir" to mean "have," that suggests that the boy merely wanted to have a penis as large and impressive as his father's, a desire to resemble physically his father. However, "avoir" can be construed as "to hold," and the previous phrase about wanting to open the fly of his trousers suggests that the boy's wish was more than merely possessing a comparable organ himself. If Rimbaud's unfulfilled wish was to grasp his father's penis, that might account for his willingness to agree to Verlaine's advances. (This is not an instance in which to apply the maxim, "A boy's reach should exceed his grasp.") The final lines in which he suggests mutual masturbation to his father confessor exceed the usual limits of adolescent fantasy. Can we credit a youth, not yet eighteen, with an insight into the latent homosexuality of some men who renounce heterosexuality and become celibate priests, or is it merely a display of his anticlericalism? Taken as a whole, *Les remembrances du vieillard idiot* indicates that Rimbaud had many deep-seated, unresolved conflicts about his prepubescent sexual impulses and a persistent sense of guilt about his own masturbation.

Rimbaud began writing *Une saison en enfer* in April 1873, probably suspended work on it when he returned to London at the end of May, then returned to it after the shooting in Brussels in July. Just how much of what he wrote in April and May he may have discarded we cannot know. If, as is commonly believed, he wrote the first section, *Mauvais sang,* before the final scene in Brussels, it indicates Rimbaud's recognition that his systematic *dérèglement des sens* had not given him the insights and inspiration he had hoped to achieve. The experiment had failed. The *inconnu* remained unknown. Perhaps the section also indicates the inevitability of his rupture with Verlaine; if so, why did he return to London? Can we attribute his leaving London in November 1872 as a sign that the relationship was even then beginning to disintegrate? Though we cannot know Rimbaud's state of mind before he went to Brussels, the picture is one of two volatile poets "dependent and almost antithetical . . . who love and hate each other, [and] at times need yet can't abide each other."[14]

When Rimbaud returned to Roche from Brussels, he began writing at fever pitch. To paraphrase da Ponte, *mille torbidi pensieri il s'aggiran per la testa,* and this was the dark night of his soul, a repudiation of what had passed, an expression of remorse, anguish, and despair. It is an *examen de conscience* cast as a complex prose poem rich in symbolic allusion and oblique metaphors, punctuated by exclamatory outbursts that verge on hysteria. Its diction, its unexpected juxtapositions, even its wildness were unlike anything written by a Frenchman before, but the hell was of Rimbaud's own making.

The psychological atmosphere of the prose poem is apparent in the second section, *Nuit de l'enfer.* Cruel as it is to cite snippets, Rimbaud tells us:

J'ai avalé une fameuse gorgée du poison. . . . Les entrailles me brûlent. La violence du venin tord mes membres, me rend difforme, me terrasse. Je meurs de soif, j'étouffe, je ne puis crier. C'est l'enfer, l'éternelle peine! . . .

C'est la honte, le reproche ici: Satan qui dit que le feu est ignoble, que ma colère est affreusement sotte.—Assez! . . . —Et dire que je tiens la verité, que je vois la justice: j'ai un jugement sain et arrêté, je suis prêt pour la perfection. . . . Orgueil.—La peau de ma tête se dessèche. Pitié, Seigneur, j'ai peur . . . —Horreur de ma bêtise . . .

Je devrais avoir mon enfer pour la colère, mon orgueil—et l'enfer de la caresse; un concert d'enfers. . . . C'est le tombeau, je m'en vais aux vers, horreur de l'horreur! Satan, farceur, tu veux me dissoudre, avec tes charmes. Je réclame, je réclame! un coup de fourche, une goutte de feu. . . . C'est le feu qui se relève avec son damné.

(I have swallowed a first-rate draught of poison. . . . My entrails are on fire. The violence of the venom wrings my limbs, deforms me, fells me. I am dying of thirst, I am suffocating, I cannot cry out. This is hell, the everlasting punishment! . . .

There is shame, reproof in this place: Satan who says that fire is disgraceful, that my wrath is frightfully foolish.—Enough!— . . . And to say that I possess truth, that I understand justice: I have a sound and steady judgment. I am prepared for perfection. . . . Pride. The skin of my head is drying up. Pity! Lord, I am terrified. . . . —The horror of my stupidity.

I ought to have my hell for wrath, my hell for pride,—and the hell of the caress; a concert of hells. . . . This is the tomb, I am going to the worms, horror of horrors! Satan, jester, you wish to undo me with your spells. I protest. I protest! one jab of the pitchfork, one lick of the flame. . . . It is the fire that rises again with the soul condemned to it.)[15]

Rimbaud impeaches himself of three of the seven deadly sins, pride, anger, and lust, and he accepts his punishment in the literal image of a medieval hell, complete with fire, brimstone, and the devil's pitchfork.

(One recalls that he spent time on the family farm.) In the next section, *Délires I,* subtitled *Vierge folle—L'Époux infernal,* he projects his relationship with Verlaine. He casts Verlaine as the foolish virgin (not accurate: Verlaine was foolish but scarcely a virgin) and himself as the infernal bridegroom (I take him at his word). Though only the first and last lines are Rimbaud speaking, he casts himself as the power of evil with Verlaine submissive to him. The bulk of the section is in Verlaine's voice, and Rimbaud gives him such lines as

Plus tard, je connaîtrai le divin Époux! Je suis née soumise à Lui.—L'autre peut me battre maintenant! . . .

Je suis esclave de l'Époux infernal, celui qui a perdu les vierges folles. C'est bien ce démon là. Ce n'est pas un spectre, ce n'est pas un fantôme. Mais moi qui ai perdu la sagesse, qui suis damnée et morte au monde,—on ne me tuera pas!—Comment vous le décrire! . . .

Je suis veuve . . . —J'étais veuve . . . —mais oui, j'ai été bien sérieuse jadis, et je ne suis pas née pour devenir squelette! . . . —Lui était presque un enfant . . . Ses délicatesses mystérieuses m'avaient séduite. J'ai oublié tout mon devoir humain pour le suivre . . . C'est un Démon, vous savez, *ce n'est pas un homme.*

(Later I shall know the divine Bridegroom! I was born submissive to Him.—The other can thrash me now!

I am the slave of the infernal Bridegroom, he who ruined the foolish virgins. He is surely that very demon. He is not a specter, he is not a phantom. But I who have lost my discretion, who am damned and dead to the world,—no one will kill me!—How am I to portray him for you! . . .

I am a widow . . . —I was a widow . . . —why yes, I was quite serious once, and I was not born to become a skeleton . . . —He was practically a child . . . His mysterious delicate ways had seduced me. I forgot every human obligation in order to follow him . . . He is a demon, you know; *he is not a man.*)[16]

But *Une saison en enfer* is more than a mere confessional poem. It is Rimbaud's elaborate exposition of good and evil, sin and repentance, a piece written to exorcise the demon within him, an atonement, an act of contrition. It was not deliberately written as Rimbaud's farewell to poetry. When he finished it in August 1873, he went to Brussels to have it published. Mme. Rimbaud paid a deposit for the typesetting and printing costs, and Rimbaud took pains to send some of his author's copies to Verlaine in prison and to his friend Delahaye, writing to him, "My fate depends upon this book." But for reasons unknown the balance of the publisher's bill was not paid, and the press run remained in his warehouse until they were discovered over a decade after Rimbaud's death, after Verlaine's *Les poètes maudits* (1884) had brought him to public notice and fame. But in the event, *Une saison en enfer* does mark the end of Rimbaud as a poet. He wrote a few more short pieces, then stopped. The poetic flame was quenched. He was a burnt-out case.

Hashish and Absinthe

The French literary tradition for describing the use of hashish (*Cannabis sativa*) seems to have originated with Gautier's *Club des haschischins* (1847) on the Île St. Louis and Baudelaire's *Paradis artificiels* (1860), in which both poets relate their sensations after using the drug. Almost surely, the young Rimbaud based his idea of becoming a *voyant* and his sytematic *dérèglement de tous les sens* on these texts, plus whatever ancillary literature he may have read on mysticism and the occult. In addition to smoking Indian hemp Baudelaire also smoked opium or drank laudanum, and he is not precise at distinguishing the effects of one from the other. Young and impressionable, Rimbaud read both texts and read them uncritically. The youth in Charleville was looking for escape, and the experience of these two distinguished poets offered him not only an easy route but the promise of insights and visions heretofore not experienced, an irresistible glimpse into the unknown.

Cannabis is not usually an hallucinogen. It is rather a mild euphoriant. Its users describe alterations in mood, a distorted sense of time, but rarely any visual, auditory, or other sensory hallucinations. With heavy use motor coordination may be impaired, and chronic users may develop a quasi-apathetic deterioration in affect. The sense of depersonalization may find its equivalent in Rimbaud's statement "*Je* est un autre," but the comment was made in his *Lettre du voyant* to Demeny in May 1871, some months before he went to Paris, met Verlaine, and had an opportunity to smoke hashish. That he might have sensed the capacity of a drug to enable him to step outside, as it were, of his persona and view himself and his reactions as objects detached from their subject is a credit to his intellect, yet there is no reason to believe he had experienced that dissociation of personality through hashish at that time.

The only documented account of the effects of hashish on Rimbaud is the report of a visit by Delahaye, who arrived in Paris one morning to find him sleeping off the effects of an evening of smoking hemp. The only visions it had induced were "some white moons, some black moons, that were chasing each other." This is unlike the hallucinations of opium use. They generally include distortions of space—vistas of boundless oceans, exotic landscapes, even faery seas forlorn—often coupled with brilliant colors like cascading jewels, brightly illuminated scenes with elaborate buildings ornately decorated, and the like. Only occasionally do opium users have dreams of terror (cf. De Quincey, Crabbe), and then only after prolonged habituation. None of these phenomena can be found in Rimbaud's poems. Fear and terror are prominent in *Une saison en enfer,* but the emotions came from the turmoil within his psyche. Hashish was rather an expensive indulgence at the time, and Verlaine and Rimbaud could probably afford it only infrequently. There is no substantive evidence that hashish had any significant effect on Rimbaud's poetry.

By contrast, absinthe could be had for fifteen to twenty centimes a shot in the sort of café that Rimbaud, Verlaine, and their friends frequented. The price was somewhat higher in fancier establishments. It was the fashionable drink of the decade and it remained popular until its manufacture in France was declared illegal in 1915. Absinthe proved to be a popular subject with artists. Manet's etching (fig. 10.5) of the solitary brooding figure with an empty bottle at his feet dates from 1862, and he later used the same figure for a life-size painting and again as a small figure in a group. Degas' painting of a seedy couple drinking absinthe in a café can be seen in the Galerie Jeu de Paumes in Paris. It dates from 1876 and was painted in the Café de la Nouvelle-Athènes in Place Pigalle. Picasso painted several canvases of absinthe drinkers, notably one dating from 1901–3 of a young woman with sunken eyes and a hectic flush on her cheekbones, and another of the poet Cornuty drinking absinthe. But his most striking absinthe icon is the set of six absinthe glasses of 1914, each different, made of metal,

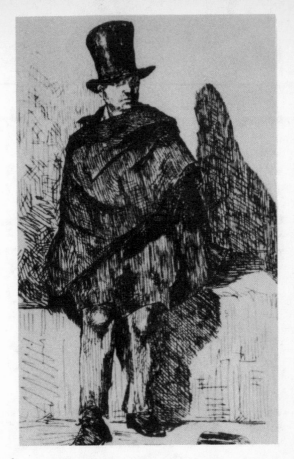

Figure 10.5. *The Absinthe Drinker*. Edouard Manet, 1862. Etching, state 2.

then painted, emphasizing the shifting axes, the curved and angular facets of form, and the stippling and hatching decorating the painted surface that are the hallmarks of Analytic Cubism.[17]

The formula for absinthe was developed by a Swiss physician who sold the recipe in 1797 to Henri Louis Pernod, who produced the liquor commercially. It was prepared by steeping an alcoholic solution of oil of wormwood (*Artemisia absinthum*) with alcoholic extracts of angelica, anise, marjoram, and other aromatic herbs, then distilling the

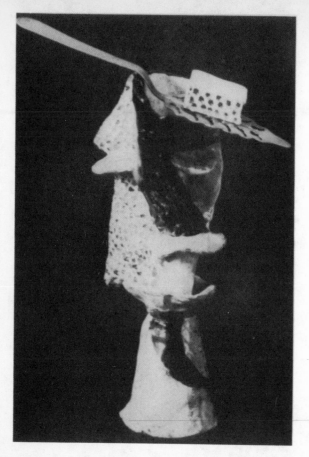

Figure 10.6. *Absinthe Glass.* Pablo Picasso, 1914. Painted metal. Courtesy of the Museum of Modern Art, New York.

fluid until it reached the desired concentration. Fairly high concentrations were needed to keep the ingredients in solution. *Absinthe ordinaire* contained about 48 percent alcohol, the *demi-fine* 68 percent, and *absinthe-Suisse* over 80 percent. Initially a drink for the lower classes, by the 1860s it became a favorite of *la vie bohème*. The boulevardiers and habitués of cafés would drink it at the end of the working day, from five o'clock to seven o'clock, in their favorite watering places, using a well-established ritual. A perforated spoon was placed over a specially designed glass. A lump of sugar and some crushed ice were placed in the bottom of the colander, and an ounce and a half of absinthe poured over them, then some anise essence. Finally, a variable amount of water would be allowed to drip slowly from the strainer into the glass, and the absinthe would change color from an emerald green to a cloudy opalescent solution. The manufacturers took special care to obtain precisely the desired green color for *l'heure verte* and to insure that the liquor "whitened" properly when the water was added. If necessary, such adulterants as indigo, tumeric, aniline green, copper sulfate, or even somewhat toxic antimony chloride were added.

The problem lay not so much with the adulterants, though they cannot be entirely exculpated, as with the wormwood (cf. the German *Vermut,* phonetically equivalent to vermouth, which contains small quantities of wormwood). Wormwood has a long tradition of being medicinally useful as a stimulant with tonic properties.

> When given in moderate doses, it promotes the appetite and digestion, quickens the circulation, and imparts to the whole system a strengthening influence. It is given in all cases requiring the administration of tonics, in dyspepsia, and other atonic states of the intestinal canal, in certain cases of amenorrhea, chronic leucorrhea, and obstinate diarrhea. . . . It is often administered in intermittent fevers with complete success.[18]

Its bitter taste was used in weaning infants from the breast; wet nurses would apply it to their nipples; recall the Nurse's speech, "And she was wean'd . . . for I had then laid wormwood to my dug" (*Romeo and Juliet* I.3.26). But its subjective affects were even more noticeable:

> [You] seem to lose your feet and you mount a boundless realm without horizon. You probably imagine that you are going in the direction of the infinite, whereas you are simply drifting into the incoherent. Absinthe affects the brain unlike any other stimulant; it produces neither the heavy drunkenness of beer, the furious inebriation of brandy, nor the exhilarating intoxication of wine. It is an ignoble poison, destroying life not until it has more or less brutalized its votaries, and made driveling idiots of them.[19]

Despite such warnings, absinthe became popular with writers, artists, musicians, and people from all walks of life. "The liqueur was popularly believed to renew activity to the brain, develop new worlds of ideas, expand consciousness, and thereby inspire noble works of the imagination in literature and art. Further, absinthe was popularly believed to have aphrodisiac properties."[20] Ernest Dowson wrote in a letter to a friend, "I understand absinthe makes the tart grow fonder."[21]

More to the point, Dowson described the hallucinogenic effects of absinthe in a prose poem:

> Green changed to white, emerald to an opal: nothing was changed.
>
> The man let the water trickle gently into his glass, and as the green clouded, a mist fell away from his mind.
>
> Then he drank opaline.
>
> Memories and terrors beset him. The past tore after him like a panther, and through the blackness of the present he saw the luminous tiger eyes of the things to be.
>
> But he drank opaline.
>
> And that obscure night of the soul, and the valley of humiliation, through which he stumbled were forgotten. He saw blue vistas of undiscovered countries, high prospects and a quiet, caressing sea. The past shed its perfume over him, today held his hand as it were a little child, and tomorrow shone like a white star: nothing was changed.
>
> He drank opaline.
>
> The man had known the obscure night of the soul, and lay even now in the valley of humiliation; and the tiger menace of the things to be was red in the skies. But for a little while he had forgotten.
>
> Green changed to white, emerald to an opal; nothing was changed.[22]

The quality of Dowson's experience has features in common with the opium-induced hallucinations of De Quincey, George Crabbe, and Francis Thompson, but he was wise enough in his folly to recognize that the effects were illusory and that "nothing was changed" in his unhappy life.

Wormwood contains a volatile oil whose chief constituent is thujone, an aromatic hydrocarbon that has a profound effect on the central nervous system. The pharmacologic properties of thujone have not been studied extensively; indeed, no studies have been carried out since the 1930s because it is not a substance likely to find a medical application. Earlier investigations showed that injecting it into animals produced marked excitation of the autonomic nervous system followed by unconsciousness and generalized epileptiform convulsions, clonic then tonic. The convulsions can be prevented by phenobarbital or bromides. The threshold for convulsions is lowered by adrenalin, nicotine, and histamine; it is raised by parasympathetic stimulants.

Absinthe was perceived as a public health menace in France and Switzerland partly because a few brutal crimes, somewhat sensationalized by the press, had been committed under its influence, partly because a progressive rise in alcohol consumption and public inebriety had given rise to a temperance movement. Absinthe, the most popular drink of the time, was the chief target of the reformers. In 1907 Switzerland prohibited its manufacture and sale. The United States declared its importation illegal in 1912. It was banned in France in 1915. Since then, Pernod Fils has manufactured Pernod, which is essentially the same anise-flavored formulation without the oil of wormwood; it contains about 40 percent alcohol. Judged by present-day standards, proof that thujone-containing oil of wormwood used under ordinary drinking conditions causes damage to the central nervous system is insufficient. Absinthe, as Rimbaud drank it, may have been less a villain than a convenient victim, and its prohibition satisfied the temperance movement by resolute legislation that did not incur serious economic penalties. What proportion of its effects on Rimbaud's poetry is due to thujone and what proportion due to its high alcohol content cannot be assayed. It may be that some of the most important poems of the 1870s, poems that influenced French poets for two generations, were written when the young poet was suffering from a simple hangover.

There is no doubt that Rimbaud and Verlaine were often in their cups. Every account of their life together described them as drinking night after night until they staggered home intoxicated. Rimbaud was fascinated by the idea of intoxication even before he met Verlaine. The use of alcohol as an escape is implicit in *Le bateau ivre,* and alcohol to liberate eroticism is explicit in *Les reparties de Nina* when the *vin du jour* induces the trembling wood to bleed with silent love and the young girl feels the quivering of her flesh. However, "l'eau verte" in *Le bateau ivre* is not to be construed as a reference to absinthe; it is the water of the river. The first poem that exhibits drug-induced imagery is the famous sonnet *Voyelles,* which begins:

> A noir, E blanc, I rouge, U vert, O bleu: voyelles,
> Je dirai quelque jour vos naissances latentes:
> A, noir corset velu des mouches éclatantes
> Qui bombinent autour des puanteurs cruelles,
>
> Golfes d'ombre; E, candeurs des vapeurs et des tentes,
> Lance des glaciers fiers, rois blancs, frissons d'ombelles;
> I, pourpres, sang craché, rire des lèvres belles
> Dans la colère ou les ivresses pénitentes; . . .
>
> (A black, E white, I red, U green, O blue; vowels,
> Some day your latent births I shall relate:
> A, black hairy corset of flies that bombinate
> Around cruel and foul
>
> Smells, gulfs of shadow; E, whiteness of tents and vapors,
> White kings, shivers of umbels, lances of proud glaciers;
> I, purples, spat blood, laughter of beautiful lips
> In anger or penitent intoxications; . . .)[23]

The trope is synaesthesia, the fusion of an image from one sensory modality with one from another, most frequently, as in this example, a fusion of a visual with an auditory image. Synaesthesia is common in drug-induced dreams and poems written by drug users. A typical example is in Francis Thompson's *Ode to the Setting Sun;* after establishing "visible music-blasts" he writes "I *see* the crimson blaring of the shawms!" Olfactory images are sometimes fused with visual and auditory images—for instance, Rimbaud's black flies buzzing around foul smells. Some biographers believe that the inspiration for *Voyelles* is Rimbaud's recollection of an alphabet book he had used as a child, and indeed suitable copies of such books have been retrieved. The notion is certainly consistent with the sort of recollection from childhood that is often evoked by drugs or alcohol. The chronology of *Voyelles* has been debated; its pronounced synaesthesia suggests a date shortly after he met Verlaine in September 1871 and had his first saturation with absinthe. Rimbaud alludes explicitly to this sonnet in *Une saison en enfer* in *Délires II,* subtitled *Alchimie du verbe:*

A moi. L'histoire d'une de mes folies . . .

J'inventai la couleur des voyelles!—A noir, E blanc, I rouge, O bleu, U vert. Je réglai la forme et le mouvement de chaque consonne, et, avec des rhythmes instinctifs, je me flattai d'inventer une verbe poétique accessible, un jour ou l'autre, à tous les sens. Je réservais la traduction.

(My turn. The history of one of my follies . . .

I invented the color of the vowels!—A black, E white, I red, O blue, U green. I established rules for the form and movement of each consonant, and, with instinctive rhythms, I flattered myself on devising a poetic language accessible, one day or another, to all the senses. I withheld the translation.)[24]

The last sentence might also be read ironically as "I reserved the translation rights," tantamount to Rimbaud's self-impeachment for inventing a private language, one he could not translate for other poets' use or for his audience. It is a confession that the alchemy, the magic, of the word had failed.

Any number of allusions to absinthe recur in Rimbaud's poems, ranging from the explicit to the indirect. In *Comédie de la soif* he writes of "L'Absinthe aux verts piliers" (Absinthe with its green pillars), but then rejects it and its effects.

> Qu'est l'ivresse, Amis?
> J'aime autant, mieux, même,
> Pourrir dans l'étang
> Sous l'affreuse crème,
> Près des bois flottants.
>
> (What's being drunk, my friends?
> I would as lief, or even prefer
> To rot in the pond,
> Under the disgusting scum
> Of floating logs.)[25]

Not perhaps the most precisely chiseled image of decay, but the tenor of his self-loathing is clear. Perhaps Rimbaud's fullest comments about his alcoholic life with Verlaine are in *Les illuminations*. (There is continued debate among scholars about the chronology of *Les illumina-*

tions, but the texts, regardless of when they were written, reveal Rimbaud's state of mind.) In the prose poem *Matinée d'ivresse* he bursts forth:

> Fanfare atroce où je ne trébuche point! Chevalet féerique! . . . Ce poison va rester dans toutes mes veines même quand, la fanfare tournant, nous serons rendu à l'ancienne inharmonie. . . . Cela commença par quelques dégoûts et cela finit,—ne pouvant saisir sur-le-champ de cette éternité,—cela finit par une débandade de parfums . . . Petite veille d'ivresse, sainte! quand ce ne serait que pour le masque dont tu nous a gratifié . . . Nous avons foi au poison. Nous savons donner notre vie tout entière tous les jours. Voici le temps des ASSASSINS.

> (Terrible fanfare of music where I never lose step! Magical rack! . . . This poison will still be in my veins even when the fanfare dies away and I return to the earlier discord . . . It all began with feelings of disgust and it ended—since I could not seize eternity on the spot—it ended with a riot of perfumes . . . Brief night of intoxication, holy night! even if it was only for the mask you bequeathed to us . . . I believe in that poison. I can give you all of my existence each day. Behold the time of the ASSASSINS.)[26]

Here again is synaesthesia, the music and the perfumes, coupled with Rimbaud's knowledge of both the pleasures and the horrors of intoxication. Even earlier, in his *Lettre du voyant,* he had predicted that when he reached the unknown through systematically deranging his senses he would end by losing the insights his visions brought him. That "assassins" is derived from "haschischins" was probably known to Rimbaud, and it is curious that he chose to use the European form rather than the word introduced into French from the Indian tongue.

Rimbaud's fascination with intoxication antedated his years with Verlaine and his actual experience of the effects of absinthe. *Le bateau ivre,* written in Charleville the summer before he met Verlaine, can be taken as an extended metaphor of the liberating effect of drink, but even in that poem there are images of menace and destruction. Perhaps when frequenting the cafés of that rather staid town he had occasionally had too much to drink, or perhaps just enough to make him feel "high," but it is doubtful that he drank regularly and to excess as he did with Verlaine. He was soon to learn that the liberation was short-lived, "the momentary quality of his exaltation and the certainty of his defeat."[27]

Une saison en enfer and *Les illuminations* are complex works with many themes that reveal the conflicts within Rimbaud's psyche—love and disgust with love, hope and despair, sin and redemption, the desire for faith and the impossibility of achieving it, beauty and squalor, and many other contrarieties—all felt under the cloud of guilt and shame, the ecstasy and the agony. The heady visions of intoxication had turned into hallucination, and the suffering was intense. Writing on the aesthetics of Rimbaud's intoxication, Enid Rhodes Peschel concludes that "after the paradise comes the fall. The beauty of his brilliant but evanescent visions is based on the continual conflict between warring contraries: strength and weakness, sanctification and damnation, hope and despair, pride and shame, self-glorification and self-condemnation. . . . The intoxicated and intoxicating quest for beauty necessarily implies love, power and poetry, as well as the antithetical grandeur of madness and defeat."[28] And, like Lucifer, his fall was of his own devising.

The Last Years

After attending to the printing of *Une saison en enfer*, Rimbaud may have written a few more poems, but they are of little consequence. The motive and the cue were lacking; he had lost his vocation. The next few years saw him wandering aimlessly around Europe, trying to find himself. He made another visit to London, this time with a young poet named Germain Nouveau. Mme. Rimbaud and his sister Vitalie visited him there after Nouveau had returned to France. Rimbaud found a job teaching French at Reading, but by the end of 1874 he was back at Charleville. He went to Stuttgart at the beginning of 1875 to study German, but after a few months wandered on foot over the Swiss Alps to Italy. The romantic critical tradition gave him the sobriquet "the man with the wind at his heels," but essentially he was a lonely drifter, a vagabond. He found occasional employment, usually at menial occupations, but he was unable or unwilling to submit to the discipline of work, and the jobs did not last for long. A social misfit, he joined the ranks of the casual proletarian work force, returning intermittently to Charleville when he ran out of money. One thinks of

Robert Frost's hired man: "Home is the place where, when you have to go there, / They have to take you in."

In 1876 he enlisted in the Dutch colonial army but soon deserted. Later that year he signed on as a sailor on a merchant vessel that took him on a long voyage around the South Seas. Part of 1877 he spent wandering in Scandinavia. Toward the end of 1879 he went to Cyprus, where he became the foreman of a construction crew. There he contracted a fever diagnosed as typhoid when he returned to Roche. However, his general health was good, and he had stopped drinking. In 1879, twenty-five years old, with no fixed occupation, no fixed address, he left Europe for the Near East, returning in 1891 to die.

In 1884, when Rimbaud was working at Aden in the commercial establishment owned by Alfred Bardey, Verlaine published the first series of *Les poètes maudits* (the other poets were Tristan Corbière and Mallarmé), which first brought Rimbaud to public notice. Two years later, believing Rimbaud had died, Verlaine published *Les illuminations* and other poems by Rimbaud in *La vogue* as the work of the "late" Arthur Rimbaud. They created a sensation; Rimbaud was hailed as the great innovator he was. The French *avant-garde* quickly recognized the evocative power of his elliptical use of language and his use of words that no longer bore only their lexical meaning but were symbols to express his unconscious feelings, his *état d'âme*.[29] Soon Rimbaud became a cult figure among the young literati, but when he was told of his fine reputation in Paris, he replied that really that sort of thing didn't interest him any more.

Details of Rimbaud's life in Aden and Harar can be found in Starkie's biography and in his letters. Apart from his last illness only two items of medical interest need be noted. Starkie informs us that circa 1889 in Harar he contracted syphilis, and that on his return from a gunrunning expedition to Abyssinia he brought back with him a slave girl whom he sent to the French mission school and intended to make his wife. Both statements are based on a letter dated 7 July 1897 from Bardey to Pierre Berrichon, who was then working with Delahaye on the first collected edition of Rimbaud's poems.[30] The contents of the letter were communicated to Starkie by M. Matrasso. This is not firm evidence. Bardey was not a physician, and there is no medical diagnosis of syphilis. Even if Rimbaud did have the disease, he may have contracted it previously from Verlaine, whom we know to have been infected, rather than as a primary lesion from a prostitute in Harar. As for the slave girl, there is no corroborative evidence. In point of fact we have no real information about Rimbaud's sexual experiences after the end of his affair with Verlaine. Every now and then in his letters home from Aden or Harar he would raise the idea of coming back to France and finding a wife, but he always gave a reason or excuse why that was not feasible. The pattern suggests he was using this as a screen or cover to pretend to himself and his family that he was normal. One can construct any number of hypotheses about Rimbaud's sexual activities, but the fact is that there is no evidence to support or refute any of them.[31]

Rimbaud worked diligently as a trader in Aden and later in Harar, where he earned a good reputation as a businessman. He lived prudently, well within his means, and when the onset of his final illness forced him to liquidate his assets, he had a net capital of 32,000 francs, perhaps a bit less than the full market value—not a fortune but a comfortable sum in those days. We first learn of his illness from a letter to his mother from Harar dated February 20, 1891. He was then in his thirty-seventh year:

> I am not well at this moment. You see, varicose veins in my right leg are very painful. . . . And these varicose veins are complicated by rheumatism. . . . For two weeks I haven't closed my eyes a minute because of the pain in this accursed leg of mine. I would leave here, and believe the intense heat of Aden would do me good, but I am owed a great deal of money, and I can't go away without losing it. I have sent to Aden for a stocking for varicose veins, but I doubt it can be found. So, will you be good enough to buy me a stocking for varicose veins, for a long thin leg (my foot takes a No. 41 shoe). The stocking must come above the knee, because there is a varicose vein above the bend in the knee.[32]

Sea mail was not rapid in the 1890s, and it was not until March 27 that his mother wrote to say she had dispatched the stocking as instructed to M. Tian in Aden, as well as some ointment for the varicose veins. During the interval Rimbaud's symptoms had become worse. The knee became greatly swollen, and the pain was constant and intense; he could no longer walk. He had constructed a special litter with sides and a canvas awning and hired sixteen men plus a train of camels for provisions to carry him from Harar to Zeyla on the coast, 200 miles across the desert, a journey of excruciating pain as his bearers stumbled over the rough, uneven trail. He left Harar on April 7, arriving at Zeyla on the seventeenth, and that day took the boat for Aden. To the medical eye the symptoms are ominous: a painful expanding mass at the knee sufficient to produce distended veins above the knee suggests a malignant tumor rather than an inflammatory reaction in the joint. The next news comes from a letter to his family dated April 30:

> I received your letter and your two stockings, but I received them under sad circumstances.
>
> Since the swelling of my right knee continued getting worse, and the pain in the joint, and unable to find a remedy or advice, because in Harar we are in a Negro colony and there are no doctors, I decided to go down to Aden. I had to give up the business, which was not easy, for my money was spread out in every direction. But finally I liquidated almost everything. For twenty days I was in bed in Harar, unable to move, suffering atrocious pain and never sleeping. . . .
>
> Once here, I went into the European hospital. . . . The English doctor, as soon as I showed him my knee, exclaimed that it is a synovitis tumor which has reached a very dangerous point. . . . He first spoke of cutting the leg off. Then he decided to wait a few days to see if the swelling, with medical care, would go down a bit. There have been six days of this with no change for the better. . . . I want to be taken to a steamship and go to France for treatment. . . .
>
> The stockings are useless. I will sell them somewhere.[33]

Rimbaud spent a few more days in Aden to settle his financial affairs, then took a steamer for Marseilles, and on May 23 was admitted to the Hôpital de la Conception. He wrote to his mother and sister: "I am very sick, very sick. I have shrunk to the state of a skeleton through this disease in my right leg which has now become huge and resembles a pumpkin. It is a synovitis, a hydrarthrosis, etc. . . . It will last a long time unless complications force them to cut off the leg."[34] Mme. Rimbaud was summoned by telegram. Amputation was carried out the day after she arrived. She stayed ten days, then returned to Roche to manage her farm. Rimbaud's convalescence was slow, and his letters to his sister Isabelle provide an account of his mental as well as his physical sufferings.[35] But wounds heal, and crutches can provide support. He was discharged on July 22 and returned to Roche the following day. He was able to stay a month, but increasing weakness and possibly some fever made it necessary for him to return to Marseilles on August 23. His sister Isabelle accompanied him and stayed with him until he died on November 10, 1891. His terminal course was marked by weakness, anorexia, weight loss, cachexia, and finally paralysis of both arms and pneumonia. He was given morphine to relieve pain, and under its influence had visions. He saw columns of amethyst, angels in marble and wood, landscapes of indescribable beauty—characteristic hallucinations of opium.

The signs, symptoms, and clinical course all point to a malignant tumor of bone, arising in either the upper end of the tibia or the lower portion of the femur. Previous biographers have called it a carcinoma or else a tumor arising as a syphilitic lesion, that is, a gumma. These diagnoses are untenable; carcinomas do not arise in the knee joint, and gummas do not progress so rapidly and are not fatal. Needless to say, Rimbaud's case was before Roentgen discovered X-rays in 1895, and it was not routine practice, as it is today, to prepare histopathologic sections of surgically excised specimens. In the absence of radiologic or pathologic information we will never know with certainty the precise nature of Rimbaud's tumor. Among the possibilities for a malignant tumor of the long bones, especially at the knee, are osteogenic sarcoma, chondrosarcoma, fibrosarcoma, and synovial sarcoma. The clinical features of these tumors are so similar that one cannot select with confidence one of them as more probable in Rimbaud's case than the others. Synovial sarcoma or chondrosarcoma are a bit more likely than osteogenic sarcoma, or fibrosarcoma. About three-fourths of the cases of osteogenic sarcoma occur before the age of twenty-five, and pure fibrosarcoma is quite uncommon, but in the absence of an X-ray film or a biopsy they are possible candidates. Classification of bone sarcomas was not so precisely delineated in the 1890s as it is today. Perhaps we ought to stand by the diagnosis made by the first doctor to see Rimbaud's tumor, the English doctor at Aden, who thought it was synovial in origin. Until recent years bone sarcomas of the lower extremity were almost invariably fatal, usually within a year, and usually with metastases to the lungs, which would explain Rimbaud's terminal "pneumonia." He survived his disease for almost ten months from the onset of symptoms and less than six months from the time of amputation, a time sequence one would expect in such tumors.

Part
Four
Materia
Medica

11
Reuben's Mandrakes:
Infertility in the Bible

*B*e fruitful and multiply, and replenish the earth and sub-due it." This was the Lord's injunction (Gen. 1:28) just after "male and female created he them" on the fifth day of Creation. He repeated the injunction in the same words to Noah (Gen. 9:1). And this is precisely what the Israelites of that generation did, even as their descendants do today in their orange groves and kibbutzim. The early Hebrews, descendants of Abraham, Isaac, and Jacob, began their tribal life in the Fertile Crescent, and, after a brief period of captivity in Egypt, the Lord guided them on their return to the Holy Land. It is self-evident in an agrarian society, with its oxen and asses, sheep and goats, and fruits of the field and vine, that fecundity is a highly prized attribute in women. Manpower was a basic necessity to tend the flocks and till the fields. Though we lack actual data, we may assume that infant mortality was high and that, despite the long years the Scriptures allot to the Patriarchs, the average life-span of adult males was short.

Deviation from the Lord's command and society's needs earned condign punishment: witness the fate of Onan (Gen. 38:7–10), who tried to circumvent the levirate law and practiced *coitus interruptus* rather than fertilize his deceased brother's wife. He spilled his seed and the Lord slew him, presumably just after *flagrante delicto;* he was cut off in the blossoms of his sin like Hamlet's father (fig. 11.1). A modern medical interpretation of the event might implicate sudden occlusion of the main stem of the left coronary artery or a cardiac arrhythmia, such as complete heart block or ventricular fibrillation, rather than the intervention of the Deity. Sudden death "in the saddle" is not unknown to modern society: witness the death of Félix Faure, sixth president of France in the Third Republic, who died in his mistress's arms in his study at the Elysée Palace, as well as the deaths of other public figures too numerous to mention. It is not an uncommon *modus moriendi,* as any medical examiner can testify, and so perhaps it was with Onan,

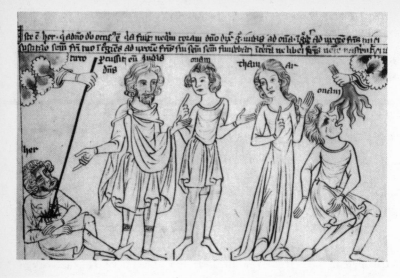

Figure 11.1. Onan and Er slain by the Lord. *Left*, Er (Her) is dispatched by a lance in the epigastrium; *center*, Judah instructs Onan to raise up a family with Tamar; *right*, Onan is slain by fire from heaven. Velisalius Bible, ca. 1350. Prague: Statni Knihovna.

who was unwilling to comply with the reproductive goals set for him by his community and the Law.

Onan and his older brother Er were the sons of Judah, who was the fourth of Jacob's sons by Leah, and Judah had arranged the marriage between Er and Tamar. But Er "was wicked in the sight of the Lord; and the Lord slew him" (Gen. 38:7–10), even as he did Onan, and using the same words. Rabbinic and Talmudic commentators have developed the argument that Er had been guilty of the same offense as Onan when Judah urged the latter to obey the levirate law and raise a family with Tamar, lest his family suffer extinction. If so, the more fool Onan, for he did not profit from the example of his brother's fate. One can understand his reason for not wishing to impregnate his sister-in-law: "the seed should not be his," that is, the children would bear Er's name, not Onan's. But what could have been Er's motive for *coitus interruptus*? The commentators suggest that he did not want pregnancy to spoil Tamar's beauty, an interesting speculation but not one supported by the received text.

Perhaps a medical explanation is possible: Both Er and Onan may have suffered from a congenital inherited defect, for example, pre-cocious arteriosclerotic plaques in the coronary artery tree, hypoplasia of one of the major arteries, or an aneurysm of the circle of Willis; the fatal event occurred just as they reached the coital climax, causing them to ejaculate just as their penes were slipping out of Tamar's introitus, while they were gasping their last. Perhaps Judah sensed this, hence his unwillingness to risk mating his third and only surviving son, Shelah, to Tamar, as required by levirate law. Thus the stage was set for Tamar, who, whether from piety or lust, "played the harlot": she disguised herself to fulfill that law and became pregnant by her unwitting father-in-law when he was en route to his sheepshearers at Timnath (Gen. 38: 11–30). Judah may be the first man recorded to have had a one-night stand with a woman he met on a business trip.

Death during sexual excitement may supervene before ejaculation takes place. One recalls the late Eric Partridge's account of the testi-mony by a London prostitute at the coroner's inquest on a client who had died in her embrace: "Seeing he was an old customer, we didn't waste time but went right on with it. He was moving along when sud-denly he gave a deep sigh, and I thought he'd come but he'd gone."

That the levirate law may impose psychological burdens upon those who observe it is not inconceivable, as the sexual peccadillos and repro-ductive performance of Henry VIII, who married his brother Arthur's widow (Catherine of Aragon) a year after his elder sibling's untimely death, might indicate. Dissatisfied with her inability—or his—to pro-duce a male heir, he broke with the papacy and founded the Church of England. Despite its superb rhetoric, the bloody events that followed that schism are among the darker pages of the history, which ultimately led to the concept of freedom of conscience.

Time has blackened and distorted the name of Onan, who had scru-ples about uncovering the nakedness of his deceased brother's wife (Lev. 18:10). No Jewish mother names her son Onan, any more than a Christian mother names her son Judas Iscariot. Precisely how Onan's name was transferred to masturbation instead of *coitus interruptus* is obscure, but the *Oxford English Dictionary* assigns the first usage of "onanism" in the sense of masturbation to Chambers' *Cyclopaedia* (1729–41), "terms which some empirics have framed to denote the crime of self-pollution." Perhaps the misapplied term became fixed in the vocabulary by the influence of the anonymous pamphlet *Onania* (1724) or Samuel Tissot's *L'Onanisme, dissertation sur les maladies pro-duite par la masturbation* (Lausanne, 1760), which went through many editions and was the precursor of a spate of later monitory tracts in English. The misuse persisted and later flourished in Victorian England. For example, see Todd's *Cyclopaedia of Anatomy* (1847–49), "a young man excessively addicted to onanism." Bucknell and Tuke's *Psychiatric Medicine* (1874) informs us that "onanism is a frequent accompaniment of insanity and sometimes causes it." Such was the lexical fate of a young man who was simply reluctant to chance reproducing his kind, despite the pressures of the society in which he lived. But the legend of his unhappy demise underscores the value the Israelites placed on fertility.

The bearing and possession of children—for children were chattel—was regarded as a gift from God: "Lo, children are a heritage of the Lord: and the fruit of the womb is his reward" (Ps. 127:3). In this context, we may recall the comment by Colonel Green-Armytage half a century ago in his address to the Royal Asiatic Society at Bengal: "This is a natural conclusion in a developing country where more hands meant better crops, and especially in the case of weak tribes, in which man-power was needed for continual wars."

Problems with infertility beset the "chosen people" from the start. Abraham and Sarah had been unable to conceive, and she suggested that he test his manliness with her Egyptian handmaid Hagar (Gen. 16:2–6). It was a challenge, and Abraham rose to the occasion with no reluctance. We may reckon this as the first clinical test for male fertility, but it was not without psychodynamic reverberations. It is not difficult to understand or sympathize with Sarah's plight. Now menopausal, for it had ceased to be with her "after the manner of women," she had no proof to leave to posterity of her muliebrity. She was probably irritable, a common symptom in perimenopausal women. But when Hagar conceived, and the onus of reproductive capacity now rested on Sarah, she responded with the jealousy born of frustration. She reproached Abraham and tried to put the blame on him: "My wrong be upon thee; I have given my maid into thy bosom, and when she saw that she had conceived, I was despised in her eye: the Lord judge between me and thee."

Wisely, the Lord did not judge between man and wife; he comforted and proteced Hagar during her pregnancy until she gave birth to Ishmael when Abraham was eighty-six years old. Some temporary reconciliation must have taken place between Sarah and Hagar, and Abraham must have been the conciliator, for they were in his household

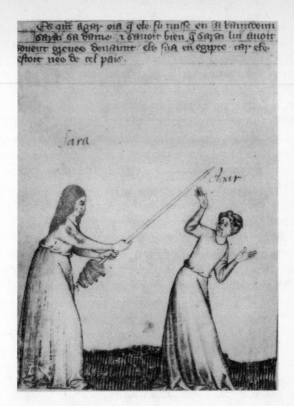

Figure 11.2. Sarah attacking Hagar. Egerton MS. 1894, Genesis, fol. 9v; first half of the fourteenth century. By permission of the Trustees of the British Library.

thirteen years later when Sarah gave birth to Isaac. Man's inhumanity to man may be great, but even greater can be woman's inhumanity to woman. It is difficult not to think of Sarah as an embittered woman who drove her pregnant handmaid into the desert and who repeatedly reproached her husband for past failures (fig. 11.2).

Sarah may have felt a burden of guilt in addition to her frustration. Not only was she barren, a reproductive failure, but she had urged her husband to have sexual relations with another woman. In biblical usage, this was not quite adultery, which was defined as cohabitation with a woman married to another man. This differs somewhat from later Western usage, which defines adultery as sexual intercourse with a partner to whom one is not married, irrespective of whether or not the partner is married. Adultery in the biblical usage was not prohibited until the time of Moses and the Ten Commandments, nor was monogamy the rule among the lusty patriarchs. But the early Hebrews did have a sense of legitimate versus illegitimate offspring, clearly related to the devolution of property. Neither Isaac nor Jacob was the firstborn son, yet each inherited his father's estate and dignity. Ishmael and Esau were in effect disinherited and treated like bastards. Esau's descendants became the Edomites, and Ishmael's progeny settled in northern Arabia, where they later became dominant in Islam. Small wonder that their twentieth-century heirs are not sympathetic to the national aspirations of Israel.

When we speculate on the possible causes for Abraham and Sarah's infertility, it is clear that conception did not occur until after her menses had apparently ceased. But occasionally a woman will experience an isolated ovulation and corresponding menstrual flow, even up to three years after her last regular period. This presents clinically as postmenopausal bleeding, and if such a patient is curetted soon after the onset of bleeding, evidence of endometrial secretion can be seen. On rare occasions such a patient will undergo laparotomy, and, if so, a recent corpus luteum can be found. That Sarah conceived after an apparent menopause can be explained on the basis of a late, isolated ovulation, the last response of her ovaries to pituitary gonadotropins. But that does not explain her failure to conceive when she was a younger woman, presumably with reasonably regular ovulatory cycles.

We must note that it was not until *after* Ishmael's birth that Abraham made his covenant with God and was circumcised at the age of ninety-nine (Gen. 17). Perhaps he was unable to impregnate Sarah because he suffered from phimosis, and once that impediment was removed, conception followed. Phimosis is not an absolute mechanical barrier to conception, only a relative one, which may explain why he had good luck with Hagar but not with Sarah. A later parallel can be found in the example of Louis XVI and Marie Antoinette, whom he married in 1770. She did not conceive until 1774, after Louis' phimosis had been surgically corrected. Whether the operation was a full circumcision or a dorsal slit is not clear, but the Dauphin was born in 1775. Parenthetically, after Abraham was circumcised, he himself circumcised all the males in his household including Ishmael, then thirteen years old, which may explain why Moslems, his latter-day descendants, circumcise at puberty or shortly before it. Abraham, of course, circumcised

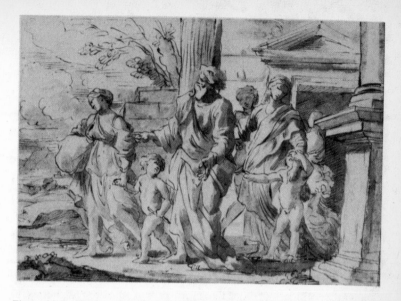

Figure 11.3. Abraham and Sarah driving out Hagar and Ishmael. Nicholas Poussin, ca. 1620. Pen and bistre wash over pencil. From the Royal Collection, Windsor; reproduced by gracious permission of Her Majesty the Queen.

himself, a painful procedure in an adult male. Perhaps the tightness of his phimosis had led to local inflammation, and he chose to relieve the pain by a single surgical procedure, painful as it must have been, rather than endure continued suffering which was aggravated during micturition and ejaculation. It may well have been an act of desperation rather than obedience to a divine injunction and covenant. Further proof of Abraham's reproductive capacity after circumcision is that after Sarah's death he married Keturah, who bore him six sons (Gen. 25:1).

It seems that Hagar and Ishmael were maintained in Abraham's household until after Isaac was born and weaned, perhaps to ensure male succession lest Sarah's infertility continue. If so, some way of legitimizing Ishmael would have been found. But after Sarah had conceived and given birth successfully, her jealousy of Hagar continued, and both the handmaid and her illegitimate son were sent away for good (Gen. 21:12–21) (fig. 11.3).

Isaac did not marry until after his mother's death, and it seems that Rebekah, his wife, also experienced difficulty conceiving: "And Isaac

entreated the Lord for his wife because she was barren . . . and Rebekah his wife conceived" (Gen. 25:21). Whatever the difficulty, it was short-lived, for she bore him twin sons, Esau and Jacob. The verse merely emphasizes the notion that children are the gift of God.

The story of Jacob and Rachel is one of the great psychological dramas of the Bible: Jacob's "love at first sight" for Rachel, Laban's underhanded dealings with him, Jacob's marriage to the two sisters (both his first cousins), their rivalry and the emotional tensions it engendered, and the birth of Jacob's twelve sons and one daughter who founded the nation of Israel. As one reads it, one thinks of classical Greek drama, Elizabethan plays, the nineteenth-century Russian novel, even an O'Neill psychodrama with dynastic overtones—but these are weak parallels. Laban insisted that Jacob marry Leah first because she was older than Rachel. Jacob accepted the subterfuge, and he treated Leah with consideration and respect even though his heart was bound to Rachel: "Leah was tender-eyed; but Rachel was beautiful and well favored" (Gen. 29:17). In swift order, Leah bore Jacob four sons—Reuben, Simeon, Levi, Judah—before his seven years of labor for Rachel were over and he could possess her. But when Jacob married Rachel, her womb was barren. We are told, "When the Lord saw that Leah was hated, he opened her womb" (Gen. 29:31); the implication is that he closed Rachel's womb because she was loved, a somewhat paradoxical arrangement of reward and punishment. When Rachel failed to conceive, she sent Jacob to Bilhah, her handmaid, who bore him Dan and Naphtali. Not to be outdone, Leah sent Jacob to *her* handmaid Zilpah, who bore him Gad and Asher.

By this time, Jacob had eight sons, but Rachel was profoundly unhappy because none of them was hers: "And when Rachel saw that she bare Jacob no children, Rachel envied her sister; and said unto Jacob, 'Give me children, or else I die.' And Jacob's anger was kindled against Rachel; and he said 'Am I in God's stead, who hath withheld from thee the fruit of thy womb'" (Gen. 30:1–2). "Or else I die" is hyperbole, an overreaction, except in the sense that unless one reproduces one's kind, there is no continuity of one's germ plasm. But this is the emotional crux of the story: Rachel, distraught with envy of Leah and shame at her own infertility, makes an agonized plea to the husband who loved her dearly, which is met with an angry rebuff and *non mea culpa* at being so challenged. Yet all the participants had behaved honorably and correctly according to the mores of the time. Leah had per-

formed her wifely duties successfully and with good will. Rachel had tried to do the same, yet, through no fault of hers or Jacob's, she failed. Their handmaids stood by in the wings ready and willing to lend their pelves and wombs to the causes. Rachel's frustration must have increased still more when Leah bore Jacob another two sons, Issachar and Zebulun, then a daughter, Dinah. At this juncture we are told that the Lord finally opened Rachel's womb, and she conceived and bore Joseph, then after an interval, Benjamin.

But the Lord's instrument seems to have been Reuben's mandrakes (Gen. 30:14–16). These fruits of the soil made their appearance after the birth of Asher, the eighth son, and it seems they were part of a bargain Rachel struck with Leah about who should share Jacob's bed on a given night. The story of the mandrakes is explicit. Reuben found them in the field at the time of the wheat harvest and brought them to Leah, his mother. For unstated reasons, Rachel asked Leah for them, but Leah, jealous because Jacob preferred Rachel, responded: "Is it a small matter that thou hast taken away my husband? And wouldst thou

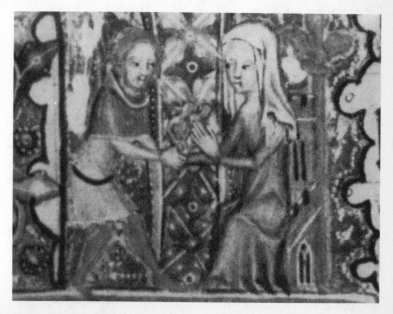

Figure 11.4. Reuben hands mandrakes to Leah. Exeter MS. 47, fol. 26v. English, before 1373. Oxford: Bodleian Library.

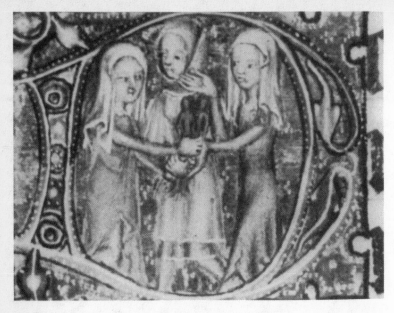

Figure 11.5. Leah hands mandrakes to Rachel. Exeter MS. 47, fol. 26r. English, before 1373. Oxford: Bodleian Library.

take away my son's mandrakes also? And Rachel said, 'Therefore he shall lie with thee tonight for thy son's mandrakes'" (Gen. 30:15). When Jacob returned from work that night, Leah claimed her rights under the bargain: "Thou must come in unto me; for surely I have hired thee with my son's mandrakes. And he lay with her that night" (Gen. 30:16). But that night's action produced Issachar, and then there were Zebulun and Dinah before Joseph was conceived—a period of no less than three years. The questions are: What do the mandrakes signify? In what way could they have reversed Rachel's infertility?

The mandrake (*Mandragora officinarum*) was well known in the ancient world. The Hebrew text of the Bible refers to them as *dudaim*, perhaps related to *dodim* (love), and though a few scholars have questioned whether *dudaim* are identical with *Mandragora*, the consensus is that they are one and the same. The plant is widely distributed throughout the Mediterranean littoral and is a member of the Solanaceae, characterized by a short stem with a tuft of ovate leaves and a thick, fleshy root that is often branched. Its purple, bell-shaped flowers are solitary and each gives rise to an orange berry. Its use in medicine dates back well over two thousand years. Hippocrates (ca. 400 B.C.) stated that "a small dose in wine, less than would produce delirium, will relieve the deepest depression and anxiety." Aristotle's *De somnia* includes mandragora along with poppies and darnel as drugs that induce sleep. In the first century, Dioscorides' *De materia medica* echoed the same properties and added that it could be used to deaden the pain from surgical procedures.

As centuries passed, a number of superstitions developed in association with the mandrake.[1] Notable among them is an assignment of gender to the plant based on the shape taken by its forked root, a unique example of androgynous anthropomorphism. Illustrations of the male and female mandrake abound in late medieval and Renaissance herbals (fig. 11.6). Another notion was that it could only be uprooted in moonlight, after appropriate prayer and ritual, by means of a black dog attached to it by a cord (fig. 11.7). When uprooted, the mandrake was supposed to give out an unearthly shriek that drove men mad, hence the term "the insane root."[2] Still another superstition was that the mandrake grew only under the gallows where a man had been hanged. Mandrake roots were often carved into human shapes, accentuating their resemblance to the male or female form, and these were carried on the person as talismans to ward off any number of misfortunes, diseases, or threats from the *malocchio*. Veiled allusions to its reputed aphrodisiacal properties can be found, and it was easy to transfer that belief into the idea that it might be of value in infertility. Such ideas may have been widespread as folklore, for both Abraham ibn-Ezra in the twelfth century and Nachmanides in the thirteenth century specifically deny it. The latter, conceding that the aroma of the mandrake's blossoms might make the marital couch more attractive, stated it had no known medical properties that would promote fertility.

By the sixteenth century, just as herbalists were beginning to cast doubt on many of these folk beliefs, Elizabethan drama and poetry became studded with allusions to its properties, some real, others fanciful. Cleopatra commands, "Give me to drink mandragora. . . . That I might sleep out this great gap of time / My Antony is away." Equally familiar is Iago's comment on the sleeplessness that jealousy has wrought in Othello: "Not poppy, nor mandragora, / Nor all the drowsy syrups of the world, / Shall ever medicine thee to that sweet sleep / Which thou ow'dst yesterday." Shakespeare was also familiar with the mandrake's

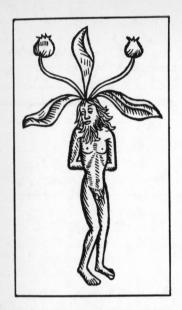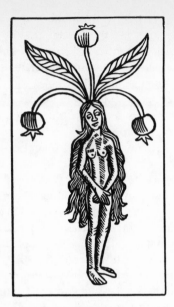

Figure 11.6. Anthropomorphic male and female forms of the mandrake root. From Johannes de Cuba, *Horta sanitatis*. Mainz, 1491.

legendary cry, hence Juliet's lines, "And shrieks like mandrakes torn out of the earth, / That living mortals, hearing them, run mad." Some writers have speculated that mandragora was in the potion Friar Laurence gave Juliet to produce a sleep that resembled death. But Shakespeare reserved the fancy of the mandrake's anthropomorphism and its reputation as an aphrodisiac for Falstaff, in his description of Justice Shallow: "When a' naked he was, for all the world like a forked radish with a head fantastically carved upon it with a knife. . . . He was the very genius of famine; yet lecherous as a monkey and the whores called him—mandrake" (*2 Henry IV* 3.2).

Other allusions to the mandrake's supposed properties occur in Marlow's *Jew of Malta,* Webster's *The Duchess of Malfi,* and Drayton's *Polyolbiol* and *Nymphal.* But most familiar of all is Donne's exhortation to an unspecified lover to "Goe and catch a falling starre, / Get with child a mandrake root. . . ." The image connotes the relation between the mandrake and fertility, but in a negative fashion: the lover can no more beget a child upon the root than he can tell where all past years are, but

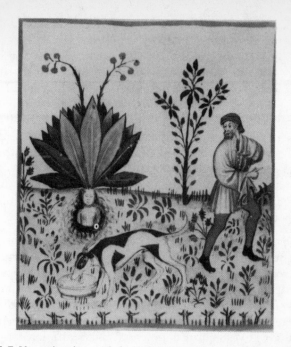

Figure 11.7. Uprooting the mandrake. A dog is attached by a rope around its neck to the neck of the "man" in the mandrake; the dog's owner holds one hand over his ear to ward off the mandrake's dreadful shriek. *Tacuinum sanitatis*, fol. 40. North Italian (Verona?), late fourteenth century. Vienna: Nationalbibliothek.

the Dean of St. Paul's does not answer the question whether the root can help a woman conceive.

By the middle of the seventeenth century, Sir Thomas Browne's *Pseudodoxia Epidemica* (1646) challenged the legend, and did so with specific reference to Rachel. "It is a common conceit that Rachel requested these plants as medicine for fecundation. . . . Which notwithstanding is very questionable, and of incertain truth." Browne's argument first questions the identity of the biblical *dudaim* with the mandrake known to later botanists, but then he continues: "It is not deducible from the Text . . . that Rachel had any such intention, and most do rest in the determination of Austin that she desired them for rarity, pulchritude or suavity. Nor is it probable she would have resigned her bed to Leah, when at the same time she had obtained a medicine to fructify herself."

Browne also raises the point that Leah conceived and bore three children between the incident of Reuben's mandrakes and Rachel's conception of Joseph. His final comment: "Although at that time they failed of this effect, yet is it mainly questionable whether they had any such vertue either in the opinions of those times, or in their proper nature." He points out that had Leah believed that mandrakes had the "vertue" of promoting fecundity, she would not have given them to her rival Rachel; as for their "proper nature," he limits the claims for the root's properties to the observation that "the Ancients have generally esteemed it Narcotick or stupefactive."

Browne closes his argument by dismissing the analogy between opium and mandragora and the claim that both promoted fertility, and for this point he reserves his most baroque prose:

> Whereas it may be thought that Mandrakes may fecundate, since Poppy hath obtained the Epithet of fruitful, and that fertility was Hieroglyphically described by Venus with a head of Poppy in her hand; the reason hereof was the multitude of seed within itself, and no such multiplying in humane generation. And lastly, whereas they may seem to have this quality, since Opium itself is conceived to extimulate unto venery, and for that intent is sometimes used by Turks, Persians, and most oriental Nations . . . they speak probably who affirm the intent and effect of eating Opium, is not so much to invigorate themselves in coition, as to prolong the Act, and spin out the motions of carnality.[3]

Mandragora was in use as a narcotic, an anodyne, and as an anesthetic until well into the fifteenth century, but as superstitious beliefs in its virtues became more elaborate, its real properties became clouded. From the sixteenth century on, authors of the great herbals wrote skeptically about it, and after Browne's day, it fell into disrepute. In 1888, Benjamin Ward Richardson published the results of some experiments with extracts of the plant. He found that the active principle was more soluble in water than in alcohol, confirming Hippocrates' suggestion that it be given in wine, a dilute aqueous alcohol medium. Perhaps the ancients first made a decoction or infusion in water, then mixed it with wine to make it palatable. Richardson's extracts produced dilatation of the pupils, paralysis of sensation and motion, excitement during the recovery phase if the dose was not lethal, and sleep and paralysis if the dose was too potent. Death was from respiratory failure; the heart continued to beat after breathing stopped. Its action seemed to be on the central nervous system. In 1889 Ahrens isolated an alkaloid from the root, and in 1901 Thoms and Wentzel showed that Ahrens' mandragorine was a mixture of hyoscine and hyosciamine, that is, scopolamine, as well as traces of other alkaloids. This accounts for its narcotic, analgesic, and anesthetic properties, but there is no pharmacologic basis for its value in infertility. One must infer that Rachel wore Reuben's mandrakes as a talisman, believing they might help her conceive, and she did.

The circumstances surrounding the conception of Samson (Judg. 13) are remarkable in that they prefigure later miraculous conceptions. Like Sarah and Rachel, the wife of Manoah the Danite was barren. The Israelites were in the hands of the Philistines, where the Lord had put them because of their evil doing, and they needed a strong man to deliver them. As befits the birth of a hero, an angel appeared to Manoah's wife, and told her she would conceive, but, "Now therefore beware, I pray thee, and drink not wine or strong drink, and eat not any unclean thing: For, lo, thou shalt conceive and bear a son; and no razor shall come on his head: for the child shall be a Nazarite unto God from the womb: and he shall begin to deliver Israel out of the hand of the Philistines." The woman promptly reported this to her husband, adding that "his countenance was like the countenance of an angel of God, very terrible." At Manoah's request the Lord sent the angel for a second visit, and he repeated the news of the impending birth as well as the instructions to avoid wine and liquor and to eat only kosher food. After some further conversation with the angel, Manoah offered a kid to the Lord, and the angel ascended in the flame from the altar. In due time, Samson was born, and his heroic deeds and sad fate are recorded in later chapters.

There is little of medical interest in the story. One cannot find a clue to the cause of Manoah's wife's infertility, nor does the couple seem to have been emotionally upset by lack of a child. But the appearance of the angel was disturbing, and this element recurs in the story of Zacharias and Elisabeth (see below).

Even more intense than Rachel's emotional outburst was Hannah's reaction to childlessness (1 Sam. 1). Like Jacob, her husband Elkanah had another wife, Peninnah, who had produced children. Though Elkanah loved Hannah deeply, "the Lord had shut up her womb." Words passed between Peninnah and Hannah, and the fertile wife provoked the infertile one to the breaking point. Together, Elkanah and Hannah repeated their annual pilgrimage to the temple at Shiloh where they consulted Eli, the high priest. So afflicted was Hannah that when she prayed, "she was in bitterness of soul . . . and wept sore." She was so distraught that "she spake in her heart; only her lips moved, but her voice was not heard." This is a description of hysterical aphonia, but Eli's first impression was that she might have been drinking to excess. Perhaps she was so upset that she was tremulous and had an unsteady gait. Fortunately, Hannah was articulate enough to clarify the matter; she told Eli, "I am a woman of a sorrowful spirit; I have drunk neither wine nor strong drink, but have poured out my soul to the Lord." Catharsis is often therapeutic in anxiety states and hysteria, and perhaps Eli recognized this, for he reassured her that the Lord would grant her petition. The combination of prayer and psychotherapy worked well. Hannah "went her way, and did eat, and her countenance was no more sad." When Elkanah returned with her to their home in Ramah, she conceived and bore Samuel (fig. 11.8).

The historical importance of the story is, of course, the vow Hannah made to consecrate her child to God if he granted her prayer. She did so gladly, and the story of Samuel as Eli's successor, his wise judgments, his role in the struggle against the Philistines, and his good counsel to Saul and David is familiar to all. Less well remembered is the fact that after Samuel's birth and weaning, Hannah bore three more sons and two daughters to Elkanah (1 Sam. 2:21). One can account for her early infertility on the basis of a serious psychological problem that got worse as she continued to try but failed. Mild anxiety may be the common lot of many men and women who find their aspirations frustrated, but when symptoms become severe, namely, anorexia and hysterical aphonia, fertility can be significantly impaired. Once Hannah had successfully borne a child, her mind was at peace with itself, and she had no further difficulty in conceiving. We often see the same profound distress in women in the twentieth century who seek medical advice for prolonged infertility. Many women who have had difficulty conceiving and proceed to adopt a child suddenly become fertile after the adoption.

Like Elkanah and Hannah, Zacharias and Elisabeth were "righteous before God," but they had no child, because Elisabeth was barren; and they were now well along in years like Abraham and Sarah (Luke 1). Zacharias was a priest in Israel, and one day it was his lot to burn the incense at the time of divine service. He must have prayed for a child,

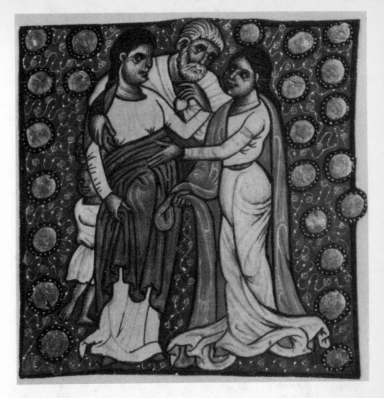

Figure 11.8. Elkanah protectively embraces Hannah while Peninnah palpates her abdomen to verify her pregnant status. The children in the background are presumably Peninnah's. Conradin Bible, south Italian, ca. 1265. MS. W.152a. Courtesy of the Walters Art Gallery, Baltimore.

for as he was swinging the censer, an angel appeared to him, told him that his prayer had been heard and that Elisabeth would bear him a son, whom he was to name John (fig. 11.9). This was the future John the Baptist, destined "to make ready a people prepared for the Lord." The text is not explicit about the quality of Elisabeth's emotional distress, but we can assume she suffered, as had Sarah, Rachel, and Hannah, for her pregnancy took away her "reproach among men." We are also told that after she conceived, she hid herself for five months.

Life was not so easy for Zacharias. When he heard the angel's news, he asked quite reasonably, "Whereby shall I know this, for I am an old

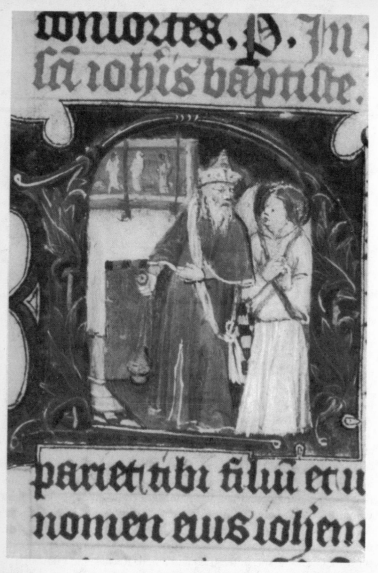

Figure 11.9. The Annunciation to Zacharias. Zacharias is shown in his priestly robes, swinging his censer. He appears well along in years and somewhat surprised as the angel informs him that Elisabeth will conceive and bear a son. Dutch Missal, ca. 1430. MS. W.174, fol. 190. Courtesy of the Walters Art Gallery, Baltimore.

man, and my wife well stricken in years?" The angel revealed himself to be the archangel Gabriel, and he punished Zacharias for not immediately accepting the glad tidings by striking him dumb. Zacharias was not even able to give his blessing to the congregation after the service, as was the custom. Punishment for even a brief hesitation in accepting divine revelation or in obeying God's dictates was swift. For the simple human gesture of turning to see her former home Lot's wife had been turned into a pillar of salt. One would have expected a masculine God like Jehovah to be more lenient with Zacharias, his priest. The natural question any man asks his wife when she tells him she is pregnant is, "Are you sure?" And had not Moses asked God for a sign when he was called to lead the people of Israel out of bondage in Egypt (Exod. 4)? In any case, Zacharias remained mute until after his son was born and ready to be circumcised. When the question of naming the baby arose, Elisabeth replied, "He shall be called John." But that simple statement did not sit well with her neighbors and cousins because she had no kinsman by that name. They signaled Zacharias, who asked for a writing tablet; on the slate he wrote, "His name *is* John." Whereupon "his mouth was opened immediately, and his tongue loosed, and he spake, and praised God."

The received text provides no information upon which to hazard a guess about the cause of Elisabeth's infertility, but Zacharias' muteness offers a chance for medical speculation. There is no reason to suspect a lesion in his organs of speech; his voice was restored intact as quickly as it had been stifled. There is nothing to suggest an organic brain lesion such as a stroke or a tumor; he continued in good health throughout Elisabeth's pregnancy, confinement, and puerperium. The most likely diagnosis is hysterical aphasia, its onset abrupt after a vision charged with profound emotion. Visions of angels were a frightening experience; Zacharias "was troubled, and fear fell upon him," even as it did to Mary at the Annunciation ("troubled . . . and cast in her mind"). The unexpected appearance of Gabriel to the aging priest, who may not have felt that his prayer would ever be fulfilled, must have been a shock, and a psychological sequela could reasonably have been predicted.

Another interesting part of the story is that the Annunciation to Mary came six months after her cousin Elisabeth had conceived. Gabriel seems to have made two round trips to Israel within that calendar year. Finding herself with child, Mary paid a visit to Elisabeth (fig. 11.10), and as she entered her cousin's house, quickening occurred

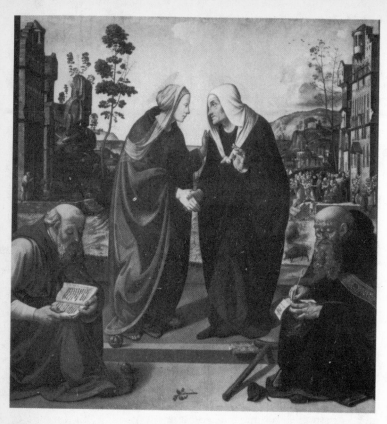

Figure 11.10. The Visitation. Piero di Cosimo, ca. 1500. Oil on wood. Elisabeth is saluting Mary at the moment of quickening. St. Nicholas of Bari, identified by his three gold balls, is seated on the left, and St. Anthony Abbott, identified by his tau staff and his pig roaming in the middle distance, is seated on the right. The Adoration of the Shepherds is shown in the left background, the Slaughter of the Innocents in the right background, and behind that, in a small chapel, the Annunciation to Mary. Courtesy of the National Gallery of Art, Washington, D.C.

within Elisabeth's womb: "the babe leaped in her womb." This event probably coincides with Elisabeth's coming out of seclusion, but why she "hid herself" is not explicit; it was neither a religious requirement nor a custom. Perhaps, being an elderly primigravida, Elisabeth took the precaution of resting at home, not venturing outside, to safeguard her much desired pregnancy by as much bed rest as possible. Mary's visit lasted three months, and she appears to have left just before Elisabeth went into labor. This seems a bit unusual; one might expect she would have stayed to help out, but apparently there were enough neighbors and kinswomen to cope. Another curious feature is God's use of Gabriel to announce to Zacharias (not to Elisabeth) that conception would take place as requested. Was he testing his powers, a dry run, so to speak, for the real Annunciation a few months later?

One of the great liturgical sequences, "*Magnificat anima mea* . . . ," comes from the episode of the Visitation. The verses are presented as Mary's reply to Elisabeth's salutation, "Blessed art thou among women." Yet the passage praising God closely resembles Hannah's joyful song, "My heart rejoiceth in the Lord, mine horn is exalted . . ." (1 Sam. 2:1-10), and it was Elisabeth's circumstance, not Mary's, that paralleled Hannah's, as in "He hath regarded the low estate of his handmaiden," that is, her childlessness, which he relieved.

Not only do these episodes from the Bible share in common the theme of the anguish of women who want to but cannot bear children, they also illustrate that barrenness was always imputed to the woman as her fault, her reproach among men. With few exceptions, it is only in the latter half of the twentieth century that infertility has been recognized as a medical condition involving couples and that, often as not, the incapacity is the man's. One such exception was the legendary eleventh-century midwife Trotula of Salerno, whose *De passionibus mulierum curandarum* discussed infertility and suggested that the urine of both male and female partners be tested to see which was at fault:

> If a woman desires to conceive, it must be first ascertained
> whether she is able to have her wish, to know if there is any fault
> in either one of them or both. It may be ascertained thus: Take
> two little pots like mustard pots, and in each . . . put wheat bran:
> . . . the man's in one . . . the woman's in the other . . . let the
> pots stand nine or more days. And if the fault is in the man . . .
> you will find worms in the urine and a terrible smell. And if the

fault is in the woman, you will find the same proof. And if worms appear in neither pot of urine, the condition of the man and the woman can be remedied, and they may have their wish with the grace of God with medicines thus: Take the testicles of a boar and dry them in a pot closed by a lid very small or pressed about the joints so that no fumes come out in an oven; when the testicles are dried, make a powder of them and let the woman drink it, after which she will have her purgation.[4]

At least this medication is hypothetically directed toward endocrinological causes for infertility and represents an advance over mandrake roots.

The gravity of a barren woman's situation in biblical times must be viewed in the context of compulsory dissolution of marriages that proved sterile. The traditions of the Mishnah and Talmud were not codified until relatively late, but the sixteenth-century 'Even Ha'ezer (cliv. 10) that forms part of the *Shulhan 'Arukh,* a codification based on the Talmud, subsequent commentaries, and Maimonides, states that it is a husband's duty to divorce his wife if she has borne him no children after ten years, excluding periods during which marital relations were impossible due to illness or separation. However, the permissible polygamy of biblical times was in effect even beyond the time of the Mishnah and Talmud. It was not until about A.D. 1000 that Rabbenu Gershom of Mainz issued an edict forbidding polygamy. This was included in later codices, but in earlier times if a man had issue from one wife, he was under no compulsion to divorce a second wife if she proved infertile. Therefore, Leah's fertility enabled Jacob to retain Rachel, and Peninnah's children enabled Elkanah to keep Hannah as his wife. Even after Rabbenu Gershom's *takanah* enforced monogamy, it is doubtful that the law was rigidly enforced, but knowledge of its provision could have done little to reduce the emotional tension of a couple who had tried repeatedly to reproduce but failed. However, the existence of such a law confirms our ideas about the high value the Israelites placed upon fecundity, even in the Diaspora.

Evidence that the Israelites might have had empirical knowledge about the optimal time for fertilization can be derived from the Talmudic tractate *Niddah,* which deals with the laws governing menstruating women. The law (*halakhah*), based on Leviticus 15:19–23 and "a running issue out of the flesh," is that sexual intercourse and intimacies that might lead to it are forbidden from the time a woman expects her menses until seven clean days have elapsed. For the purposes of the *halakhah,* a minimum of five days is fixed for the menses themselves. The minimum period of sexual abstinence is twelve days after the onset of flow. Twentieth-century studies indicate that ovulation is most likely to occur at mid cycle, or the fourteenth day. Resumption of intercourse after twelve days certainly allows for replenishment of adult spermatozoa and a maximum volume of ejaculate just before and during mid-cycle, and after such abstinence libido ought to be strong. There is no written evidence that the Israelites examined the question systematically; in fact, they probably did not. However, repeated observations about the time of coitus and subsequent conception, handed down from one generation to another in a closely knit, tribal society, may have made this part of an oral tradition that gradually became custom, and from custom came oral law, which during the period in question had the force of written law.

12

The Plague at
Granada, 1348–49:
Ibn al-Khatib
and Ideas of Contagion

*H*istorical relations between cause and effect can be difficult to ascertain, especially when an event identified as a single effective cause produces a variable effect. The Black Death of 1348–49 devastated Western Europe. Most authorities concur that the Black Death was the death knell of Siena as an important city, but Florence survived to flourish again.[1] Mute testimony of Siena's decline are the remains of the walls of the unfinished enlargement of its cathedral—"Bare ruined choirs where late the sweet bird sang." Yet the same epidemic of bubonic plague struck Granada a few weeks later, and the Moors were able to complete the Alhambra during the reign of Mohammed V (1354–59 and 1362–91). We lack information upon which to calculate the mortality rate at Granada; many records were destroyed when Ferdinand and Isabella ousted the Moors in 1492 after their hegemony of two and a half centuries.[2] Only a few Islamic manuscripts survived at the end of the fifteenth century; most of them were in the library of Phillip II's Escorial.

Ultrachristian Spain had little interest in Islamic culture, and not until 1863 did M. J. Müller, a German scholar, bring Ibn al-Khatib's manuscript on bubonic plague to the notice of the scholarly world.[3] But Müller's call went unheard, possibly because he issued it at a meeting of the philosophy and philology section of the Royal Bavarian Academy of Science. At that time Pasteur's theory that germs cause disease was still unsettled. It was only a few years before Koch announced his postulates. It was the dawn of the modern era in bacteriology. Investigation of epidemics and how diseases spread were a major concern of medical scientists the world over, but their eyes were on the new discoveries of the present, not the past. The notion that a fourteenth-century Moorish statesman-physician-poet could tell them anything of value was, to put it kindly, information they did not wish to have. Even today, Ibn al-Khatib's ideas are known only to a few scholars in medieval Islamic culture.

Lisan-ad-Din Ibn al-Khatib (1313–75) came from a family that migrated from Syria to Iberia during the eighth century. His father died at the battle of Salado in 1340, and shortly thereafter the young man, whose educational attainments at Granada had marked him as promising, entered the service of Yusuf I as secretary under the vizier Ali b. al-Djayyab. When the latter died of plague in January 1349, Ibn al-Khatib was appointed head of the royal chancery with the title of vizier. He retained this office when Mohammed V succeeded Yusuf I in 1354. When Mohammed V was deposed from 1359 to 1362, Ibn al-Khatib was imprisoned, then set free to join his leader in exile in Morocco. He returned to power with Mohammed V in 1362 as vizier and chief dignitary of the court. He continued in office until 1372, when a cumulation of intrigues against him made it convenient to take advantage of an inspection tour of fortifications in western Granada and slip across the border to Ceuta. His enemies had charged him with heresy as well as other crimes against the state. He remained safe at Ceuta for a few years, but ultimately his enemies at Granada proved too powerful. He was returned there, imprisoned, and tried before a private court. No conclusive verdict was pronounced, but he was secretly strangled in prison in 1375. Such were the risks of power in fourteenth-century Islamic Spain, to say nothing of any number of contemporary Christian states.

Ibn al-Khatib was a polymath. Distinguished in many branches of learning, he wrote on history, philosophy, mysticism, and medicine, as well as producing a considerable amount of poetry. His monograph *Al-Ihata fi ta'rikh Gharnata* is a valuable source for the early history and topography of Granada, and his *Djaysh al-tawshih* is considered a fine anthology of poetry. Of even greater importance is his treatise on bubonic plague, *Muqni'at as-sa'il 'an marad al-ha'il* (Escorial MS. No. 1785, fols. 39a–48b), probably written between 1359 and 1362 during his exile in Morocco. It was certainly written after 1352 because it mentions Ibn Battutah's account of the plague in the Middle East, written after that savant's visit to Granada in 1349–52.

Greek and Roman medical writers had explained epidemics of infectious disease by the concept of miasma, noxious pollution of the atmosphere (cf. the etymology of *malaria*). Varro may have been prescient during the first century B.C. when in *De re rustica* he considered that placement of a country house should take into account:

[Q]uod crescunt animalia quaedam minuta, quae no possunt oculi consequi, et per aera intus in corpus per os ac nares perveniunt atque efficiunt difficiles morbos.

(Because certain tiny animals grow, which the eyes cannot detect and which pass through the air and into the body through the mouth and nostrils and produce refractory diseases.) [4]

In the next century Columella echoed these ideas, advising that farm buildings be situated at a distance from marshland because the marshes emit a harmful virus (*noxium virus*) that breeds swimming and crawling pets that produce human disease. Such tentative modifications of the miasma theory could not be tested until the latter half of the nineteenth century, and it would be claiming too much to suggest that Varro's idea of living, airborne, invisible animal infectious agents foreshadowed modern bacteriology or that Columella's *virus* bore a conceptual relationship to the viruses that twentieth-century scientists have detected. Although the seeds of the animalcule theory of infection can be read into the text today, later Greek and Roman writers generally adhered to miasma theory, an idea that coincided neatly with the humoral theory of disease, popularized in the continuing Galenic tradition that dominated both Christian and Moslem medicine until the seventeenth century.

The miasmal theory of plague was congenial to Moslem theology, which held that the disease is a martyrdom, a mercy from God for a Moslem, and a punishment for an infidel. It followed that a Moslem should neither enter nor flee from a plague-stricken place, and that there was no contagion. Orthodox Islamic medical thought accepted the premise and the reasoning from it. Bound with Ibn al-Khatib's *Muqni'at* in Escorial MS. No. 1785 are two other Andalusian treatises on the plague. The first is *Tahsil al-gharad al-qasid fi tafil al-marad alwafid* by Ahmad ibn Ali ibn Khatimah, a physician and poet from Almeria; probably written early in 1349, it has been described as the fullest contemporary medical explanation of plague written in Arabic.[5] The other treatise, *Tahqiq an-naba' 'an amr al-waba'* (fols. 106a–11a), is a layman's guide to treating plague victims written by Mohammed ibn Ali ash-Shaquri, a physician of Granada who was one of Ibn al-Khatib's pupils. Both of these subscribe to the miasmal theory without reservation. It has been suggested that Ibn al-Khatib wrote his *Muqni'at* as a rebuttal to Ibn-Khatimah's treatise, a plausible but undocumented theory.

Medieval man feared sudden death and death at an early age much as twentieth-century man fears nuclear catastrophe and old age. It was easy for the faithful to ascribe pestilence to divine wrath and punishment upon a sinful people, a feeling greatly reinforced by the evident impotence of human efforts to control the spread of the disease. Other supernatural causes were invoked to account for epidemics of plague and notable astrological portents, and such ideas were often combined. The *Compendium de epidemica,* prepared in 1348 for Philip IV by the Paris College of Physicians, a faculty noted for its orthodoxy, presented a mixture of astral and miasmal doctrine. Hirst summarizes it briefly, if not intelligibly, for modern readers: "[T]he state of heavenly bodies led to a pernicious corruption of the air through vapours drawn up from the southern seas and carried as a fog, with great dampness and heat, to many places on the earth. The poisonous activity lasted as long as the sun remained in the sign of the Lion."[6] Shakespeare echoes this idea in *Timon of Athens,* written in the first decade of the seventeenth century; the misanthrope tells Alcibiades to "Be as a planetary plague, when Jove / Will o'er some high-viced city hang his poison / In the sick air" (4.3.109–11). Regardless of religious orthodoxy, fourteenth-century physicians had an implicit idea that plague was communicable. The medical faculty of Paris warned healthy citizens to avoid the poisoned air exhaled by the sick and to keep a distance from them. Gentile de Foligno, who died of the disease in 1348, noted that plague passed from one person to another. So even did Ibn-Khatimah, whose orthodoxy compelled him to ascribe the disease to the will of Allah. It remained for Ibn al-Khatib to make the idea of contagion explicit and to base his argument on personal, empirical observation rather than received orthodox beliefs.

The *Muqni'at* provides a clear clinical description of the plague, explaining (as one would expect) the clinical features of the disease, especially predisposition to it, in terms of the prevailing humoral theories of the era. Ibn al-Khatib distinguished between the bubonic and pneumonic forms of the infection and recommended a number of measures for prophylaxis and treatment, none of which differs materially from those advised by other late medieval writers. What distinguishes his treatise is his emphasis on contagion (*al-adwa*). Freely translated, the passage reads:

> It becomes clear to anyone who has diagnosed or treated the disease that most of the individuals who have had contact with a plague victim will die, whereas the man who has had no exposure will remain healthy. A garment or vessel may carry infection into a house; even an earring (*al-halak*) can prove fatal to the man who has put it in his ear. The disease can make its first appearance in a single house of a given town, then spread from that focus to other persons—neighbors, relatives, visitors. The disease can break out in a coastal town that had been free of the disease until a plague victim landed there, coming across the sea from a town where plague is raging. The date at which plague appears in the town coincides with [i.e., occurs a few days after] the debarkation of this carrier.
>
> Many people remained in good health who kept themselves in isolation from the outside world, for example the pious Ibn Abi-Madyan in Salé. He believed in contagion; therefore he laid by a store of provisions and bricked up his house, sequestering his large family. The town was severely stricken, but no one in his household took ill. There are many accounts of communities remote from highways and commerce that remained unscathed. There is also the remarkable example of the prisoners in the Arsenal at Seville who were unaffected even though the city itself was hard hit. Other reports tell us that itinerant nomads who live in tents in North Africa remained free of disease because the air is not shut in, and the corruption from it is only mildly infectious.

This is a coherent, internally consistent description of the transmission of disease by human contact. It relates contagion from a single infected person to a large number, at first within a given household, then more widely to people exposed to that household. That the initial infection appeared in seaports and was transmitted by sailors from commercial ships coincides with the known distribution of the plague's attack, first appearing at Messina in Sicily in October 1347, then more or less simultaneously at Genoa and Venice, with a third portal of entry at Pisa a few weeks later. Ibn al-Khatib also cites several examples of how infection was avoided by one or another form of isolation. The image of an earring as an object that could carry infection is characteristically Levantine.

What is lacking, of course, is identification of the organism that caused the disease, the insect vector (fleas), and the animal reservoir (rats). Varro's notion of "tiny animals . . . that the eye cannot detect" was unknown to Ibn al-Khatib. Latin literature was then as closed a book to Islamic scholars as Islamic medical writings were to nineteenth-century bacteriologists and epidemiologists. Not until 1546 with Frascastorius' *De contagione* was a unified theory of infection and contagion broached, and it was not until 1658 that Athanasius Kircher observed bacilli in the blood of plague victims through a primitive microscope.[7]

In the fourteenth century the most striking contrast was not that between religious and secular views of disease but between Christian and Islamic attitudes toward it. When confronted by plague, Islam adopted a fatalistic response. No effort was made to take precautions, to isolate victims, or to prevent transport of the infection. Indeed, the very idea of contagion was strenuously denied. The teachings of the Prophet dictated three principles: Plague was a mercy and a martyrdom sent by God; plague could not be contagious because disease came directly from God; no Moslem should flee from a plague-stricken city. Conversely, Christians saw it as a punishment for sin.

How did Ibn al-Khatib reconcile his idea that plague was transmissible with the orthodox view, the revealed work (*ash-har'*), that plague was not contagious? He replied: "That infection exists is confirmed by experience, investigation, insight, personal observation, and reliable reports. These are the elements of proof."[8] He was confident that received doctrine could be refuted by empirical observations if they were carefully made and confirmed by their recurrence and by independent observers. But he was experienced enough a diplomat and dialectician to anticipate the form that rebuttal from strict constructionists would take. He continued: "One may not ignore the principle that a proof taken from tradition (*Hadith la-adwa*), if observation and inspection show the contrary, must be interpreted allegorically." To the fundamentalist mind, allegorical interpretation of what it perceives as literal truth is anathema. To the orthodox mind, applying the test of reason to faith is likewise anathema. In an authoritarian-fundamentalist society that is enough for a charge of heresy.

Precisely why Ibn al-Khatib was secretly strangled in a Granada prison cell in 1375 is not known, but the charge of heresy was probably supplemented by charges of malfeasance in office. Lest we judge his executioners too harshly, we should recall that Christians burnt Michael Servetus at the stake in 1553 and dealt with Giordano Bruno in like fashion in 1600. The difference seems to be that Christians barbecued their heretics in public and called it an *auto da fé*—an act of faith.

13

The Trial of
Spencer Cowper:
Expert Witnesses
to the Rescue

*T*he charge was murder. The time and place were July 18, 1699, at the Hertford Assizes. Spencer Cowper, a thirty-year-old barrister, was charged with killing Sarah Stout, a young unmarried Quaker, on the night of March 13. The case was a *cause célèbre* in its day, and it was fully reported in Cobbett's *State Trials*.[1] So important was it that Macaulay devoted a chapter to it in his *History of England* (1855).[2] Yet most twentieth-century readers are unfamiliar with it, and the story bears retelling.

The Cowpers were an influential Whig family in Hertfordshire. Spencer Cowper's older brother William, later Lord Chancellor as Earl Cowper, was already a prominent M.P. Spencer himself, educated at Westminster School and called to the bar, was an active member of the home circuit and was prospering in his profession. Happily married since 1688, he was the father of two sons, William (born 1689) and John (born 1694); John was later the father of William Cowper, the poet.

Many of the facts in the case were not in dispute. On March 13 Spencer Cowper had ridden up from London to Hertford to attend a session of the assizes with three colleagues, Ellis Stephens, William Rogers, and John Marson; at the trial those three stood in the dock with him, also charged with murder. They arrived at their lodgings together, but Cowper had an errand to perform: he was to turn over to Sarah Stout some money he had collected on her behalf, interest on a mortgage. Sarah lived with her mother, the widow of a well-to-do Quaker maltster, in a good-sized house alongside the millstream, a quarter of an hour's walk from the center of town. Sarah had invited Cowper to spend the night there as their guest, but he had made arrangements through his brother to let a room in the home of a couple named Barefoot who frequently provided lodgings for members of the circuit. However, Cowper did accept an invitation to supper.

The prosecution established that after supper Cowper and Sarah Stout sat together in the parlor until nearly eleven o'clock. At eleven she instructed Sarah Walker, the housemaid, to warm a bed for Mr. Cowper. The prosecutor's charge claimed:

> The maid of the house, gentlemen, upon this went up stairs to warm his bed, expecting the gentleman would have come up and followed her before she had done; but it seems while she was warming his bed, she heard the [front] door clap together; and the nature of the door is such, that it makes a great noise and the clapping of it to, that anybody in the house may be sensible of any one's going out. . . . [S]he came down, but there was neither Mr. Cowper nor [Miss] Stout; so that we suppose, and for all we can learn, they must go out together. After their going out, the maid and the mother came into the room; and the young gentlewoman not returning, they sat up all night in the house. . . . The next morning . . . the first news . . . was that she lay floating and swimming in the water by the mill dam. . . . There she lay with her petticoats and apron, but her night rail and morning gown were off, and one of them was not found until some time after.

Sarah Walker's direct testimony confirmed this part of the charge; Mrs. Stout, unable to take an oath because she was a Quaker, could not testify. The prosecution followed with a series of witnesses who had been present when the body was removed from the water. They agreed that at the milldam the stream was about six feet deep and that Sarah Stout was found floating on her right side just below the surface of the water, with her right arm caught between two of the stakes used to keep weeds from drifting into the mill. Other witnesses added that her head was also trapped in the gate formed by the stakes. The point of this evidence was to establish that there was nothing to prevent the body from sinking to the bottom.

The next witnesses were the three women who had prepared the body for burial. They stated that when the clothing was removed the body showed no swelling and that there were a few bruises on the trunk but no mark around her neck. Their evidence was corroborated by John Dimsdale, Jr., a surgeon, whom Mrs. Stout had summoned to examine the body. Then Sarah Peppercorn, a midwife, testified that she had been asked to inspect the body because a rumor had started that Sarah Stout was pregnant; she found no external sign of pregnancy, but she did notice a small amount of froth at the mouth.

The body of the unfortunate young lady was duly buried, but rumors continued to fly. These were supported by reports of conversation among the three men charged with Cowper as they were drinking wine that evening. They had been overheard, as Macaulay puts it,

> talking about the charms and flirtations of the handsome Quaker girl in the light way in which such subjects are discussed even at the circuit tables and mess tables of our more refined generation. Some wild words, susceptible of a double meaning, were used about the way she had jilted one lover, and the way in which another lover would punish her for her coquetry. On no better grounds than these, her relations imagined that Spencer Cowper had, with the assistance of these three retainers of the law, strangled her, and thrown her corpse into the water. (*HE*)

The matter did not rest there. Political and sectarian considerations intervened, and the case commanded wide public attention: "The Quakers and the Tories joined to raise a formidable clamour. The Quakers had, in those days, no scruples about capital punishments. They would, indeed, as Spencer Cowper said bitterly, but too truly, rather send four innocent men to the gallows than let it be believed that one who had their light within her had committed suicide. The Tories exulted in the prospect of winning two seats from the Whigs" (*HE*). Accordingly, on April 28, more than six weeks after the drowning, Mrs. Stout had the body exhumed and dissected.

The autopsy was a collaborative effort. Most of the prosecution seems to have been carried out by, or at least under the supervision of, Dr. Coatsworth, a surgeon, but the uterus was removed by Dr. Phillips. Also present were other local physicians, Drs. Nailor, Woodhouse, and Bide, as well as Mr. Camblin and Dr. John Dimsdale, Sr., the father of the surgeon who had examined the body soon after it was removed from the millstream. Dr. Coatsworth presented most of the medical evidence for the prosecution:

> Her face and neck, to her shoulders, appeared black, and so much corrupted, that we were unwilling to proceed any further;

but, her mother would have it done, and so we did open her; and as soon as she was opened, we perceived the stomach and guts were as full of wind as if they had been blown by a pair of bellows; we put her guts aside, and came to the uterus, and Dr. Phillips shewed it [to] us in his hand, and afterwards cut it out and laid it on the table, and opened it, and we saw into the cavity of it, and if there had been any thing in it as minute as a hair, we might have seen it, but it was perfectly free and empty; and after that, we put the intestines into their places; and we bid him open the stomach, and it was opened with an incision-knife, and it sunk flat, and let out wind but no water; afterwards we opened the breast and lobes of the lungs, and there was no water; then we looked on each side, and took up the lobes of the lungs too, to see if there was no water in the diaphragm, and there was none, but all dry. Then I remember I said, this woman could not be drowned, for if she had taken in water, the water must have rotted all the guts. (*ST*)

The autopsy clearly established that Sarah Stout was not pregnant, and the doctors signed an affidavit to that effect: "We . . do find the Uterus perfect and empty, and of the natural Figure and Magnitude as usually in Virgins; we found no Water in the Stomach, Intestines, Abdomen, Lungs, or Cavity of the Thorax."[3] Cautiously, they did not commit themselves in writing to an opinion whether the cause of death was drowning.

Dr. John Dimsdale, Sr., followed Dr. Coatsworth in the witness box and supplied the opinion the prosecution needed: "[W]e held a consultation to consider, whether she was drowned or not drowned; and we were all of an opinion, that she was not drowned; only Mr. Camblin desired he might be excused from giving his opinion . . . but all the rest of us did give our opinions, that she was not drowned" (*ST*). When asked by Baron Hatsell, who was the judge at the Assizes, how he could tell after so many weeks whether she had met death by drowning or not, Dimsdale replied, "for if she had been drowned, there had been some sign of water; and if there had been a pint of water, it would have rotted her lights and her guts; and that is done in a week's time by fermentation" (*ST*).

The substance of the prosecution's medical evidence was that Sarah Stout had neither drowned nor been drowned because there was no water in her stomach, lungs, or pleural cavities, but there is no indication that the local surgeons opened the trachea and bronchi or examined the cut surface of the lungs. Nor did their postmortem examination supply a cause of death.

Next the prosecution attempted to account for the fact that the body had been found floating rather than at the bottom of the millstream. An unexpected witness was Edward Clement, a seaman, who had had some experience with seeing men drown:

> [I]n [the] Beachy fight, I saw several thrown over-board during the engagement, but one particularly I took notice of, that was my friend, and killed by my side; I saw him swim [i.e., float] for a considerable distance from the ship. . . . I saw several dead bodies floating at the same time; likewise in another engagement, where a man had both his legs shot off, and died instantly, they threw over his legs; though they sunk, I saw his body float. . . . I have seen men when they have been drowned, that they have sunk as soon as the breath was out of their bodies, and I could see no more of them. (*ST*)

The sailor elaborated under further question: "Men float with their heads just down, and the small of their back and buttocks upward" (*ST*). A further question by Mr. Jones, the prosecutor, resolved any ambiguity in the testimony:

> Q: Then you take it for a certain rule, that those that are drowned sink, but those that are thrown over-board do not?
> A: Yes, otherwise why should the government be at that vast charge to allow threescore and fourscore of weight of iron to sink every man, but only that their swimming [i.e., floating] about should not be a discouragement to others. (*ST*)

The prosecutor pointed out to the jury that all this testimony indicated that Sarah Stout did not drown herself but that her body had been placed in the millstream after she had been killed. However, he did not comment on how she might have been killed. At this point he digressed and made a strong psychological point against Spencer Cowper. Apparently, in spite of the amicable feelings between the Cowpers and the Stouts, when he heard of Sarah's death the following morning, he expressed no word of sadness or sorrow, did not call on the bereaved mother, gave his evidence at the coroner's inquest with the utmost coolness, and the next day proceeded on circuit as if nothing unusual had happened.

At this point, perhaps we may digress and turn to Sir Thomas Browne's *Pseudodoxia Epidemica* (1646) and see what seventeenth-century erudition brought to bear upon the questions raised by the prosecution's evidence. Browne tells us:

> That Men swim naturally, if not disturbed by fear; that Men being drowned and sunk, do float the ninth day when their gall breaketh; that Women drowned, swim prone, but Men supine, or upon their backs; are popular affirmations, whereto we cannot assent. . . . For the time of floating, it is uncertain according to the time of putrefaction, which shall retard or accelerate according to the subject and season of the year. . . . Such as are fat do commonly float soonest, for their bodies soonest ferment. . . . Lastly, that Women drowned float prone, that is with their bellies downward, but Men supine or Upward, is an assertion where the *hoti* or point it self is dubious; and were it true, the reason alleged for it, is of no validity. The reason yet current was first expressed by Pliny, *veluti pudori defunctorum parcente natura,* nature modestly ordaining this position to conceal the shame of the dead. . . . For first, in nature the concealment of secret parts is the same in both sexes, and the shame of their reveal equal: so Adam upon the first taste of the fruit was ashamed of his nakedness as well as Eve. . . . While herein we commend the modesty, we condemn the wisdom of nature: for that prone position we make her contrive unto the Woman, were best agreeable to the Man, in whom the secret parts are very anteriour and more discoverable in a supine and upward posture.[4]

It is unlikely that the sailor had dipped into Browne's *Vulgar Errors,* and in fact he was repeating one of them. The bench was of no help; Baron Hatsell had remarked earlier that he did not understand Browne's chapter. The remainder of the prosecution's case was an effort to implicate Stephens, Rogers, and Marson. Their frivolous conversation at the Glove and Dolphin was duly introduced into the proceedings, but no witness placed them in the vicinity of the Stouts' home.

Spencer Cowper mounted a vigorous defense. In his opening remarks to the jury he pointed out that the stakes in the millstream were one foot apart and that by holding the right arm between them they could easily have prevented the body from sinking. He stated:

> [E]very one knows, that though a drowned body will at first
> sink, yet it is buoyant, and does not go downright and rest in one
> place like lead; for a human body is seldom or never in a stream
> found to lie where it was drowned; a body drowned at Chelsea
> has been often found by fishermen at London. . . . Now, if a
> body is so buoyant, and that it is driven down by the impellent
> force of the current. . . . [I]t seems a consequence, that when it
> comes to be stopped or resisted by the stakes, which lie with
> their heads downward, inclining with the stream, the stream
> bearing the body against the stakes, must needs raise it upwards.
> (*ST*)

He also commented on the absence of water in the body at autopsy: "I
think it hardly deserves a physician to prove that a body may be drowned
with very little water" (*ST*). Yet he did not hesitate to call several distinguished physicians to support the point. He also gave the jury an account of his movements on the fatal day and evening of March 13 and
stated baldly that the prosecution had been instigated by malice.

Cowper's first witnesses were Robert Drew, the parish officer, and
the constable, Mr. Young. These were the men who had supervised the
removal of the body from the water. They testified that the body was
partly submerged, with only the clothing at the surface, that it was
partly held upward by the stakes, and that abundant froth was issuing
from the mouth. Young added that he had measured the depth of the
water on the morning of the trial and had found it to be four feet two
inches deep; it had been about the same on the morning of March 14.
The water's depth was not an important point, but Young's accurate
measurement cast doubt on the accuracy of previous testimony by the
Crown's witnesses.

Cowper's next witnesses were medical experts who testified on the
forensic aspects of drowning. The first physician was Hans Sloane
(1660–1753), created baronet in 1716. Sloane was a dominant figure
in London medicine. He had been a Fellow of the Royal College of
Physicians since 1687 (later its president, 1719–35) and a Fellow of
the Royal Society since 1685 (later its secretary, 1693–1712, then its
president, 1712–41). His collections formed the nucleus from which
the British Museum was formed. His magisterial manner was impressive. He commented on the absence of water in the stomach:

> [I]f a great quantity of water be swallowed by the gullet into the
> stomach, it will not suffocate or drown the person. Drunkards

who swallow freely a great deal of liquor, and those who are
forced by civil law to drink a great quantity of water . . . have no
suffocation or drowning. . . . But on the other hand, when any
quantity comes into the windpipe, so as it does hinder or inter-
cept the respiration, or coming in of air . . . the person is suffo-
cated. . . . [I]t is very likely that when one struggles he may (to
save himself from being choked) swallow some quantity of water,
yet that is not the cause of his death, but that which goes into the
windpipe or lungs. (*ST*)

Cowper asked Sloane whether it was possible for water to pass into the
thoracic cavity. Sloane replied that it would be impossible without
force and violence because of the membranes that cover the lungs (i.e.,
visceral pleura). Cowper asked Sloane whether it would be possible to
find water in a drowned body six weeks after death. To this Sloane replied that if there was any in the lungs, "the sponginess would suck up
some part of it," and that with respect to the stomach, "if there was a
great fermentation, a great deal of it would rise up in vapours or
steams."

Cowper's next medical expert was Samuel Garth (1661–1718), one
of London's most popular physicians. Garth had been a Fellow of the
Royal College of Physicians since 1693, had delivered the Harveian ora-
tion in 1697, and was the author of "The Dispensary," a long satire
defending the College's founding of a free dispensary against the attack
by the Royal Society of Apothecaries. Garth was prominent in literary
and artistic circles, was a member of the Kit-Cat Club, and was later to
organize Dryden's funeral and deliver the Latin eulogy. Asked by Cowper to express his opinion of the evidence offered by the medical witnesses for the Crown, Garth replied:

[T]he first gentleman called for the king . . . was Mr.
Coatsworth: He saith he was sent for to open her, upon an as-
persion of her being said to be with child. I agree with him in
what he speaks to that point, but must differ with him where he
infers she was murdered because he found no great quantity of
water in her. . . . I think it is not much material whether there be
any water or no in the cavities of the body; if water would hasten
putrefaction, it would do it as well in the lungs as otherwise. . . .
The next was Mr. Dimesdale. . . . [H]e laid the stress of his opinion upon the mortification of the head, which I think is not at all

material, no more than what they infer from her floating; it being impossible the body should have floated, unless it has rested, or had been entangled among the stakes, because all dead bodies (I believe) fall to the bottom. . . . The witnesses all agree she was found upon her side, which to suppose her to float in this posture, is as hard to be conceived, as to imagine a shilling should fall down and rest upon its edge rather than on its broad side; or that a deal board should rather float edgeways than otherwise; therefore it is plain she was entangled, or else the posture had been otherwise. . . . I doubt not, but that some water fell into her lungs . . . but if we consider the windpipe with its ramifications as one cylinder, the calculation of its contents will not amount to above twenty-three or twenty-four solid inches of water, which is not a pint, and which might imperceptibly work and fall out. (*ST*)

Justice Hatsell asked Garth to comment on the testimony of the sailor to the effect that bodies thrown overboard will float unless weights are tied to them. Garth disposed of it adroitly:

My lord, in this they are mistaken. The seamen are a superstitious people, they fancy that whistling at sea will occasion a tempest. I must confess I never saw any body thrown over-board, but I have tried some experiments on other dead animals, and they will certainly sink. . . . [W]e have reason to suspect the seaman's evidence; for he saith that threescore pound of iron is allowed to sink the dead bodies, whereas six or seven pounds would do as well. I cannot think the commissioners of the navy guilty of so ill husbandry. . . . (*ST*)

Then followed Christopher Morley, a Fellow of the Royal College of Physicians since 1686 and author of *Collectanea chemica Leydensia* (1684). He concurred with the opinions expressed by Sloane and Garth and added some experimental evidence:

We last night drowned a dog, and afterwards dissected him, and found not a spoonful of water in his stomach, and, I believe, about two ounces in his lungs. . . . [W]e drowned another, and he lay at the bottom and did not float; no more would he have done, if he had been hanged before thrown into the water; we took him up, and opening him, we found much the same quantity of water in his lungs, and little or none in the stomach. They both froth'd at nose and mouth, because the water coming into the little bladders of the lungs, and there meeting with air, a commotion arose between that water and air, which caused froth. (*ST*)

Morley's empirical evidence was followed by testimony from Dr. John Wollaston, whose Utrecht degree had been incorporated by the Royal College of Physicians in 1693 and who had been admitted a Candidate in 1696. He recounted his experience at examining the bodies of two men who had been drowned from the same boat. The bodies were recovered the following day: "[O]ne of them was indeed prodigously swelled, so much that his clothes were burst in several places. . . . [H]is hands and fingers were strangely extended; his face was almost all over black. . . . [T]he other was not swelled in any part, nor discoloured; he was as lank, I believe, as ever he was in his life-time; and there was not the least sign of any water in him, except the froth at his mouth and nostrils" (*ST*).

The next important medical expert for the defense was William Cowper (1666–1709), a surgeon and one of the best-known English anatomists of the period, author of *The Anatomy of Humane Bodies, with figures drawn after the life by some of the best masters in Europe, and curiously engraven in 114 copperplates* . . . (1696). He was not related to the defendant. His rhetoric was prolix, but he testified that

> when the head of an animal is under water, the first time it is obliged to inspire . . . the water will necessarily flow into its lungs, as the air would do if it were out of water; which quantity of water (if the dimensions of the windpipe and its branches in the lungs be considered) will not amount to three inches square, which is about three ounces of water. Nor is a greater quantity of water in the windpipe necessary to choak any person, if we do but reflect what an ebullition is caused by its meeting with the air which remained in the lungs, whereby a small quantity of water is converted into froth, and the channel of the windpipe, and those of the bronchi, are filled with it, insomuch that no air can enter the lungs for the office of respiration. (*ST*)

Mr. Cowper stated he had been present with Drs. Sloane and Morley at the experiments on dogs the previous evening and confirmed their ob-

servations. With respect to the issue of sinking or floating he testified: "Dead bodies necessarily sink in water, if no distention of their parts buoy them up. . . . This enlargement of them is caused by a rarefaction of the humours within the cavities, and the bodies necessarily rise to the surface. . . . Your lordship may infer this from what the seaman told you; and the great weight they use to fasten to their bodies that die of diseases, was not of such use to sink them, as it was to prevent their floating afterwards" (*ST*).

The last medical expert mentioned in the transcript was Dr. Crell, perhaps the same physician listed in *Munk's Roll* as Jodocus Crull, a native of Hamburg who had been a Fellow of the Royal Society since 1681 and a Licentiate of the Royal College of Physicians since 1692. He agreed that three ounces of water would suffice to fill the windpipe and stop breathing. He also cited Ambroise Paré's observation that froth around the mouth and nostrils was a common finding in bodies recently drowned. This ended the parade of medical experts for the defense.

Cowper's next witnesses were a succession of young ladies and gentlemen who had been on friendly terms with Sarah Stout. They testified that she had been melancholy for the past year. One of them, Mrs. Low, testified that she had taxed Sarah with being in love and that Sarah had admitted it but had told her she was in love with a man she could not marry. Finally, the defense played its trump card. With a show of reluctance, Cowper introduced into evidence letters written to him in London by Sarah Stout, one of which at least was extremely damaging to her reputation. It read in part: "I will assure you I know of no inconveniency that can attend your cohabiting with me, unless the grand jury should thereupon find a bill against us; but I won't fly for it, for come life, come death, I am resolved never to desert you" (*ST*).

Cowper explained that he had allowed the maidservant to go up to warm his bed so that he could talk privately with Sarah and assure her he had no intention of cohabiting with her. It was plain to the jury that Sarah had tried to persuade Cowper, a married man, to have an affair with her. When he rejected her, he left the house abruptly and was followed by Sarah; finding her desires thwarted, she then flung herself into the millstream. As the trial drew to a close, Sarah's brother tried to call witnesses to vouch for her spotless reputation, but Baron Hatsell, perhaps wearied by the lengthy proceedings, would not allow such evidence: "I believe no body disputest that she might be a virtuous woman, and her brains might be turn'd by her passion, or some distemper"

(*ST*). The jury was out for half an hour and returned a verdict of not guilty.

The matter did not die there. Pamphlets and broadsides were issued by the Tories and the Quakers, and in the next election the two Whig seats went to the Tories. But Spencer Cowper's career did not suffer. He was appointed King's Counsel in 1715 and Chief Justice of Chester in 1717; when he died in 1728 he was a Judge of Common Pleas at the King's Bench in London.

It is difficult to gauge the effect of the testimony by experts on the jury and its verdict. The most damning evidence against Spencer Cowper was that he had been the last person to see Sarah Stout alive and that on hearing of her death the following morning he had simply ridden away, despite the long acquaintance between her family and his. Without the evidence of her melancholy and her compromising letters there could easily have been room for adverse speculation about his motives and actions. But that is circumstantial rather than substantive evidence.

The indictment had charged that Cowper and his three friends had placed "a certain rope of no value, around the neck of the said Sarah then and there feloniously and of your malice aforethought, did put, place, fix and bind . . . the neck and throat . . . and did hold, squeeze, and gripe . . . and did choak and strangle [her] . . . then secretly and maliciously did put and cast [into a certain river . . . called the Priory River] to conceal and hide the said Sarah Stout, so murdered" (*ST*). In other words the Crown alleged that Sarah Stout had been strangled first and then her dead body had been placed in the millstream. Yet there was no mark of a rope on her neck; the prosecution's witnesses saw at most some discoloration of the neck ascribed to settling of blood and a small bruise on the left arm. The local surgeons who dissected the body six weeks later did not examine the neck organs for signs of strangulation, and needless to say, no rope was ever found. They testified that her death was not due to drowning. Was the jury to infer that if she had not drowned, she must have been strangled? Certainly the prosecution did not offer proof of the charge as given in the indictment.

It is curious that Dimsdale and Coatsworth concluded she had not been drowned because of the absence of water in the lungs, stomach, or pleural cavities. But they did not open the tracheobronchial tree, nor, so far as their direct testimony goes, examine the cut surface of the lungs. The jurors were from Hertfordshire, then a farming community, and many would have been acquainted with the anatomy of slaughtered animals and could have known that there is no natural passage between the trachea and pleural cavities. They were likewise familiar with drowned animals and could be expected to know that upon drowning they first sink to the bottom, only to surface after the gases of decomposition cause them to rise. Even more curious was the Crown's indictment of Cowper's three colleagues, whom no witness placed at the scene of the alleged crime and whom the Crown's own witnesses placed at a tavern in the town at the time the crime was supposed to have been committed. Even an uncritical juror must have recognized that the Crown's witnesses had not substantiated the charges in the indictment. The obvious insufficiency of the Crown's case lends support to Cowper's claim that the indictment was brought about by malice and that it was a political and factional trial.

Judged by twentieth-century standards the expert witnesses for the defense acquitted themselves well. It is curious that the transcript does not indicate that Cowper, who conducted his own defense, asked questions so that the jury might hear their impressive qualifications. Perhaps the transcriber omitted this for the sake of brevity, though the witnesses for the prosecution readily supplied their occupations. The names and achievements of Hans Sloane, Samuel Garth, and William Cowper may be familiar to medical historians, but that is no guarantee that their reputations were known to the Hertfordshire yeomen of the jury. However, the role of the expert witness was not well defined in the seventeenth and eighteenth centuries, and courtroom procedures for qualifying them as such had not been developed. The five physicians Cowper brought up from London were unanimous in testifying that dead bodies sink to the bottom, that death from drowning is the result of a sufficient quantity of water in the trachea and bronchi to prevent air from having access to the lungs, and that only a small quantity of water is required. They all pointed out that there is no natural connection between the windpipe (trachea) or gullet (esophagus) with the thorax (pleural cavities), thereby invalidating one of the points raised by the local surgeons. They all stated or implied that the amount of water in the stomach was unimportant and varied from case to case. All of them commented on the presence of froth at the mouth and nostrils as an important sign that death was due to drowning. What they could not have known at the time was that the froth is not merely the result of "ebullition" or "commotion" of air mixing with aspirated water but is the fluid of pulmonary edema. In addition, they bolstered their testimony about drowned human bodies by supplying experimental evidence from the two dogs they had drowned and dissected the night before the trial. This is certainly the effect of the Royal Society, which had been founded in 1662, and the developing emphasis on experimental evidence. Such a test would not have occurred to physicians of the previous generation.

To a modern forensic physician the case of Sarah Stout is an example of fresh-water drowning. Because of its low sodium content fresh water is absorbed rapidly into the circulation, where it produces hemolysis and hemodilution and increases the blood volume. Extrapolating from animal models, the blood volume can be increased by as much as 30 percent in a minute. The heart is quickly overcome by this increased load, and pulmonary edema can develop after only a minute of submersion in fresh water. Death usually occurs in three to five minutes and is the result of a terminal cardiac arrhythmia.

A modern textbook tells us that "no reliable tests permitting an unequivocal diagnosis of drowning are available. Thus, the central question in the case of a body recovered from water is whether the individual was alive at the time he entered the water. The scene, the circumstances surrounding the incident with all available background information, the decedent's clothing, all play a significant role in this determination."[5] In the case of Sarah Stout the prosecution alleged that the body had been strangled and was dead before it entered the water, but the evidence to support that claim was insubstantial. The expert witnesses for the defense were well informed. The text goes on to inform us that "from a practical standpoint, the presence of water in the lungs and stomach of a drowning victim is of no real significance. Water may well reach these organs after death. . . . At autopsy, the lungs of a drowning victim resemble those seen in deaths associated with pulmonary edema. . . . [T]he presence of foam in the airway indicates beyond doubt that the victim was alive at the time of submersion."

Modern attempts to establish that death was due to drowning by analyzing blood for variations in electrolytes have proven unreliable. Microscopic examination of sections of bone marrow for diatoms that have entered the victim's circulation from the water are diagnostic when present, but they cannot be demonstrated consistently. We have little to add to the expert witnesses of 1699.

14
Notes on Placentophagy

In a recent Swiftean satire, a modest proposal was made that the human female might prevent choriocarcinoma by emulating placentophagous viviparous mammals that eat the placenta.[1] At that time only one case of choriocarcinoma in an animal had been reported, specifically in an armadillo.[2] Shortly thereafter, an example of choriocarcinoma was reported in a rhesus monkey.[3] It was with some dismay that the writer of the modest proposal learned of an instance of human consumption of a term placenta following natural childbirth by a member of the counterculture.[4] A young woman living in a commune had natural childbirth assisted by friends. After delivery the placenta was steamed, and she shared it with those who stayed behind. She described the aftereffects as "wonderfully replenishing and delicious." In today's Western society human placentophagy is as taboo as cannibalism, and it was with astonishment that the modest proposer learned from a Czechoslovakian medical officer that circa 1960 placentophagy was being practiced by midwives and obstetrical nurses in Vietnam.

The text of this communication seems worth recording, and has prompted a search for evidence of placentophagy in other cultures.

I was working as head of the Pathology Department at the Hospital of Czechoslovak-Vietnamese Friendship at Haiphong from September 1958 to December 1960. The group of Czechoslovak specialists . . . including physicians, nurses, laboratory technicians, engineers, and administrators. Soon after my arrival, I was told by the Czech chief nurse-midwife from the Ob-Gyn Department that "they eat placentae." After my inquiry I got the following explanation: Several Vietnamese male and female nurses (mid-wives) in the department used to eat placentae, delivered by patients. They would not eat any placenta, but only those delivered by a young, apparently healthy and handsome mother. They stripped the membranous parts away and chopped the cotyledons in small pieces and fried them in a pan, usually together with onions. The Czech nurse . . . showed me the pan with a few pieces of dark brown placental tissue mixed with onions. The ethnic background of those practising this was not Vietnamese; they belonged to the "minorities" group, tribes of Chinese and Thai origin inhabiting the mountains of North Vietnam.

I asked several Vietnamese doctors in the hospital about it, but they were very reluctant to give me any information, since they already knew the aversion of Czech personnel toward the practice. Actually, Vietnamese doctors in the Ob-Gyn Department tried to suppress any information about it and also tried to prevent their personnel from eating placentae. . . . I am not really able to tell whether the observed placentophagy was a widespread cultural habit among these tribes nor whether placentae were also eaten by the mothers who had delivered them.[5]

It is tempting to consider that the placenta was eaten to supply additional protein to a protein-poor diet in underdeveloped areas. Perhaps protein was more limited in the mountains whence these nurse-midwives originated than in plains where cattle might graze or in coastal regions where fish and seafood would be available. If so, the practice might have the sanction of regional mores. But evidence for placentophagy is scanty. Annalists and chroniclers accepted childbirth as a natural quotidian event and did not record the circumstances connected with it. Moreover, parturition was the quintessence of muliebrity, and, partly from superstition, partly as a defense against a male-dominated society, women tended to exclude men from its mysteries. Most ancient medical writings supply only superficial, often inaccurate and misleading accounts of obstetrical phenomena. Not until the sixteenth century do we find iconographic representation of a woman in labor, and even then much is concealed by drapery. Archeological materials furnish only limited insight. A statuette of the Aztec birth goddess Tlazoteotl correctly shows the squatting posture in delivery, but surely the intercrural face presentation is the sculptor's distortion of nature. Likewise, literary allusions are few and indirect. Reliable ethnographic evidence was not collected until the mid-nineteenth century,

and even in that corpus data relating to childbirth and the fate of the placenta were not usually recorded.

The earliest known representation of the placenta is seen on the frequently reproduced palette of King Narmer, a well-preserved stele found at Hierankopolis at the end of the nineteenth century. The uppermost panel on the reverse side shows Narmer in ceremonial procession preceded by royal standards; to the right are piled decapitated bodies of his enemies. The standard nearest the king has the shape of a bilobate disc with a streamer hanging down; it has been interpreted as the king's placenta and umbilical cord, the prototype of flags carried into battle with their streamers of red, white, and blue.[6] As did many primitive people, the ancient Egyptians believed that a child was formed in its mother's womb from blood not shed during gestation and that accumulated unused blood formed the afterbirth or placenta, a reserve of vital material. From this belief stemmed the idea that the placenta was the child's "secret helper," a quasi twin; hence it would be reasonable for a king or his troops to carry a representation of it into battle. King Narmer was a predynastic ruler during the transition period between Neolithic and Chalcolithic settlements and the First Dynasty. He followed such cultures as the Tasian, Badarian, Amratean, Gerzean, and Semainian, and his palette dates from the dawn of history, probably between 3500 and 3100 B.C. We know little about these cultures and nothing about their obstetrical practices, let alone the fate of their placentas. What may be relevant is that they did practice human sacrifice; cannibalism and even placentophagy, especially in an agrarian society, would be a logical sequel.

More specific allusion to the ancient practice of placentophagy is found in Deuteronomy 28 (Authorized Version). The chapter begins with fourteen verses describing the material blessings that will befall the Israelites if they hearken diligently unto the voice of the Lord their God. The concluding fifty-four verses warn them of the condign punishments they will incur if they do not observe the Lord's commandments and statutes. Verses fifty-two to fifty-seven admonish the Israelites of what will happen when their cities are besieged and the enemy within their gates—namely, the men will practice cannibalism: "And thou shalt eat the fruit of thine own body, the flesh of thy sons and thy daughters," and the women will practice placentophagy: "The tender and delicate woman among you, which would not adventure to set the sole of her foot upon the ground . . . her eye shall be evil toward the husband of her bosom, and toward her daughter. And toward her young one that cometh out from between her feet, and toward her children which she shall bear; for she shall eat them for want of all things secretly in the siege and straitness. . . ."

Choosing the *Targum of Aquila* as their authority, the translators of the Authorized Version employed the trope of euphemism. In the Greek text the phrase "that cometh out from between her feet" is written as *chorion,* and in the Vulgate it appears as *secundinae partes,* clearly the placenta. In Aramaic codices the phrase is *u:ve-shilyatah,* from the root *shilya* which means "placenta"; cf. *uvishphir shilyeta* (placenta and membranes) in the *Targum of Jerusalem,* which is translated as "that which issues forth from the place of shame at the time of birth." (For "the place of shame," cf. *pudenda.*) The 1917 translation of the Jewish Publication Society of America, based on the Masoretic text, correctly uses the word "afterbirth."

What Jehovah seems to be telling the Israelites is that if they do not obey him, he will reduce them to the level of the beasts. If we accept the idea that biblical imagery and metaphor reflect the culture of the time and place, it is reasonable to infer that the passage refers to a remote tribal memory, now suppressed, of a period when placentas were eaten, at least in times of famine. We have no written record of the customs of such coexistent tribes as the Hittites, the Moabites, the Ammonites, the Amalekites, or even of the Philistines, but one may speculate whether this practice was not uncommon in the prehistory of the Levant and Mesopotamia, where drought and crop failure were familiar and recurrent events, even as in the Nile basin. Anthropologists have often posed the question of what distinguishes humans from beasts. Several criteria have been proposed, the most popular that we have the power of symbolic speech. But this is not an absolute distinction, for many animal species have been shown to possess elaborate systems of communication. An equally plausible distinction might be that humans, that is, civilized humans, do not eat human placentas.

Hunger pangs may not be the only motive and cue for placentophagy. The placenta has both medicinal and magical properties, and its ingestion may be connected with either or both. Considering the many priorities assigned to Chinese civilization, it is not surprising that the *Great Pharmacopoiea of 1596* by Li Shih-chen recommended a mixture of human milk and placental tissue for an ailment known as *ch'i* exhaustion, an ill-defined entity characterized by anemia, weakness of the extremities, and coldness of the sexual organs with involuntary ejaculation of semen.[7] The Chinese *ch'i* was a vital force very much like the Egyptian vital material inherent in the placenta, though not necessarily derived from accumulated blood. The recommended treatment gave on alternate days doses of Virtuous Birth Elixir followed by Connected Destiny Elixir. The latter consisted of three wine-cups of human milk into which a dried, powdered human placenta was stirred and warmed in a saucer by exposure to sunlight. Precisely how old and traditional this remedy was in 1596 is not known, but it was no less effective than medications offered a few decades earlier by Paracelsus in Western Europe.

The magical properties of the placenta have been widely known since Frazer's magisterial summary appeared just before World War I.[8] But none of Frazer's examples cited eating or ingesting placentas or placental extracts. Later ethnographers reported isolated instances of placentophagy by primitive people, and in the light of the above exposition it seems now convenient to review them.

A few points of congruence and a pattern of behavior emerge from this literature. In parts of Indonesia the placenta is thought to be a "younger brother" (cf. "secret helper") and is buried with care.[9] It is preserved during the first year of life for use in case of sickness to supply the missing life force. In primitive societies the placenta is quite commonly buried, often by the father, sometimes by the midwife, often with ceremony approaching ritual, sometimes secretly and silently. The usual explanation for burial is to prevent its being eaten by animals, in which case the life or health of the child would be imperiled. An unusual variation is the custom in parts of Java in which the placenta, decorated with flowers and little lights, is set afloat on the river at night as food for crocodiles.[10] In some cultures the placenta or a segment of umbilical cord is preserved as a protective amulet or good luck charm. In parts of rural Poland peasants "dry it and use it in powdered form as medicine, or the dried cord may be saved and given to the child when he goes to school for the first time, to make him a good scholar."[11]

In at least one culture the flavor of the placenta was valued. The Kurtachi of the Solomon Islands preserved it in the lime pot that contained the mother's supply of powdered lime for chewing with the areca nut.[12] But in a larger number of cultures the placenta's medicinal value was prized. The Mirebalais in Haiti buried the placenta itself but preserved part of the cord. If the child became ill, the cord was boiled and the supernatant broth given as medicine.[13] Somewhat less specific is a report that among the Sierra Tarascan Indians the cord, too, is usually buried, but one midwife asserted that it was preserved and used for unspecified remedies in case of illness.[14] More specific is Robert Redfield's study of Topotzlan, a Mexican village, in which the umbilical cord was used as a remedy for eye trouble.[15] Two decades later Oscar Lewis confirmed Redfield's observation and noted that the same practice prevailed in nearby Mitla.[16] Perhaps related to this is Loeb's earlier observation that Pomo Indians in California keep a remnant of the cord as medicine for the child and find it especially useful for snakebites.[17]

Crossing from the North American mainland into the Caribbean and South America, we learn that in Jamaica the placental membranes (caul) were used to prevent convulsions ascribed to irritation of the child by a ghost.[18] In this instance the tissue was carefully parched over a hot brick and a bit put into the infant's tea. The Araucanian Indians of Argentina dried the umbilical cord, ground it to a powder, and gave a little to the child whenever it was sick.[19] A much earlier report from Peru noted the tribal custom of letting an ailing infant suck on the preserved cord.[20] Adults who fell ill were given the cord to chew, but it was important that it be the patient's own cord; another person's was not considered effective.

Moving eastward across the Atlantic, we learn that in Tanganyika the Chaga continue what may be a survival of parental cannibalism. The placenta is put into a receptacle and placed for two months in the attic to dry. Then it is ground with eleusine (a plant) into a flour from which a porridge is made. This is consumed by the old women of the family, who claim that it is a way of preserving the child's life.[21] Further to the East, the Kol tribe in Central India relates the placenta to reproductive function. A childless woman, by eating a portion of either the placenta or umbilical cord, may dispel the influences that keep her barren, but in so doing injury or even death may occur to the family from which she received by stealth the required parts.[22]

Apart from the Vietnamese nurse-midwives mentioned earlier, none of the other examples of placentophagy indicate that it was eaten with gusto and relish. For the Israelites it was a punishment, and in primitive societies magico-medical motives prevail. What may be the future of placentophagy? One recalls Aldous Huxley's *Brave New World* (1932), in which fertilization and gestation were accomplished *in vitro* and there were no placentas. Does the recent delivery of a "test tube baby" presage a gestation carried to term entirely outside a womb and without the need of a placenta? But Huxley was aware that, given sufficient motivation, humankind will eat anything. Less than a decade later, in *After Many a Summer Dies the Swan* (1939), Jo Stoyte, the archetypical American tycoon, was willing to emulate the fifth Earl of Gonister and ingest triturated raw carp entrails as an elusive elixir in his quest for longevity. Advertising copy for a cosmetic cream now in the marketplace advises us that "we have added, at the behest of our researchers, a pure organic placenta composite. Placenta contains concentrated levels of hormones, nutrients, and natural protective agents."[23] Another company manufactures not only a skin-moisturizing cream containing Vitamin E and placental extract but also a shampoo, a hair conditioner, a "Placentene" hair-setting product, and a "Gift of Life" face cream. There are at least twenty-nine different cosmetics on the market in which human placental extracts are used. Some are named Placenta plus, Golden Placenta, and Placentally Yours. The active ingredient is often lyophilized bovine placental tissue. These commercial products are expensive, but it may be only a question of time before American consumers put their mouths where their money is.

But hunger is probably the strongest motive for eating what under normal circumstances would be considered inedible. Perhaps if the ominous prognostications of pundits terrified by untrammeled population growth come true, one can imagine a world in which each member of humanity crouches on a sternly allotted sandpile and presents a plastic card at the state-controlled commissary for the weekly ration of fish protein. At such a time the placenta may well become a delicacy of haute cuisine. In that far-off day we may find useful the valedictory used by the Toradja natives of the Celebes, who hang the placenta in the fork of a large *Ficus* tree and on departing address it: "You, after-birth, do not say that I do not love you; we love you. Do not tickle the soles of the feet of your little brother (sister) and do not pinch his (her) stomach."[24]

Notes

1. Bottoms Up! The Fine Arts and Flagellation

1. I. Gibson, *The English Vice* (London: Duckworth, 1978), facing p. 52.

2. W. B. Ober, "Swinburne's Masochism: Neuropathology and Psychopathology," in *Boswell's Clap and Other Essays* (Carbondale: Southern Illinois University Press, 1979), 43–88.

3. R.O. Rubinstein, "A Bacchic Sarcophagus in the Renaissance," in *British Museum Yearbook I: The Classic Tradition* (London: British Museum Publications, 1976), 103–56.

4. G. Sarton, "Aristotle and Phyllis," *Isis* 14 (1930), 8–19.

5. M. Baxandall, *Painting and Experience in Fifteenth-Century Italy* (Oxford: Oxford University Press, 1972), 3–13.

6. D. Kraus and H. Kraus, *The Hidden World of Misericords* (London: Michael Joseph, 1975), 122.

7. W. A. Cooper, *A History of the Rod in All Countries* (London: John Camden Hotten, 1867), facing p. 395.

8. *Bilderlexikon der Erotik* (Wien/Leipzig: Verlag der Kulturforschung, 1928–31), 4 vols.; E. Fuchs, *Illustrierte Sittengeschichte* (Munich: Albert Lange, 1912), 6 vols.; E. Fuchs and A. Kind, *Die Weiberherrschaft in der Geschichte der Menschheit* (Munich: Albert Lange, 1914), 3 vols.; E. Schertel, *Der Flagellantismus als literarisches Motiv* (Parthenon, 1930–32), 4 vols.; L. Schidrowitz, *Sittengeschichte des Lasters* (Wien/Leipzig: Verlag der Kulturforschung, 1928–30).

9. A. J. V. Cheetham and D. Parfit, *Eton Microcosm* (London: Sidgwick and Jackson, 1964).

10. *The World of Hogarth: Lichtenberg's Commentaries on Hogarth's Engravings,* trans. Innes and Gustave Herdan (Boston: Houghton Mifflin, 1966), 29–30.

11. *Madam Birchini's Dance* (London: George Peacock, 1783).

12. Fuchs and Kind, *Die Weiberherrschaft,* between pp. 192–93.

13. D. Hill, *Mr. Gillray the Caricaturist* (London: Phaidon, 1965).

14. H.S. Ashbee [Pisanus Fraxi], *Catena librorum tacendorum* (London: privately printed, 1885), 425.

15. Hill, *Mr. Gillray,* 10–11.

16. Hill, *Mr. Gillray,* 16.

17. Hill, *Mr. Gillray,* 142.

18. O. Lancaster, "The Face of Caricature," *The Spectator,* June 4, 1965, pp. 724–25.

19. G. W. Peck, *Peck's Bad Boy and His Pa* (Chicago: Belford, Clarke, 1883), 129.

20. A. L. Guptill, *Norman Rockwell, Illustrator* (New York: Watson-Guptill, 1946), 105, 128.

21. A. L. Guptill, *Norman Rockwell: A Sixty Year Retrospective* (New York: Abrams, 1972), 61.

22. R. Dirks, *The Katzenjammer Kids* (rpt., New York: Dover, 1974), 17.

23. J. D. Meibom, *De flagorum usū in re veneria & reumque officio* (Leyden, 1629).

2. Robert Musil: What Price Homosexual Sadism?

1. W. B. Ober, "A Few Kind Words about W. Somerset Maugham (1874–1965)," *New York State Journal of Medicine* 69 (1969), 2692.

2. R. Musil, *Young Törless,* trans. E. Wilkins and E. Kaiser, with an afterword by John Simon (New York: Pantheon, 1955).

3. F. Kermode, preface to *Tonks and Other Stories,* by Robert Musil (London: Martin Secker, Warburg, 1965).

4. F. Kermode, "A Short View of Musil," in *Puzzles and Epiphanies* (New York: Chilmark Press, 1962).

5. S. J. Elliot, "*The Man Without Qualities:* An Interpretation," ms. in possession of the author, 1972.

3. Carlo Gesualdo, Prince of Venosa: Murder, Madrigals, and Masochism

1. C. Gray, "The Life of Carlo Gesualdo," in *Carlo Gesualdo, Prince of Venosa, Musician and Murderer,* ed. C. Gray and P. Heseltine (London: Curwen & Sons, 1926), 11–12.

2. Gray, "Life of Carlo Gesualdo," 18–19.

3. Gray, "Life of Carlo Gesualdo," 11–12.

4. Gray, "Life of Carlo Gesualdo," 18–19.

5. Gray, "Life of Carlo Gesualdo," 18–19.

6. C. Gray, "Carlo Gesualdo Considered as a Murderer," in *Carlo Gesualdo,* ed. Gray and Heseltine, 72.

7. Gray, "Life of Carlo Gesualdo," 42–43.

8. Gray, "Life of Carlo Gesualdo," 42–43.

9. Gray, "Life of Carlo Gesualdo," 50.

10. T. Campanella, *Medicinalium, juxta propria principia.*

11. F. Vatielli, *Il Principe di Venosa e Leonora d'Este.*

12. P. A. Heseltine, "Gesualdo the Musician," in *Carlo Gesualdo,* ed. Gray and Heseltine, 123–24.

13. D. B. Rowland, *Mannerism: Style and Mood* (New Haven, Conn.: Yale University Press, 1964).

14. A. Huxley, "Gesualdo: Variations on a Musical Theme," in *Tomorrow and Tomorrow and Tomorrow* (London: Chatto and Windus, 1956).

15. Heseltine, "Gesualdo the Musician," 123–24.

16. A. Einstein, *The Italian Madrigal* (Princeton, N.J.: Princeton University Press, 1949) 2:715.

17. Einstein, *The Italian Madrigal* 2:715.

4. The Sticky End of František Kočžwara, Composer of The Battle of Prague

1. *Modern Propensities, or, an Essay on the Art of Strangling, &c. Illustrated with Several Anecdotes. With Memoirs of Susannah Hill, and a Summary of her Trial at the Old Bailey on Friday, September 16, 1791, on the Charge of Hanging Francis Kotzwarra, at her Lodging in Vine Street, on September 2* (London: J. Dawson, 1791).

2. A. Loesser, *Men, Women and Pianos* (New York: Simon & Schuster, 1954), 167–74, 243–44.

3. T. Fawcett, *Music in Eighteenth-Century Norwich and Norfolk* (Norwich: University of East Anglia, 1979), 51.

4. H. C. R. Landon, *Haydn in England, 1791–1795,* vol. 3 of *Haydn: Chronicle and Works* (London: Thames & Hudson, 1976), 97.

5. Landon, *Haydn* 1:181ff.

6. R. J. Wolfe, "The Hang-Up of Franz Kotzwara and Its Relationship to Sexual Quackery in the Late Eighteenth Century" (Paper delivered at the Eleventh Annual Janus Foundation Lecture on the History of Medicine, San Francisco, January 15, 1980).

7. J. C. Rupp, "Autoerotic Asphyxia," in *Modern Legal Medicine, Psychiatry and Forensic Science,* ed. W. J. Curran, A. L. McGarry, and C. S. Petty (Philadelphia: F. A. Davis, 1980), 584–87.

8. P. E. Dietz, "Recurrent Discovery of Autoerotic Asphyxia," in *Autoerotic Fatalities,* ed. R. R. Hazelwood, P. E. Dietz, and A. W. Burgess (Lexington, Mass.: D.C. Heath, 1983), 13–44.

9. B. S. Abeshouse and L. H. Tankin, "True Priapism: A Report of Four Cases and a Review of the Literature," *Urologic and Cutaneous Review* 54 (1950), 449–65; R. deV. White and H. M. Nagler, "Priapism" (in press).

10. J. H. Jackson, "Cervical Fracture-Dislocations," *Lancet* i (1897), 18–24; rpt. in *Neurological Fragments* (London: Oxford University Press, 1925).

11. F. Wood-Jones, "The Ideal Lesion Produced by Judicial Hanging" *Lancet* i (1913), 53; see also ensuing correspondence, pp. 193–94, 639–40.

12. A. W. Burgess, P. E. Dietz, and R. R. Hazelwood, "Study Design and Sample Characteristics," in *Autoerotic Fatalities,* ed. Hazelwood, Dietz, and Burgess, 45–53.

13. Rupp, "Autoerotic Asphyxia."

5. Weighing the Heart against the Feather of Truth

1. D. Guthrie, "History of Medicine," *Encyclopaedia Britannica,* 14th ed. (1966), 15.

2. J. Milton, *Areopagitica,* in *Milton's Prose* (London: Oxford University Press, 1925), 311.

3. R. O. Faulkner, *The Ancient Egyptian Coffin Texts* (Warminster, England: Aris & Phillips, 1977) 2 : 181.

4. P. Ghalioungi, *Magic and Medical Science in Ancient Egypt* (London: Hodder & Stoughton, 1963), 159.

5. C. Seeber, *Untersuchungen zur Darstellung des Totengerichts im alten Ägypten,* vol. 35 of *Münchner Ägyptologische Studien* (Munich: Deutscher Kunstverlag, 1976).

6. The papyri described in the above paragraphs are catalogued as follows: Ani (British Museum [BM] EA10470.3); Nedjmet (BM EA 10541); Entinuny (Metropolitan Museum of Art 30.3.1); Nestanbtashru (BM EA10544.63); Anhai (BM EA10412.4); Tameniu (BM EA10008.3/Barker 210.III); Kerasher (BM EA 9995); Hor-Netzi-Atef-Ef (Pierpont Morgan Library, Amherst 35).

7. Museum of Fine Arts, Boston 08.205.

8. BM B-639.

9. Metropolitan Museum of Art 47.11.5.

10. Bodleian Library MS. Douce 180, fol. 15, ca. 1270. See also the Hamburg altarpiece ascribed to Master Bertram, 1479–83 (Victoria and Albert Museum 5490-1859), and the Cloisters *Apocalypse.*

11. S. Schoenbaum, *Shakespeare, the Globe and the World* (New York: Oxford University Press, 1979), 40–41.

12. Pierpont Morgan Library, Coptic Theological Texts, Crum Theological Papyrus, fols. 1v, 7v.

13. E. Mâle, *Religious Art in France: Thirteenth Century,* trans. Dora Nussey (London: J.M. Dent; New York: E.P. Dutton, 1913), 374–83.

14. T. S. R. Boase, *Death in the Middle Ages: Mortality, Judgment and Remembrance* (London: Thames & Hudson, 1972), 34–35.

15. Among the many variations on the theme of St. Michael with the scales of judgment are some notable examples: (1) a colorful thirteenth-century Spanish primitive painting by the Master of Soriguerola in the Episcopal Museum at Vichy;

(2) one figure in a polyptych of saints by Simone Martini in the Fitzwilliam Museum at Cambridge; (3) a side panel in a fourteenth-century altarpiece by the Croatian painter Dobrivcevic in the Dominican church at Dubrovnik; (4) a panel by Giovanni di Francesco dated ca. 1439 at the J. Paul Getty Museum at Malibu, California; (5) an illumination in the Sforza Book of Hours, BM, add. MS. 34298, fol. 186v; (6) an Andrea della Robbia lunette in relief in the Sternberg Palace at Prague; (7) a painting by the Züricher Nelkenmeister dated ca. 1500 in the Kunsthaus at Zürich; (8) a brilliantly decorated panel by the fifteenth-century Villa Roya Master in the Art Museum at Princeton University showing the damned being cast into the mouth of hell, which is represented by the gaping mouth of a whale; and (9) an elaborately robed floating figure of the archangel in a Last Judgment at the Hospice de Beaune by Roger van der Weyden.

16. W.-H. Hein, *Christus als Apotheker* (Frankfurt-am-Main: Govi-Verlag, 1974).

17. T. Kerkring, *Spicilegium anatomicum continens observationum anatomicum rarorum, &c.* (Amsterdam: Frisii, 1670), 39.

18. J. Bouillaud, *Traité clinique des maladies du coeur* (Paris: Ballière, 1835), 25–72.

19. J. Cruveilhier, *Essai sur l'anatomie pathologique en general, et sur les transformations et productions organiques en particulier* (Paris: L'Auteur, 1616), 1:184–85.

20. J. Lobstein, *Lehrbuch der pathologischen Anatomie* (Stuttgart: Broadhag, 1835), 2:360–62; J. Clendinning, "Facts and Inferences Relative to the Condition of the Vital Organs and Viscera in General, as to Their Nutrition in Certain Chronic Diseases," *Medical-Chirurgical Transactions* 21 (1838), 33–68; J. Reid, "On the Measurements of the Heart," *Monthly Journal of Medical Sciences* 3 (1843), 295–323, 411–12; T. B. Peacock, "On the Weight and Development of the Human Heart in Health and Disease," *Monthly Journal of Medical Science* 19 (1854), 193–214, 313–23, 403–27.

21. C. Rokitansky, *A Manual of Pathological Anatomy* (London: Sydenham Society, 1853) 4:150–71; R. Virchow, *Die Sektions-Technik im Leichenhause* (Berlin: Hirschwald, 1875).

22. W. Müller, *Die Massenverhältnisse des menschlichen Herzens* (Hamburg and Leipzig: Voss, 1883).

23. F. Albright, "Some of the 'Do's' and 'Do-nots' in Clinical Investigation," *Journal of Clinical Investigation* 23 (1944), 921–26.

6. Can the Leper Change His Spots? The Iconography of Leprosy

1. The text in Numbers 12:10 informs us that "behold, Miriam became leprous, white as snow." If she was protesting against Moses' wife's blackness, Jehovah's punishment carries a note of irony: "You don't like black? Then be white." A talmudic gloss states that to be smitten with leprosy was a punishment for gossip.

Perhaps this explains Jehovah's displeasure; Miriam had made a private peccadillo a matter of public clamor. But were such the case, the punishment seems excessive for the offense.

2. B. Narkiss, *Hebrew Illuminated Manuscripts* (New York: Leon Amiel, 1969), 56, 66.

3. B. Berenson, "Italian Illustrators of the *Speculum Humanae Salvationis*," in *Studies in Medieval Painting* (New Haven, Conn.: Yale University Press, 1930).

4. A. Mieli, *Panorama general de historia della ciencia. La epoca medieval: Mundo islamico y occidente cristiano* (Buenos Aires: Aspara-Calpe, 1946), 134–35.

5. B. Rama Rao, personal communication.

6. N. R. Banerjee, personal communication.

7. L. Goldman and A. R. Sawyer, "Ancient Peruvian Medicine," *Journal of the History of Medicine and Allied Sciences* 13 (1958), 10–14.

8. D. D. Vérut, *Pre-Columbian Dermatology and Cosmetology in Mexico* (Bloomfield, N.J.: Schering Corp., 1973).

9. S. N. Brody, *The Disease of the Soul: Leprosy in Medieval Literature* (Ithaca, N.Y.: Cornell University Press, 1974).

10. Rabanus Maurus, "De universo," in *Patrologiae cursus completus: Patrologia Latina*, ed. J. P. Migne (Paris: 1844–64), vol. 111 (1856), 501–3.

11. Richard of St. Victor, "Allegoriae in Novum Testamentum, II, xvi," in *Patrologia Latina*, ed. Migne, vol. 175 (1861).

12. C. A. Robson, *Maurice of Sully and Medieval Vernacular Homily* (Oxford: Oxford University Press, 1952), 91.

13. K. Weitzmann, *The Miniatures of the "Sacra Parallela," Parisinus Graecus 923* (Princeton, N.J.: Princeton University Press, 1979).

14. W. Strohn, *Lepradorstellung in der Kunst des Rheinlandes* (Berlin: Junker & Dünnhaupt, 1936), 29–40.

15. T. K. Penniman, *A Hundred Years of Anthropology* (New York: William Morris, 1974), 31–32.

16. C. H. Talbot, "Medicine and Miracles," *St. Mary's Hospital Gazette* 66 (1960), 182–96.

17. M. Meiss, *Painting in Florence and Siena after the Black Death* (Princeton, N.J.: Princeton University Press, 1951), 74–78.

18. S. Morpurgo, "Le epigrafi volgari in rima del Trionfo della Morte," *L'Arte* 2 (1899), 51–87.

19. L. D. Ettlinger, *The Sistine Chapel before Michelangelo* (Oxford: Oxford University Press, 1965), 89–90.

20. K. Grön, "Leprosy in Literature and Art," *International Journal of Leprosy* 41 (1973), 249–83.

21. J.-K. Huysmans, "The Grünewalds in the Colmar Museum," in *Grünewald*, trans. Robert Baldick (Oxford: Phaidon, 1976). Huysmans' essay was first published in *Trois primitifs* (1905).

22. W. H. McNeill, *Plagues and People* (New York: Doubleday, 1976), 174–81.

23. P. Richards, *The Medieval Leper and His Northern Heirs* (Cambridge: D.S. Brewer, 1977), 103–20.

24. D. C. Danielssen and C. W. Beck, *Om spedalskhed,* (Bergen: Gröndahl, 1847), vol. 2.

7. *The Iconography of* Fanny Hill: *How to Illustrate a Dirty Book*

1. J. Cleland, *Memoirs of a Woman of Pleasure,* ed. P. Sabor (Oxford: Oxford University Press, 1985); *Fanny Hill, or Memoirs of a Woman of Pleasure,* ed. P. Wagner (Harmondsworth, Mdx.: Penguin, 1985).

2. *Records of the Most Ancient and Puissant Order of the Beggar's Benison and Merryland, Anstruther* (Anstruther: privately printed, 1892; rpt., Edinburgh: Paul Harris, 1982), p. 23, supp. p. 15.

3. *Memoirs,* ed. P. Sabor, xiv.

4. C. H. Rolph, ed., *The Trial of Lady Chatterley* (Harmondsworth, Mdx.: Penguin, 1961), 144–45.

5. C. Rembar, *The End of Obscenity* (New York: Random House, 1968).

6. D. Foxon, *Libertine Literature in England, 1660–1745* (New Hyde Park, N.Y.: University Books, 1965), 54–55.

7. Drybutter is as elusive as G. Fenton. The first reference to his conviction dates from 1864, a century later, in a note added by Bohn to his edition of Lowndes' *Bibliographer's Manual,* but no contemporary documentation of it, nor even of his existence, has come to light.

8. *Commonwealth v. Holmes,* 17 Mass. 336. Holmes was convicted in the Court of Common Pleas. The citation is the opinion of the Supreme Judicial Court of Massachusetts denying reversal and stating that the Court of Common Pleas as Successor to the Court of Sessions had jurisdiction of the offense of publishing libels. The opinion also held that in an indictment it was sufficient to give a general description of a book or print without copying the book or minutely describing the print "to aver their evil tendency."

9. H. S. Ashbee [Pisanus Fraxi], *Catena librorum tacendorum* (London: privately printed, 1885), 60–61.

10. Foxon, *Libertine Literature,* 59–63.

11. Cleland, *Memoirs,* ed. Sabor, 91.

12. Sabor, introduction to Cleland, *Memoirs,* xx.

13. *The Private Case: An Annotated Bibliography of the Private Case Erotica Collection in the British (Museum) Library* (London: Jay Landesman, 1981), 136–42. The illustrated editions comprise the following:

(1) *Memoirs of a Woman of Pleasure* (*MWP*). "From the original corrected edition." 2 vols. London, 1766. Two frontispieces and thirty plates ascribed to Gravelot. P.C.30.k.27.

(2) *Nouvelle traduction de Woman of Pleasur [sic] ou Fille de joye de M. Cleland.* Londres: Chez G. Fenton dans le Strand, 1770. "Avec XV planches en taille-douce." P.C.30.d.12.

(3) Another edition of 2. Londres, 1776. P.C.30.g.37.

(4) *La fille de joie, par M. Cleland.* Londres, 1776. Fifteen plates engraved by Elluin after designs by Borel. P.C.30.g.38.

(5) *La fille de joie.* Paris: Chez Madame Gourdan, 1786. Frontispieces and tail-pieces added to plates engraved by Elluin after designs by Borel as in 4. P.C.30.e.8.

(6) Another edition of 4. Londres, 1776 (Paris?, ca. 1830). Frontispiece and seven plates from 4. P.C.30.g.39.

(7) Variant of 6. Eight plates. P.C.30.g.36.

(8) Variant of 6 and 7. Eight plates. P.C.30.b.7.

(9) *La meretrice inglese.* Batavia, ca. 1840. Engraved frontispiece. P.C.29.b.69.

(10) *La meretrice inglese, o Aventure de Fanny Will [sic].* Parigi, 1861. Four woodcuts. P.C.30.b.10.

(11) *Die Memoiren der Fanny Hill.* Paphos, Im Jahr der Cythere, 1906. Vienna: C.W. Stern. Eight plates by Franz von Bayros. P.C.17.b.32.

(12) *Memoirs of Fanny Hill.* "A new and corrected edition." N.p.: privately printed (Paris: Charles Hirsch, 1923?). Frontispiece and ten plates by Paul Avril(?). Text contains sodomy episode. P.C.13.h.3.

(13) *Mémoires de Fanny Hill, femme de plaisir, &c.* "Introduction et essai bibliographique par Guillaume Apollinaire. Ouvrage orné de six compositions d'après la suite gravée par William Hogarth: La Destinée d'une courtisane." Paris: Bibliothèque des Curieux, 1933. P.C.15.a.2.

(14) *Die Memorien der Fanny Hill.* Vienna, Munich, and Basel: Kurt Desch, 1964. Sixteen plates plus vignettes by Lilo Rasch-Nägele. P.C.29a.72.

(15) *Memoiren eines Freudenmädchens.* Hamburg: Gala Verlag, 1964. Frontispiece, three facsimiles, and thirty-four plates. P.C.19.b.26.

(16) Prospectus for *Mémoires de Fanny Hill, femme de plaisir.* A sample of the text, together with reproductions of the title page and two plates by Edouard Chimot. Paris, ca. 1955. P.C.19.b.21.

14. Editions at other libraries are as follows:

(1) Library of Congress: *MWP.* "Edition arranged and designed, numbered and signed by John J. Jamieson, Jr. Printed for subscribers." New York: Satyr Press, 1938. Vignettes only.

(2) Library of Congress: *MWP.* N.p.: Rare Book Co., 1949.

(3) Beinecke Library (Yale): *MWP*. Seventeenth ed. "With plates designed and engraved by a master of the Royal Academy." [London:] G. Fenton, 1813. Frontispiece and three plates. The copy is defective: pages 123–54 and 189–208 have been torn out.

(4) Firestone Library (Princeton): *MWP*. Hoboken, N.J., 1929. Frontispiece plus five plates. Text contains sodomy episode.

(5) Dr. Basker's copy: title page missing. Internal evidence and costume suggest publication in London ca. 1820. Ten colored plates. Sodomy episode not in text.

(6) Olin Library (Cornell): *Memoirs of Fanny Hill*. "A genuine reprint of the rare edition of 1749." Paris and Benares: The Kamashastra Society, 1907. Three illustrations. Traces of a frontispiece, now missing, are visible, as well as traces of illustrations removed at pp. 48, 120, and 184.

15. H. Amory, personal communication.

16. R. Pearsall, *The Worm in the Bud* (London: Weidenfeld & Nicolson, 1969), 103.

17. *Sex or Symbol: Erotic Images of Greece and Rome* (Austin: University of Texas Press, 1982), 10.

8. Johnson and Boswell: "Vile Melancholy" and "The Hypochondriack"

1. T. Bright, *A Treatise of Melancholie* (London: Vautrollier, 1586), 102.

2. T. Willis, *Two Discourses concerning the Soul of Brutes, &c.*, trans. S. Pordage (London: Dring, Harper, and Leigh, 1683), 188. (A translation of *De Anima brutorum*, 1672.)

3. Anne, Countess of Winchilsea, *The Spleen, a Pindarique Ode* (London: Hills, 1709). (First published anonymously, 1701.)

4. G. Cheyne, *The English Malady; or, a Treatise of Nervous Diseases of all Kinds, as Spleen, Vapours, Lowness of Spirits, Hypochondriachal and Hysterical Distempers, &c.* (London: Strahan, 1733), i–ii.

5. Letter to Thomas Wharton, May 24, 1771, in D. C. Tovey, ed., *The Letters of Thomas Gray* (London: Bell, 1912) 3:320; letter to Richard West, May 27, 1742, in Tovey, *Letters* 1:102.

6. W. Cowper, *The Task* 4:582; letter to Mrs. King, August 4, 1791, in T. Wright, ed., *Correspondence of William Cowper* (New York: Dodd Mead, 1904) 4:104.

7. A. L. Reade, "A New Admirer for Dr. Johnson," *London Mercury* 21 (1930), 243–53.

8. *Boswell's Life of Johnson,* ed. G. B. Hill, rev. L. F. Powell (Oxford: Clarendon Press, 1934), 1:63.

9. *Life of Johnson* 1:65.

10. W. J. Bate, *Samuel Johnson* (New York: Harcourt Brace Jovanovich, 1977), 118–19.

11. J. Hawkins, *The Life of Samuel Johnson, LL.D.,* ed. B. H. Davis (New York: Macmillan, 1961), 122.

12. Letter 56 in R. W. Chapman, ed., *The Letters of Samuel Johnson* (Oxford: Clarendon Press, 1952) 1:61. The quotation, from Euripides' lost play *Bellerophon,* is given in Greek in the original letter.)

13. Letter 57 in Chapman, *Letters of Samuel Johnson,* 1:62.

14. *Diaries, Prayers, and Annals,* vol. 1 of *The Works of Samuel Johnson* (New Haven, Conn.: Yale University Press, 1958), 69.

15. M. Waingrow, ed., *The Correspondence and Other Papers of James Boswell Relating to the Making of the "Life of Johnson,"* Yale Edition of the Private Papers of James Boswell (New York: McGraw-Hill, 1969), 2:24.

16. K. Balderston, "Johnson's Vile Melancholy," in *The Age of Johnson,* ed. F. W. Hilles (New Haven, Conn.: Yale University Press, 1949), 3–14.

17. Chapman, *Letters* 1:307.

18. Bate, *Samuel Johnson,* 384–88.

19. Hawkins, *Life of Samuel Johnson* 3:175–76.

20. Hawkins, *Life of Samuel Johnson* 5:215.

21. F. A. Pottle, *James Boswell: The Earlier Years, 1740–1769* (New York: McGraw-Hill, 1966), 1–6.

22. Pottle, *James Boswell,* 21.

23. Pottle, *James Boswell,* 1–6.

24. Pottle, *James Boswell,* 1–6.

25. Pottle, *James Boswell,* 1–6, 32.

26. Pottle, *James Boswell,* 32.

27. Pottle, *James Boswell,* 34.

28. Pottle, *James Boswell,* 130.

29. Hawkins, *Life of Samuel Johnson* 2:317.

30. S. Johnson, *Lives of the Poets (1778): William Collins* (Oxford: Oxford University Press, 1787–89) 2:380–84.

31. Hawkins, *Life of Samuel Johnson* 5:215.

32. M. Bailey, ed., *Boswell's Column, 1777–1783* (London: William Kimber, 1951).

33. A. Ingram, *Boswell's Creative Gloom: A Study of Imagery and Melancholy in the Writings of James Boswell* (London: Macmillan, 1982), 25.

34. Bright, *Melancholie,* 102.

35. F. Brady, *James Boswell: The Later Years, 1769–1795* (New York: McGraw-Hill, 1984), 176, 269.

9. *Margery Kempe: Hysteria and Mysticism Reconciled*

1. From *Guide to the Ruins* (1947), in *The Collected Works of Howard Nemerov* (Chicago: University of Chicago Press, 1977), 53. Copyright © 1977 by Howard Nemerov. Reprinted by permission of Howard Nemerov.

2. *The Book of Margery Kempe: A Modern Version by W. Butler-Bowdon* (London: Oxford University Press, 1936), 15. All subsequent quotations from the *Book* are from the 1954 World's Classics edition of this version and are cited parenthetically in the text.

3. S. B. Meech, introduction to *The Book of Margery Kempe: The Text from the Unique MS. owned by Colonel W. Butler-Bowdon*, ed. S. B. Meech and H. E. Allen (1940; rpt., London: Oxford University Press, 1961), xxxii.

4. Quoted in H. E. Allen, prefatory note to *The Book of Margery Kempe*, ed. Meech and Allen, lxv.

5. Allen, *The Book of Margery Kempe*, ed. Meech and Allen, lvii, lx–lxi.

6. M. Thornton, *Margery Kempe: An Example in the English Pastoral Tradition* (London: Society for Promoting Christian Knowledge, 1960), 3–4.

7. D. Knowles, *The English Mystical Tradition* (London: Burnes and Oates, 1961), 139.

8. Knowles, *The English Mystical Tradition*, 143.

9. It had been only as recently as 1401 that Parliament had passed the statute *De heretico comburendo* and William Sawtrey had been burned as the first Lollard martyr in England.

10. R. B. Carter, *On the Pathology and Treatment of Hysteria* (London: John Churchill, 1853), 43 and passim.

11. R. A. Knox, *Enthusiasm* (London: Oxford University Press, 1950), 41–42. Knox recognized the value of the mystical tradition and was in part sympathetic to it. But as a proper churchman, he circumspectly kept his distance: from the slow, calm waters of the Isis he described with Oxonian detachment the modern revival meetings of the Anglo-Saxon plebs as "some countryside Bethel at the height of a Welsh revival."

12. Knox, *Enthusiasm*, 36.

13. R. C. Zaehner, *Drugs, Mysticism and Make-Believe* (London: Collins, 1972), 68.

14. I. Veith, *Hysteria: The History of a Disease* (Chicago: University of Chicago Press, 1965), 1.

15. W. James, *The Varieties of Religious Experience: A Study in Human Nature* (New York: Modern Library, 1929), 421, 422–23.

16. James, *Varieties*, 371–72.

17. James, *Varieties*, 25–26.

18. W. H. Auden, introduction to *The Protestant Mystics*, ed. A. Fremantle (Boston: Little, Brown, 1964), 11.

10. All the Colors of the Rimbaud

1. A. Rimbaud, *Oeuvres complètes,* ed. A. Adam, Bibliothèque de la Pléiade (Paris: Gallimard, 1972); E. Starkie, *Arthur Rimbaud* (New York: New Directions, 1961).

2. Conflated from W. Fowlie, *Rimbaud: Complete Works, Selected Letters* (Chicago: University of Chicago Press, 1966), 75–78, and P. Schmidt, *Arthur Rimbaud: Complete Works* (New York: Harper & Row, 1974), 77–79.

3. Schmidt, *Rimbaud,* 10.

4. Fowlie, *Rimbaud,* 81–82. The word "plundered," substituted for "stolen," is taken from E. R. Peschel, *Four French Symbolist Poets* (Athens: Ohio University Press, 1981), 194–95. In this passage dealing with Rimbaud's first sexual experience, I have qualified it by writing of it as "supposed" and stating that it "may have" taken place because there is no documentation of it. However, it is a well-established item in the biographical myth, and I do believe it actually occurred and that the sixteen-year-old boy was buggered, perhaps more than once, and none too gently at that. Otherwise, I find his conduct on returning to Charleville and *Le coeur volé* inexplicable. Not uncommonly in historiography we have to infer causes from their effects. The word *chique,* translated as "quid," refers to a plug or "chaw" of tobacco.

5. Fowlie, *Rimbaud,* 304–7.

6. E. R. Peschel, *Flux and Reflux: Ambivalence in the Poems of Arthur Rimbaud* (Geneva: Droz, 1977), 15–16.

7. J. Richardson, *Paul Verlaine* (London: Weidenfeld & Nicolson, 1971), 3–11, 27.

8. Fowlie, *Rimbaud,* 318–23.

9. Starkie, *Rimbaud,* 279.

10. Fowlie, *Rimbaud,* 318–23.

11. Medical examination of Verlaine before the trial revealed a relaxed anal sphincter, which the physicians interpreted as evidence of passive sodomy. The probative value of this observation is inconclusive. Today's terminology would be "consistent with but not diagnostic of." Also, the Mautés' legal representatives appeared in court and insinuated that the relationship between Verlaine and Rimbaud involved "unnatural acts." It is doubtful whether such evidence would be admissible in an American or British court today. The allegations were taken into account in sentencing Verlaine, and the two years in prison reflect the court's repugnance toward homosexuality. Curiously, the same sentence was meted out to Oscar Wilde in England two decades later, when the charge was actually sodomy rather than assault with a dangerous weapon. Courts are somewhat less homophobic these days, as is evident in the following quip, which was current in London shortly before the Wolfenden report: A newly appointed judge asked the advice of a senior colleague—"What do you give a man for buggery?" To which the senior is supposed to have replied, "Oh, a pound note or two—whatever you have in your pocket."

12. Rimbaud, *Oeuvres complètes,* 1050–54. A. Adam's editorial note explains the origin and nature of the *Album Zutique,* its contents, and its subsequent literary and bibliographical history.

13. Fowlie, *Rimbaud,* 160–63.

14. E. R. Peschel, personal communication, March 12, 1985.

15. A. Rimbaud, *A Season in Hell & The Illuminations,* trans. E. R. Peschel (Oxford: Oxford University Press, 1973), 60–75.

16. Rimbaud, *Season in Hell,* 60–75.

17. B. Adams, *"Picasso's Absinthe Glasses: Six Drinks to the End of an Era," Artforum* 18 (1980), 30–33.

18. W. Beach, *The Family Physician* (New York: James M'Allister, 1847), 680.

19. W. Beach, "Absinthe," *American Journal of Pharmacy* 40 (1868), 356–60.

20. D. D. Vogt and M. Montagne, "Absinthe: Behind the Emerald Mask," *International Journal of Addictions* 17 (1982), 1015–29.

21. D. Flower and H. Maas, eds., *The Letters of Ernest Dowson* (London: Cassell, 1967), 441.

22. E. Dowson, *The Poems of Ernest Dowson,* ed. M. Longaker (Philadelphia: University of Pennsylvania Press, 1968), 143.

23. E. R. Peschel, *Symbolist Poets,* 196–97.

24. Rimbaud, *Season in Hell,* 76–77.

25. Fowlie, *Rimbaud,* 132–33.

26. Fowlie, *Rimbaud,* 232–33.

27. Peschel, *Flux,* 53–61.

28. Peschel, *Flux,* 53–61.

29. Starkie, *Rimbaud,* 355.

30. Starkie, *Rimbaud,* 361. The first collected edition of Rimbaud's poems was published in 1898, edited by Paterne Berrichon (né Pierre Dufour)—who married Rimbaud's sister Isabelle in 1897, ten years before Mme. Rimbaud's death in 1907—and Ernest Delahaye, Rimbaud's classmate and friend since childhood.

31. Here are six statements about Rimbaud's sexuality, all possible, none verifiable:

(1) Rimbaud's homosexuality was fixed in boyhood or early adolescence. The incident in the Rue Babylon confirmed it, and the affair with Verlaine was its fruition.

(2) Rimbaud's sexuality in 1870–71 was ambivalent and unfixed. The incident in the Rue Babylon was an unfortunate accident. He consented to a homosexual relationship with Verlaine to experience "all forms of love," but his heterosexuality asserted itself, and he found the relationship unsatisfactory.

(3) After the break with Verlaine, Rimbaud had no more homosexual experiences and slowly established heterosexual competence.

(4) After the break with Verlaine, Rimbaud had occasional homosexual experiences as the opportunity presented and his needs required.

(5) After the break with Verlaine, Rimbaud had casual affairs with both male and female partners.

(6) After the break with Verlaine, Rimbaud's sexuality was inhibited and he became completely asexual.

32. Fowlie, *Rimbaud,* 357.
33. Fowlie, *Rimbaud,* 359–61.
34. Fowlie, *Rimbaud,* 359–61.
35. Rimbaud, *Oeuvres complètes,* 670–93.

11. Reuben's Mandrakes: Infertility in the Bible

1. C. J. S. Thompson, *The Mystic Mandrake* (London: Rider, 1934).
2. G. W. T. H. Fleming, "The Insane Root," *Journal of Mental Science* 99 (1958), 638–53.
3. T. Browne, *Pseudodoxia epidemica,* vol. 2 of *The Works of Sir Thomas Browne,* ed. G. Keynes (London: Faber & Faber, 1928), 499–503.
4. B. Rowland, ed., *Medieval Woman's Guide to Health: The First English Gynecological Handbook* (Kent, Ohio: Kent State University Press, 1981), 169. This early-fifteenth-century manuscript (British Library Sloane MS. 2463) is in Middle English and is derived from the eleventh-century manuscript traditionally assigned to Trotula. This modern transcription is accompanied by a facing-page translation in modern English. It antedates by about a century *The Byrth of Mankynde.*

12. The Plague at Granada, 1348–49: Ibn al-Khatib and Ideas of Contagion

1. W. M. Bowsky, "The Impact of the Black Death upon Sienese Government and Society," *Speculum* 39 (1964), 1–34. Bowsky calculates the mortality at Siena as on the order of 50 percent of the population, but recovery from the effects of such a loss depends not only upon the actual number of survivors but also upon the stability of local government, capacity for economic reconstruction, and general social morale. In *Painting in Florence and Siena after the Black Death* (Princeton, N.J.: Princeton University Press, 1951), Millard Meiss furnishes a detailed account of the impact of the epidemic on the psychology of the survivors and its effect on the visual arts. Florence flourished and Siena declined because socioeconomic factors favored the former.
2. A. Ibn Khatimah, *Tahsil al-gharad al-qasid fi tafsil al-marad al-wafid,* Escorial MS. No. 1785, fols. 49a–115b. According to Ibn Khatimah there were seventy deaths daily at Almeria at the peak of the epidemic, compared to seventeen hun-

dred a day at Valencia. Ibn al-Khatib, based at Granada, provides no specific figures for the death rate in his city but claims that seven-tenths of mankind perished, probably an exaggerated figure. Mortality may well have been higher at Granada than in other cities of Andalusia, but perhaps the truth lies in between.

3. M. J. Müller, "Ibnulkhatibs Bericht über die Pest," *Sitzungsber. königl. bayer. Akad. Wissensch.* 4 (1863), 1–34. Müller provides a transcription of Ibn al-Khatib's text and his own comments, but not a translation.

4. S. Jarcho, "Medical and Nonmedical Comments on Cato and Varro, with Historical Observations on the Concept of Infection," *Transactions of the College of Physicians of Philadelphia* 43 (1976), 372–78.

5. M. W. Dols, *The Black Death in the Middle East* (Princeton, N.J.: Princeton University Press, 1977), 320–35.

6. L. F. Hirst, *The Conquest of Plague: A Study of the Evolution of Epidemiology* (Oxford: Clarendon Press, 1953), 26. According to the astrological-humoral model, there had been a conjunction of Saturn, Jupiter, and Mars in the house of Aquarius. The conjunction of Saturn and Jupiter notoriously caused death and disaster, while the conjunction of Mars and Jupiter spread pestilence in the air. Jupiter, being warm and humid, was calculated to draw up evil vapors from the earth and water which Mars, hot and dry, then kindled into infective fire.

7. A. Kircher, *Scrutinium physico-medicum contagiosae luis: quae dicitur pestis, &c.* (Rome: Mascardi, 1658). There is reasonable doubt that Kircher's 32-power lens system could have shown him the microorganism *Pasturella pestis*, though he may well have seen red and white blood cells. However, he was the first to write of *contagium animatum*, or infection by a living organism. Frascastorius' term *seminaria contagionum* was described and defined in physical terms. The decision of priority depends upon whether the arbiter is a materialist or a vitalist.

8. Müller glosses this text as follows: "Die Existenz der Ansteckung steht fest durch die Erfahrung, die Forschung, die Sinneswahrnehmung, die Autopsie und verbürgte Kunden." "Autopsie" does not imply postmortem dissection ("Sektion") but must be translated in its etymological sense, "to see for one's self." This usage was common in the mid-nineteenth century. The sightseeing omnibus from London to Brighton was known as the "autopsy bus."

13. The Trial of Spencer Cowper: Expert Witnesses to the Rescue

1. W. Cobbett, *Complete Collection of State Trials, from the Earliest Period to 1783* (London: Longmans, 1816) 13:1106–1250. Hereafter cited parenthetically in the text as *ST*.

2. T. B. Macaulay, *History of England* (London: J. M. Dent, 1906) 4:489–93. Hereafter cited parenthetically in the text as *HE*.

3. *Some Observations on the Tryal of Spencer Cowper, J. Marson, E. Stevens, W. Rogers,*

That Were Tried at Hereford, about the Murder of Sarah Stout, Together with Other Things Relating Hereunto (London, 1701), 13.

4. T. Browne, "Of Swimming and Drowning," in *Pseudodoxia Epidemica,* vol. 2 of *The Works of Sir Thomas Browne,* ed. G. Keynes (London: Faber & Faber, 1928), 287–90.

5. W. U. Spitz and R. S. Fisher, *Medicolegal Investigation of Death,* 2d ed. (Springfield, Ill.: Charles C. Thomas, 1980), 351–66.

14. Notes on Placentophagy

1. W. B. Ober, "A Modest Proposal for Preventing Choriocarcinoma among Innocent Mothers," *Obstetrics and Gynecology* 31 (1968), 866–69.

2. M. Marin-Padilla and K. Benirschke, "Thalidomide Induced Alterations in the Blastocyst and Placenta of the Armadillo, *Dasypus novemcinctus mexicanus,* Including a Choriocarcinoma," *American Journal of Pathology* 43 (1963), 999–1016.

3. J. R. Lindsey, L. R. Wharton, J. D. Woodruff, and H. J. Baker, "Intrauterine Choriocarcinoma in a Rhesus Monkey," *Pathologia Veterinaria* 6 (1969), 378–84.

4. W. B. Ober, letter, *Obstetrics and Gynecology* 41 (1973), 317.

5. K. Jindrak, personal communication, May 23, 1974.

6. G. E. Smith, *Human History* (New York: Norton, 1929), 304–21.

7. W. C. Cooper and N. Sivin, "Man as a Medicine: Pharmacological and Ritual Aspects of Traditional Therapy Using Drugs Derived from the Human Body," in *Chinese Science: Explorations of an Ancient Tradition,* ed. N. Nakamaya and N. Sivin (Cambridge: MIT Press, 1973), 221, 227–28.

8. J. G. Frazer, *The Golden Bough: A Study in Magic and Religion,* 3d ed. (New York: Macmillan, 1911–15), 1:182–201.

9. B. Alkema and T. J. Bezemer, *Beknopt Handboek der Volkenkunde van Nederlandsch-Indië* (Haarlem, Netherlands: Tjeenk Willink & Zoon, 1927), 358.

10. G. A. Wilken, *Handleing voor de Vergelijkende Volkenkinde van Nederlandsch-Indië* (Leyden: Brill, 1893), 231.

11. S. Benet, *Song, Dance and Customs of Peasant Poland* (New York: Roy, 1951), 196–97.

12. B. Blackwood, *Both Sides of the Buka Passage: An Ethnographic Study of Social, Sexual and Economic Questions in the Northwest Solomon Islands* (Oxford: Clarendon Press, 1935), 160.

13. M. J. Herskovitz, *Life in a Haitian Valley* (New York: Knopf, 1937), 92–93.

14. R. L. Beals, *Cheran: A Sierra Tarascan Village,* Smithsonian Institution Institute of Social Anthropology Publication no. 2 (Washington, D.C., 1946), 184.

15. R. Redfield, *Tepotzlan, a Mexican Village: A Study of Folk Life* (Chicago: University of Chicago Press, 1930), 135–36.

16. O. Lewis, *Life in a Mexican Village: Tepotzlan Restudied* (Urbana: University of Illinois Press, 1951), 215.

17. E. M. Loeb, *Pomo Folkways* (Berkeley: University of California Press, 1926), 250.

18. M. W. Beckwith, *Black Roadways: A Study of Jamaican Folk Life* (Chapel Hill: University of North Carolina Press, 1929), 57.

19. M. I. Hilger, *Araucanian Child Life and Its Cultural Background*, Smithsonian Miscellaneous Collections, vol. 133 (Washington, D.C., 1957), 248.

20. G. de la Vega, *El Inca: The Royal Commentaries of the Yncas,* trans. C. R. Markham, Hakluyt Society Publications, series 1, vol. 41 (London, 1869), 447.

21. O. F. Raum, *Chaga Childhood: A Description of Indigenous Education in an East African Tribe* (London: Oxford University Press, 1940), 86.

22. W. G. Griffiths, *The Kol Tribe of Central India,* Royal Asiatic Society of Bengal Monograph Series, vol. 2 (Calcutta, 1946), 59.

23. Advertisement for Dermatein, *Mainliner Magazine* (United Airlines), November 1977.

24. N. Adriani and A. C. Kruty, *De Bare'e Strekende Toradjas van Midden-Celebes (Oost-Toradjas)* (Amsterdam: Noord Hollandsche Uitg. Mij., 1950–51), 376. (Anonymous translation in Human Relations File at the Graduate Center, City University of New York.)

William B. Ober, M.D., is Director Emeritus of Pathology at the Hackensack Medical Center, Hackensack, New Jersey, Visiting Professor of Pathology at the New Jersey College of Medicine, and Assistant Medical Examiner of Bergen County. He was for many years Pathologist at the Beth Israel Medical Center in New York and Professor of Pathology at Mount Sinai School of Medicine. He has published over two hundred medical articles; his previous book, *Boswell's Clap: Medical Analyses of Literary Men's Afflictions,* was published by Southern Illinois University Press in 1979. Dr. Ober resides in Tenafly, New Jersey.